GOLDEN YEARS?

GOLDEN YEARS?
SOCIAL INEQUALITY IN LATER LIFE

Deborah Carr

A Volume in the American Sociological Association's
Rose Series in Sociology

Russell Sage Foundation • New York

Library of Congress Cataloging-in-Publication Data
Names: Carr, Deborah S., author.
Title: Golden years? : social inequality in later life / Deborah Carr.
Description: New York : Russell Sage Foundation, [2018] | Includes
   bibliographical references and index.
Identifiers: LCCN 2018038709 (print) | LCCN 2018041063 (ebook) | ISBN
   9781610448772 (ebook) | ISBN 9780871540348 (pbk. : alk. paper)
Subjects: LCSH: Older people—United States—Social conditions. |
   Aging—United States. | Equality—United States.
Classification: LCC HQ1064.U5 (ebook) | LCC HQ1064.U5 C356 2018 (print) |
   DDC   305.260973—dc23
LC record available at https://lccn.loc.gov/2018038709

Copyright © 2019 by the American Sociological Association. All rights reserved. Printed in Canada. No part of this publication may be reproduced, stored in a retrieval system, or transmitted in any form or by any means, electronic, mechanical, photocopying, recording, or otherwise, without the prior written permission of the publisher.

Reproduction by the United States Government in whole or in part is permitted for any purpose.

The paper used in this publication meets the minimum requirements of American National Standard for Information Sciences—Permanence of Paper for Printed Library Materials. ANSI Z39.48-1992.

Text design by Suzanne Nichols.

RUSSELL SAGE FOUNDATION
112 East 64th Street, New York, New York 10065
10 9 8 7 6 5 4 3 2 1

The Russell Sage Foundation

The Russell Sage Foundation, one of the oldest of America's general purpose foundations, was established in 1907 by Mrs. Margaret Olivia Sage for "the improvement of social and living conditions in the United States." The foundation seeks to fulfill this mandate by fostering the development and dissemination of knowledge about the country's political, social, and economic problems. While the foundation endeavors to assure the accuracy and objectivity of each book it publishes, the conclusions and interpretations in Russell Sage Foundation publications are those of the authors and not of the foundation, its trustees, or its staff. Publication by Russell Sage, therefore, does not imply foundation endorsement.

BOARD OF TRUSTEES
Claude M. Steele, Chair

Larry M. Bartels
Cathy J. Cohen
Karen S. Cook
Sheldon Danziger
Kathryn Edin

Jason Furman
Michael Jones-Correa
Lawrence F. Katz
David Laibson
Nicholas Lemann

Sara S. McLanahan
Martha Minow
Peter R. Orszag
Mario Luis Small
Hirokazu Yoshikawa

EDITORS OF THE ROSE SERIES IN SOCIOLOGY

Amy Adamczyk
Richard D. Alba

Lynn S. Chancer
Nancy Foner

Philip Kasinitz
Leslie S. Paik

THE ROSE SERIES IN SOCIOLOGY EDITORIAL BOARD

Peter Riley Bahr
Joyce M. Bell
Irene H.I. Bloemraad
Susan K. Brown
Shelly Brown-Jeffy
Pawan H. Dhingra
Cybelle Fox

Sylvia A. Fuller
Shannon Marie Gleeson
Rosanna Hertz
Alexandra Hrycak
Shawna Hudson
Tomas R. Jimenez
Nikki Jones

Mary Ellen Konieczny
John T. Lang
Brian Mayer
Lori Peek
Andres Villarreal
Sara Wakefield
Geoff K. Ward

Previous Volumes in the Series

American Memories: Atrocities and the Law
Joachim J. Savelsberg and Ryan D. King

America's Newcomers and the Dynamics of Diversity
Frank D. Bean and Gillian Stevens

Beyond the Boycott: Labor Rights, Human Rights, and Transnational Activism
Gay W. Seidman

Beyond College For All: Career Paths for the Forgotten Half
James E. Rosenbaum

Changing Rhythms of the American Family
Suzanne M. Bianchi, John Robinson, and Melissa Milkie

Counted Out: Same-Sex Relations and Americans' Definitions of Family
Brian Powell, Lala Carr Steelman, Catherine Bolzendahl, and Claudi Giest

Divergent Social Worlds: Neighborhood Crime and the Racial-Spatial Divide
Ruth D. Peterson and Lauren J. Krivo

Egalitarian Capitalism: Jobs, Incomes, and Growth in Affluent Countries
Lane Kenworthy

Ethnic Origins: History, Politics, Culture, and the Adaptation of Cambodian and Hmong Refugees in Four American Cities
Jeremy Hein

Family Consequences of Children's Disabilities
Denis Hogan

Good Jobs, Bad Jobs: The Rise of Polarized and Precarious Employment Systems in the United States, 1970s to 2000s
Arne L. Kalleberg

The Long Shadow: Family Background, Disadvantaged Urban Youth, and the Transition to Adulthood
Karl Alexander, Doris Entwisle, and Linda Olson

Making Hate a Crime: From Social Movement to Law Enforcement
Valerie Jenness and Ryken Grattet

Market Friendly or Family Friendly? The State and Gender Inequality in Old Age
Madonna Harrington Meyer and Pamela Herd

Nurturing Dads: Social Initiatives for Contemporary Fatherhood
William Marsiglio and Kevin Roy

Passing the Torch: Does Higher Education for the Disadvantaged Pay Off Across the Generations?
Paul Attewell and David Lavin

Pension Puzzles: Social Security and the Great Debate
Melissa Hardy and Lawrence Hazelrigg

A Pound of Flesh: Monetary Sanctions as Punishment for the Poor
Alexes Harris

Sites Unseen: Uncovering Hidden Hazards in American Cities
Scott Frickel and James R. Elliott

Social Movements in the World-System: The Politics of Crisis and Transformation
Dawn Wiest and Jackie Smith

They Say Cut Back, We Say Fight Back! Welfare Activism in an Era of Retrenchment
Ellen Reese

Trust in Schools: A Core Resource for Improvement
Anthony S. Bryk and Barbara Schneider

Forthcoming Titles

Collateral Damages: Saving and Losing the City
Meredith Greif

Family Relationships Across the Generations
Judith A. Seltzer, Emily Wiemers, and Suzanne M. Bianchi

Interracial Romance and Friendship in Adolescence and Adulthood
Grace Kao, Kara Joyner, and Kelly Stamper Balistreri

Race and Gender Discrimination and the Stalled Revolution
Reginald A. Byron and Vincent J. Roscigno

Who Benefits from College?
Jennie E. Brand

The Rose Series in Sociology

The American Sociological Association's Rose Series in Sociology publishes books that integrate knowledge and address controversies from a sociological perspective. Books in the Rose Series are at the forefront of sociological knowledge. They are lively and often involve timely and fundamental issues on significant social concerns. The series is intended for broad dissemination throughout sociology, across social science and other professional communities, and to policy audiences. The series was established in 1967 by a bequest to ASA from Arnold and Caroline Rose to support innovations in scholarly publishing.

AMY ADAMCYZK
RICHARD D. ALBA
LYNN S. CHANCER
NANCY FONER
PHILIP KASINITZ
LESLIE S. PAIK

EDITORS

This book is dedicated in loving memory to my parents, Raymond H. Carr and Naomi Bojar Carr. While they did not live to enjoy their own "golden years," they made every sacrifice so that their five children might.

Contents

	List of Illustrations	xiii
	About the Author	xv
	Acknowledgments	xvii
CHAPTER 1	Golden Years? An Introduction	1
CHAPTER 2	Older Adults in the Contemporary United States: A Snapshot	13
CHAPTER 3	Life-Course Perspectives on Social Inequalities in Later Life: A Brief Overview	36
CHAPTER 4	The Fit and the Frail: Physical Health Among Older Adults	51
CHAPTER 5	The Satisfied and the Sorrowful: The Mental Health of Older Adults	86
CHAPTER 6	The Loved and the Lonely: Social Relationships and Isolation in Later Life	112
CHAPTER 7	The Home Front: Residential and Community Experiences of Older Adults	149
CHAPTER 8	Is Death the Great Equalizer? Disparities in Dying	179
CHAPTER 9	Conclusion: Future Trends and Policy Considerations for the Twenty-First Century	210
	Notes	247
	References	289
	Index	345

List of Illustrations

Figure 2.1	The Projected Shift in the Ethnic and Racial Composition of the U.S. Population Age Sixty-Five and Older, by Race and Hispanic Origin, 2014–2060	19
Figure 2.2	Educational Attainment Among U.S. Adults Age Sixty-Five and Older, by Race, 2015	21
Figure 2.3	Marital Status of U.S. Men Age Sixty-Five and Older, by Age Group, 2015	22
Figure 2.4	Marital Status of U.S. Women Age Sixty-Five and Older, by Age Group, 2015	23
Figure 2.5	Living Arrangements of U.S. Men Age Sixty-Five and Older, by Race, 2015	24
Figure 2.6	Living Arrangements of U.S. Women Age Sixty-Five and Older, by Race, 2015	25
Figure 2.7	Labor Force Participation of U.S. Adults Age Sixty-Two and Older, by Age and Sex, 1965–2015	27
Figure 2.8	Poverty Among U.S. Adults Age Sixty-Five and Older, by Sex, Race-Ethnicity, and Household Structure, 2014	31
Figure 2.9	Income Sources for Households Headed by U.S. Adults Age Sixty-Five and Older, by Household Income Level, 2014	33
Figure 4.1	Estimated Share of Contribution to Premature Death in the United States, 2007	53
Figure 4.2	Death Rates for U.S. Adults Age Sixty-Five and Older, by Disease, 1981–2014	64
Figure 4.3	Male and Female Age-Adjusted Death Rates, by Age, 1955–2014	67
Figure 4.4	Life Expectancy at Birth, by Race and Sex, 1970–2015	68

xiv List of Illustrations

Figure 5.1	U.S. Adults Age Fifty-One and Older with Clinically Relevant Depressive Symptoms, by Sex and Age Group, 2014	91
Figure 5.2	Quality of Treatment Received by Persons with a Depressive Disorder in the Past Twelve Months, by Race-Ethnicity, 2001–2003	92
Figure 5.3	Suicide Rates over the Life Course, by Race and Sex, 2010	95
Figure 6.1	Marital Status of U.S. Men Age Sixty-Five and Older, by Race, 2010	116
Figure 6.2	Marital Status of U.S. Women Age Sixty-Five and Older, by Race, 2010	116
Figure 6.3	Children Under Age Eighteen Living with a Grandparent, by Race-Ethnicity and the Presence of Parent(s), 2012	127
Figure 7.1	Older Adults Living in Long-Term Care, Community Housing with Services, or Traditional Community, by Age Group, 2013	151
Figure 7.2	Adults Age Sixty-Five and Older Living Alone, with Nonrelatives, with Other Relatives, or with a Spouse, by Age and Sex, 2014	152
Figure 7.3	Neighborhoods with Street and Sidewalk Lighting and Sidewalks, by Neighborhood Income Level, 2012	167
Figure 8.1	Proposed Trajectories of Chronic Illness and Death	187
Figure 8.2	Medicare Hospice Enrollees, by Ownership of Hospice Provider, 2000–2011	195
Figure 8.3	Durable Power of Attorney for Health Care Appointments Among Wisconsin Longitudinal Study Respondents, by Marital and Parental Status, 2003–2004	208
Figure 9.1	U.S. Income Inequality, 1967–2016	214
Figure 9.2	Opioid and Heroin Overdose Death, 2002–2015	219
Figure 9.3	Projected Number of Persons Age Sixty-Five and Older with Alzheimer's Disease, by Age Group, 2010–2050	225
Figure 9.4	Projected Ratio of Caregivers to Care Recipients, 1990–2050	227

About the Author

Deborah Carr is professor and chair in the Department of Sociology at Boston University and editor in chief of the *Journal of Gerontology: Social Sciences*.

Acknowledgments

I am grateful to my colleagues, family, and friends who provided the wise insights, emotional and social support, and good humor that helped me to produce this book. I am indebted to participants at an April 2017 workshop at the Russell Sage Foundation (RSF), who offered feedback on an early draft of this book and brainstormed about ways to strengthen it. A sincere thank-you to Toni Antonucci, Sheldon Danziger, Mary Gatta, Mary Clare Lennon, Dawne Mouzon, and Julie Phillips. The ASA Rose Series editorial team at Rutgers University, Lee "Chip" Clarke, Judith Gerson, Lauren Krivo, Paul McLean, Patricia Roos, and Lindsay Stevens, have helped to guide this project since the earliest days of the proposal. I also benefited from the creative input and enthusiastic encouragement of Amy Adamcyzk, Leslie Paik, and their colleagues at the CUNY Graduate Center, who now edit the ASA Rose Series.

My sincere gratitude to Suzanne Nichols, RSF's director of publications, who supported this project from the start and provided the right mix of encouragement, cheerleading, and deadline enforcement when I needed it most. Her assistance in navigating the revision process was invaluable. The three anonymous reviewers of the manuscript provided tough, thoughtful, and tremendously helpful feedback that forced me to dig into nuances more deeply, scrutinize policies more thoughtfully, and sing out my message more clearly. The book is stronger because of their knowledge and insights.

For fifteen years, I had the good fortune of working with superb, smart, and kind colleagues in the Sociology Department and the Institute for Health, Health Care Policy, and Aging Research at Rutgers University. I am grateful for their brilliance and friendship, especially Sharon Bzostek, Ira Cohen, Phaedra Daipha, Judy Gerson, Emily Greenfield, Allan Horwitz, Ellen Idler, Lisa Iorillo, Laurie Krivo, David Mechanic, Jane Miller, Dawne Mouzon, Julie Phillips, Pat Roos, Kristen Springer, and Eviatar Zerubavel. My new colleagues at Boston University have provided a warm, welcoming, and intellectually stimulating professional home.

A hearty thank-you to Amanda Kaplan, who took time from her busy schedule as a Rutgers sociology graduate student to meticulously compile and edit the book's extensive list of references. Elizabeth "Libby" Luth provided research support for chapter 8 at precisely the same time she was polishing up her own terrific dissertation at Rutgers. Her knowledge and insights into end-of-life decision-making were essential to this chapter.

If uplifting social relationships are the key to well-being, then I have it made. Although siblings (and siblings-in-law) account for just a tiny fraction of scholarly research on social ties, I can attest to their value in enriching our lives. My gratitude goes out to siblings Tracy, David, Shellie, and Danny, Team C siblings-in-law Mark, Sandy, Francois, and Yumi, and Team Z siblings-in-law Rebecca, Val, John, Kim, Marc, and Linne, and a heartfelt thank-you to my parents-in-law Rissy and Joe, who offered love, support, and regular chicken dinners while I finished writing this book. They exemplify the notion of "golden years" and graciously and generously share their happiness and good fortune with others. Last but not least, my endless gratitude to Sam, who gets full credit for any and all insights into oral health in this book. More importantly, he simply makes my life and work much better.

Chapter 1

Golden Years? An Introduction

Susannah Mushatt Jones was the oldest living person in the United States on May 11, 2016. At 116 years old, Jones had defied all the odds. Born in Alabama in 1899 to African American sharecroppers, she was the third of eleven children. As a teenager, Jones worked in the fields alongside her parents and siblings, but she was determined to do more with her life. She graduated from high school in 1922 and was accepted into Tuskegee Institute's Teachers Program. Although her parents could not afford her tuition, Jones remained intent on seeing the world beyond rural Alabama, even if she couldn't go to college. She moved to Harlem in 1923 and found work as a nanny to wealthy families. Although Jones was married for a brief spell, she never had children of her own. Still, she enriched the lives of her friends and relatives (including more than 100 nieces and nephews), even sending money back to her Alabama high school to establish a scholarship fund so that younger generations could live out her dashed dream of a college education.

Jones died on May 12, 2016, and the distinction of being the oldest living person in the United States was passed on to Goldie Korash Michelson, age 113. Michelson was born in Russia in 1902 to a Jewish doctor and his wife. Michelson, her parents, and two siblings emigrated to Worcester, Massachusetts, when she was two years old. She enjoyed many privileges that Jones did not. In 1924, Michelson graduated from Pembroke College, the former women's college that is now part of Brown University. She received her bachelor's degree in sociology and eventually earned a master's degree from Clark University. She was married to her real estate developer husband David for nearly forty years, until his death. The mother to one daughter, Michelson was an enthusiastic supporter of the arts, establishing scholarship programs for theater students at Clark and teaching theater to teens at her local synagogue. When Michelson died at home on July 8, 2016, one month short of her 114th birthday, 113-year-old Adele Dunlap stepped into the position of oldest living American.

Living to age 100, never mind age 116, is a rare feat. Fewer than 0.02 percent of all Americans will celebrate their 100th birthday. Centenarians are held up as inspirations and role models. Books with titles like *If I Live to Be 100: The Wisdom of Centenarians* and *How to Achieve Healthy Aging: Effortlessly Form the Habits of a Centenarian* offer readers hope that they too can live a long and purposeful life. When centenarians are asked to divulge the secrets to their longevity, they invariably mention two factors: good genes and healthy living. Jones clearly possessed good genes; her grandmother reportedly survived until age 117. Both Jones and Michelson told journalists that they never touched alcohol or cigarettes. Michelson was also an avid walker, until she became too frail. As she told a newspaper reporter, "I was a great walker—four or five miles every morning, weather permitting. I never used a car if I could walk."[1]

When scientists are asked to share the secrets of longevity, their responses echo those of the centenarians, up to a point. Researchers working on projects like the Georgia Centenarian Study and the New England Centenarian Study have tracked hundreds of exceptionally long-lived older adults and find that genes and a healthy lifestyle, especially a nutritious diet, contribute to longevity.[2] Sex also matters; it's no coincidence that both Jones and Michelson are women. Of the twenty-five oldest living Americans as of August 2018, twenty-four were women; 112-year-old Richard Overton was the only man who cracked the list.

Yet when scientists dig more deeply into their data, they find that social factors spanning a lifetime, including how much money and education our parents had when we were growing up, how far we went in school, the jobs we hold, the salary and savings we have to live on, the social ties we rely on, the kinds of stressors we face (and how we cope with them), and where we live are powerful predictors of how long we live. Even after taking into account how often we smoke, drink, or take daily five-mile walks, researchers consistently find that race and socioeconomic status (SES)—key dimensions of social inequality in the United States—predict our life span. Susannah Mushatt Jones defied the odds by living to 116, but she also defied the odds by surviving into old age at all. Old age is a milestone that African Americans, those from poor families, and unmarried people are less likely to attain, relative to whites, those from privileged backgrounds, and married people, like Goldie Michelson. Blacks die roughly five years younger than whites in the United States today. Women who drop out of high school die about twelve years younger than women who go on to graduate school, while the gap for men is a remarkable sixteen years.[3] Geography also matters:

residents of states with generous health and welfare spending, like Michelson's home state of Massachusetts, live six years longer on average than those hailing from states that spend little on social programs, like Jones's birthplace of Alabama.[4]

The most profound social disadvantages exact the heaviest personal tolls and generate the widest disparities. A homeless person living on the streets today survives until age sixty-four on average, about sixteen years less than the average U.S. life expectancy.[5] Being homeless in old age, like many other late-life struggles, is the end result of experiences that have accumulated over years, if not decades. That was the case with Michael Leslie, who died prematurely while living on the streets of Washington, D.C. Leslie's early life was marked by seemingly endless misfortunes: he had a difficult childhood, was bullied, dropped out of school by the sixth grade, battled alcoholism and poverty, and was in and out of jail before ending up destitute and living on the streets.[6]

Impoverished men in the bottom 1 percent of the income distribution die fifteen years younger than men in the top 1 percent, while the comparable gap for women is ten years.[7] The epidemiologist Sandro Galea and his colleagues have gone so far as to argue that poverty kills more Americans each year than automobile accidents, high school dropout is linked with more deaths than heart attacks, and racial segregation outranks cerebrovascular disease as a root cause of death.[8] These statistics convey the magnitude of social disparities in survival. Yet they reveal just one of the myriad ways in which symptoms of social inequality, like poverty, racial segregation, hazardous work conditions, social isolation, discrimination, and strained interpersonal relationships can undermine the quality of older adults' lives.

Social policies can help to chip away at disparities in older adults' well-being, arguably more so than at any other point in the life course. Social Security provides a guaranteed monthly income for most older adults, while Supplemental Security Income (SSI) provides an added boost for low-income older adults. Medicare covers the costs of many of the health care needs of older adults, while Medicaid helps to cover long-term care expenses. Yet each of these programs also has well-documented limitations, so some older adults' financial, medical, caregiving, and housing needs may not be met adequately. And because so many later-life hardships are a consequence of adversities that have accumulated gradually throughout youth, adolescence, and the working years, the benefits provided by old-age policies may be "too little too late" to meet the needs of the most disadvantaged Americans, whose bodies and minds may start to falter in their fifties and sixties, or even younger.

The Aims of *Golden Years*

The goal of this book is to reveal the complex, surprising, and often heartbreaking ways in which social inequalities affect nearly all aspects of older adults' lives, including how long they live; how much money they have in their retirement years; the quality of their physical and emotional health, social relationships, housing, and neighborhood conditions; and whether they have the privilege of dying with dignity. Old age can be the best of times, marked by good health, unprecedented longevity, happiness, a comfortable home, a carefree retirement spent volunteering, the pursuit of hobbies, enjoyable time spent with loved ones, and the sense of equanimity, contentedness, and wisdom that comes from a lifetime of experience. For most Americans, old age can be aptly described as the "golden years." More than three-quarters of Americans age sixty-five and older say they are in good or excellent health. Studies consistently show that happiness levels peak in our sixties and seventies, and more than two-thirds of older adults say they are very happy with their family, friends, and homes.[9]

Yet old age also can be the worst of times, marred by illness, compromised physical functioning, cognitive decline, loneliness, poverty, unsafe housing, and mistreatment at the hands of the very people who should be providing care and protection. Millions of older adults are living under difficult conditions that would be trying even for a young and healthy person. For an older adult with fading health and physical strength, these adverse conditions can be devastating and potentially deadly. Consider a few statistics about older adults in the United States today:[10]

- An estimated 165,000 adults age fifty-five and older are in prison.
- More than 306,000 adults age fifty and older are homeless or living in shelters.
- Two million older adults age sixty-five and older are homebound.
- An estimated 7.1 million older adults age sixty-five and older live in poverty.[11]

Taken together, these counts eclipse the 72,000 centenarians who are celebrated on the local news and featured in inspirational self-help books. Yet these disadvantaged older adults, some without homes and some who either cannot leave or are afraid to leave their homes, are invisible to most of us. Our social lives are structured such that frail, lonely, and impoverished older adults are out of our sightlines. Contemporary social life is highly age-segregated, so that most adults live, work, and socialize with people their own age and many never come into contact with older adults outside of their own families. This invisibility is compounded by the fact that some older adults, especially those who have difficulty walking, driving, or taking public transit, do not stray far from their immediate environs. One recent study found that one in five older adults had not left their city, town, or county in the past two months because they were incapable of traveling or lacked the friends and family to help them navigate beyond the neighborhood they call home.[12] It is not only physical challenges that keep vulnerable older adults sequestered away: some are afraid to leave their homes, fearful of crime victimization in their neighborhoods.

The media are complicit in keeping images of older adults' suffering out of our sight lines. The public messages we receive about old age have shifted dramatically over the past half-century, a consequence of public policies, scientific advances, cultural expectations, and market forces. Older adults were once treated as a population deserving of concern and support. As recently as the mid-1960s, nearly one in three adults age sixty-five and older lived in poverty. In a now-legendary broadcast, Walter Cronkite described the plight of impoverished older adults who had no choice but to eat dog food because they could not afford groceries.[13] It was against this backdrop that President Lyndon B. Johnson, as part of his Great Society program, expanded Social Security benefits so that they lifted millions of older Americans out of poverty.

In stark contrast, contemporary news coverage of older adults favors feel-good stories about super-agers, those who inspire us with their feats of atypical strength, vigor, longevity, or mental acuity. During a single week in March 2017, *NBC Nightly News* aired a feature on Tão Porchon-Lynch, who, at age ninety-nine, still teaches eight yoga classes a week and does ballroom dancing, while *CBS Evening News* introduced viewers to seventy-seven-year-old Jacinto Bonilla, a prostate cancer survivor and personal trainer who was the oldest competitor in the physically grueling 2017 CrossFit Games. NBC's *Today Show* showcased a group of septuagenarians and octogenarians whose brains resembled those of people in their twenties, an advantage attributed to their physical fitness, stimulating hobbies like playing piano and doing crosswords, and active social lives.

These inspiring portrayals of the triumph of the human spirit over senescence attract enthusiastic viewers. The 75 million baby boomers born between 1946 and 1964 are marching into old age, and these can-do media images may appeal to generations who pride themselves on being agentic change-makers. The youthful generation who protested to lower the legal voting age from twenty-one to eighteen in 1970 is now mobilizing to transform our notions of old age. Boomers are also a highly sought-after consumer market, spending billions each year on health foods, fitness programs, anti-aging products, and other products and services that might help them to someday be featured on a super-agers news segment.[14]

The scientific community also is committed to showing that old age can and should be a time of good health, youthful vigor, and unprecedented longevity. In 2016, the National Academy of Medicine unveiled its Healthy Longevity Grand Challenge, an initiative that invites scientists to contribute to "an explosion of potential new medicines, treatments, technologies, and preventive strategies that could help revolutionize the way we age."[15] Silicon Valley moguls jumped on this bandwagon, contributing billions of dollars toward research in quest of a cure for aging and death. The ultimate goal, in the words of Martine Rothblatt, founder of a successful biotech firm, is to make death and aging "optional."[16] An unintended consequence of this single-minded focus on optimal aging, however, is that the spotlight is cast on people like the seventy-seven-year-old CrossFit champion for whom old age is the best of times—leaving millions of unhealthy, poor, socially isolated, victimized, incarcerated, and otherwise struggling older adults in the shadows.

In this book, I explore why there is such a vast divide between older adults like Ivy League graduate Goldie Michelson, who enjoyed more than a century of health, wealth, and purpose, and people like Michael Leslie, who died prematurely after struggling with poverty, health problems, homelessness, and substance use. I argue that whether old age is marked by vigor or infirmity, social integration or loneliness, opulence or scarcity, or purpose or despair is guided in large part by an individual's social location, including SES, race, and gender. Socioeconomic status, race, and gender are the three main axes of difference that social scientists study because they are tightly linked to the opportunities and constraints that individuals encounter throughout life. SES encompasses many dimensions, from socioeconomic resources while growing up, such as parents' education, occupation, or poverty status, to attainments in adulthood like years of schooling completed, job status or prestige, income, wealth (the value of savings and possessions), and reliance on public programs for basics like food, shelter, and access to health care. Race and gender also are tightly tied to social and economic opportunities, especially among current cohorts of older adults who grew up in an era before the civil rights and women's rights movements opened up new educational and career possibilities.

Race, gender, and SES profoundly shape how a person ages because they influence the obstacles (or benefits) in childhood, adolescence, and adulthood that set the course for how he or she grows old. These three social markers are linked to level of schooling, marital status, the kind of jobs a person holds, access to health insurance, the quality of care received from medical professionals, assistance received (or not) when struggling with difficult caregiving chores, life stressors, and ways of coping with those stressors. Late-life disparities rarely emerge anew upon one's sixty-fifth birthday. Rather, these inequities are the result of slowly unfolding, cumulative processes that can span decades, like a lifelong smoking habit, persistent workplace discrimination, or long-term exposure to neighborhood pollution.

Federal programs like Social Security and Medicare have been tremendously effective in improving the overall health and economic well-being of older Americans over the past half-century—so much so that some policy experts have questioned heavy public investment in programs that benefit older adults when children today are more likely to live in poverty.[17] Yet that claim is undermined by two important considerations. First, while official measures of poverty generated by the Census Bureau show that just 10 percent of older adults, yet nearly 20 percent of children, live in poverty, newer measures suggest that old and young Americans are equally likely to be poor, both with rates of about 15 percent. The newly developed Supplemental Poverty Measure (SPM) is considered a more accurate and realistic snapshot of late-life poverty because it takes into consideration older adults' very high out-of-pocket health care expenses, among other factors.[18]

Second, these overall statistical snapshots conceal persistent and vast inequalities among older adults. For instance, black and Latino women living on their own are nearly five times as likely as married white men to be poor. This divide is explained in part by the structure of Social Security benefits, which essentially penalize those with short-term (or no) marriages as well as those in dual-earner couples, experiences that are especially common among women of color.

Likewise, Medicare, which provides health care coverage to nearly all older adults, is one of the most successful social programs in U.S. history. However, this federal health insurance program does not cover all of beneficiaries' health expenses.[19] Well-off older adults can make up the gap with their savings, and very low-income older adults can supplement their Medicare coverage with Medicaid. But older adults living just above the poverty line must either scrape together money for additional insurance or else forgo those medications or assistive devices they cannot afford. And access to health care alone cannot resolve problems like the implicit biases that may lead health care providers to treat black and white older patients differently, or economic factors that limit access to healthy foods, neighborhoods, and lifestyles.[20] A theme throughout this book is that public policies play a major role in helping to even out the playing field in later life, but they cannot fully eradicate disparities in older adults' well-being because these chasms are so deep-seated and their roots so multifaceted.

A further goal of this book is to reveal the powerful ways in which old age intensifies the harmful consequences of social and economic disadvantage, and conversely, how the "normal" and anticipated complications of old age, like a weakening immune system and an unsteady gait, are particularly threatening for those aging under adverse conditions. Shoddy housing with sporadic heating in the winter and unreliable air conditioning in the summer is uncomfortable for anyone, but it can sicken older adults, who are particularly susceptible to hypothermia and hyperthermia. Natural disasters like hurricanes and floods, which disproportionately affect poor areas with substandard housing, can be life-altering or even lethal for frail or isolated older adults who lack the wherewithal to evacuate. Homelessness and imprisonment are difficult for anyone, but can be devastating for older adults. Sleeping on a thin mattress with a threadbare blanket in a homeless shelter can be painful for older adults' frail and arthritic bodies. Incontinence and the need for help with dressing and toileting may leave an older prisoner vulnerable to victimization at the hands of predatory cellmates. Old age intensifies the indignities of disadvantage, just as disadvantage amplifies the indignities of aging.

Sociological theories of cumulative inequality conceptualize old age as an end product of the accumulating experiences that came earlier in life. I show how the accumulation of misfortune (or good fortune) continues and may even escalate after one reaches old age. For instance, social isolation makes an older adult especially vulnerable to abuse and financial exploitation. This mistreatment, in turn, intensifies older victims' isolation, either because they are fearful and embarrassed to show their bruises and scrapes to others, or because their abusers cut them off from the outside world. Ageism, which encompasses mistreatment or discrimination on the basis of age, poses a steep hurdle to older adults who want or need to go back to work.[21] People who have had hardscrabble lives are even more vulnerable to ageism than their well-off counterparts because they tend to be younger when they develop visible signs of aging like gray hair, wrinkled skin, a slower gait, tooth loss, or stooped shoulders. Even in old age, adversity can beget further adversity, widening the divide between those who age well and those who do not.

The final goal of the book is to identify potential strategies, including public policies, community initiatives, and cultural and attitudinal shifts, that may help to ensure that all people have an opportunity to age well. The plight of Americans growing old under conditions of poverty and social isolation demands the attention of researchers, policymakers, practitioners, business leaders, and the general public. Understanding late-life social inequalities is important not just because the suffering of older adults violates our belief that our elders should be respected and cared for, or because the thought of older adults going without adequate food, heat, or medication tugs at our heartstrings today, just as it did during Walter Cronkite's emotional broadcasts five decades ago. Vast numbers of Americans are growing old under disadvantageous circumstances, and thoughtful policy solutions and community interventions are required. Older adults will account for an unprecedented 21 percent of all Americans by the year 2030, with their ranks projected to top 74 million. If the current old-age poverty rate prevails, even using the conservative estimate of 10 percent, more than 7 million older adults in 2030 will struggle to afford basic essentials.[22] Alongside population aging, levels of income inequality—or the gap between the haves and have-nots—have escalated dramatically since the 1980s and may lead to even wider disparities in health and well-being as the baby boom cohort and subsequent generations reach old age.

Throughout the book, I synthesize the results of rigorous research based on high-quality data to describe the complex ways in which socioeconomic status, race, and gender shape multiple aspects of older adults' lives. I describe the measures and methods that social scientists use to study aging and older adults' well-being, and I show how potential sources of bias in these measures may lead to inaccurate or misleading conclusions about late-life disparities. I draw on evidence from sociology, epidemiology, medicine, psychology, public health, economics, and gerontology to provide a more comprehensive analysis of later-life inequalities than can be captured with any one disciplinary approach. By adopting a multidisciplinary approach, I hope to reveal the complex biological, psychosocial, behavioral, environmental, and policy mechanisms that explain, intensify, or help to resolve disparities in the quality of older adults' lives.

An Overview of the Book

Before delving into how and why older adults' lives diverge so starkly on the basis of SES, race, and other social factors, it is important to first provide a demographic and conceptual foundation for understanding older Americans today, including who they are, why there are so many of them, and why some possess the economic resources necessary to enjoy their golden years while others do not. Chapter 2 provides a statistical snapshot of the older adult population in the United States today, describing how and why population aging happens, the demographic and economic characteristics of the sixty-five-and-older population in the contemporary United States, and the social, economic, historical, and public policy factors that have contributed to the makeup of today's older population.

Chapter 3 gives an overview of the theoretical perspectives that help us understand why and how experiences in childhood, adolescence, and adulthood leave such a powerful imprint on how we age. I draw on life-course perspectives in sociology, which emphasize that our experiences in later life are not solely a response to immediate circumstances but rather are the end product of long-standing social, economic, and interpersonal forces. Taking this long-term view, I describe conceptual models of cumulative inequality that show how accumulating experiences of good fortune can put one on track to a happy and healthy old age, whereas snowballing hardships may set one on a course toward disease and despair in late life. That's not to say that a blissful childhood guarantees a golden old age, or that early struggles destine a child to a life of illness and sorrow. Life-course perspectives also reveal the ways in which personal choices, supportive social relationships, coping strategies, fortuitous historical circumstances, and innovative public policies and social programs can help to redirect one's fortunes.

The next five chapters dig deeply into domains that are essential to older adults' well-being: their physical health (chapter 4), mental health (chapter 5), social relationships and integration (chapter 6), homes, living conditions, and neighborhoods (chapter 7), and end-of-life care (chapter 8). These chapters show the complex ways in which race, SES, and gender shape nearly every aspect of older adults' lives. They also underscore that while many strains of aging—like health declines, caregiving demands, bereavement, and encounters with ageism—are universal and inevitable, the extent to which they undermine older adults' well-being depends on their other social and economic resources.

Chapter 4 explores disparities in older adults' physical health, focusing on their risk of death, disease, and disability. The story of older adults' health and longevity over the past century is largely a good news story: life span has increased, and rates of most diseases have declined.[23] Yet, as with poverty rates, these statistical snapshots conceal stubborn and substantial disparities. Blacks consistently fare worse than whites; those with fewer socioeconomic resources experience more illness and disability and earlier death than their better-off counterparts; and women generally have worse health, although longer life spans, than men. I focus on three main mechanisms that contribute to these disparities: stress, health behaviors, and access to care. An overarching theme is that biological aging is inevitable, yet stress can speed up these processes such that disadvantaged older adults suffer earlier onset of symptoms and ultimately earlier death.

Chapter 5 investigates older adults' mental health, including symptoms of depression, anxiety, substance use, and suicidal tendencies, and shows the complex ways in which stress and coping resources render an individual vulnerable to (or resilient in the face of) mental health threats. Mental health poses a particularly intriguing topic when studying inequalities in later life, because different disparities emerge for different outcomes. Older women are more depressed than men, yet men are more likely to kill themselves. Blacks and whites are similar when it comes to depression rates, yet blacks are less likely than whites to receive the mental health treatments they need to address their symptoms. These complex and even paradoxical findings shed light on how structural and interpersonal factors contribute to late-life mental health disparities. In chapters 4 and 5, I underscore that risk factors for compromised or inadequately treated physical and mental health are modifiable, and I show how current public policies and health care innovations may help to narrow the health divide in later life.

Chapter 6 describes how older adults experience key social relationships (or the lack thereof), including marriage and romantic partnerships, parenthood and grandparenthood, and friendships. I highlight race, gender, and socioeconomic differences (and similarities) in these experiences and show the importance of social ties in contributing to (or mitigating against) disparities in older adults' well-being and financial security. I then explore the dark side of older adults' social relationships, shedding light on three common problems: social isolation and loneliness, elder mistreatment, and intensive caregiving. I show that all older adults are at risk of these experiences, yet for those who are already physically, psychologically, or economically vulnerable, this risk is most acute and makes them even more susceptible to further isolation, distress, and ultimately premature death. Social relationships are a key mechanism driving cumulative disadvantages, yet they also can be a source of protection that mitigates against growing inequities in health and well-being in late life.

Chapter 7 shows that the dramatic variation in where, with whom, and how comfortably older adults live is a consequence of their earlier experiences, including wealth accumulation, residential discrimination, and social ties. I describe older adults' living arrangements, the personal and public policy factors that shape these arrangements, and the impact of older adults' homes and neighborhoods on their health, well-being, and social integration. As the chapter illustrates, how and where older adults live is a function not only of personal preferences and resources but also of public policies dictating the type of long-term care services covered by Medicare and Medicaid. I hone in on four aspects of place that sustain and exacerbate disparities in older adults' well-being: compositional factors (who lives in their neighborhood), physical aspects of the built environment, crime and neighborhood disorder, and vulnerability to disasters. I conclude by focusing on a small yet growing group of older adults who have fallen through the cracks and are living on the streets, in shelters, or in prison. Older prisoners and homeless persons provide an especially devastating example of how cumulative disadvantages over the life course can threaten well-being and personal dignity in late life.

Chapter 8 focuses on the final stage of older adults' lives: the days and weeks leading up to their deaths. While chapter 4 describes social inequalities in older adults' risk of death, this chapter investigates social inequalities in the process of dying. I provide a historical sketch of death and dying in the United States and suggest reasons why inequalities in older adults' dying experiences are a uniquely contemporary phenomenon. I describe the core components of good versus bad deaths and show how these experiences are linked to race, socioeconomic status, gender, and social integration (or isolation). I also argue that while death is inevitable, a bad death is not—not even for older adults experiencing persistent disadvantages over the life course. I describe individual strategies that may help older adults die peacefully and on their own terms, like advance care planning, while also delineating the ways in which public policies, especially Medicare enrollment criteria and reimbursement practices for hospice care, may contribute to disparities in end-of-life care.

Finally, chapter 9 provides a glimpse into the future, describing the ways in which current social, economic, and political trends are setting the stage for the aging experiences of the large cohort of baby boomers and for the Generation X and millennial cohorts that follow. In speculating about how late-life inequalities might diminish (or widen) in the future, I identify five social and economic patterns that may influence how future cohorts age: rising levels of income inequality; the lingering impact of the Great Recession; escalating rates of obesity and opioid addiction; dramatic changes in family structure; and the challenges and opportunities associated with extreme longevity. These forces could create an even larger bifurcation between the haves and have-nots among future cohorts of older adults if public policies and social programs do not target the roots of these disparities. I conclude by suggesting broad public initiatives that may help to uphold the quality of life of all Americans as they transition into old age, and that recognize, promote, and celebrate the important contributions of older adults to society as citizens, volunteers, workers, family members, and caregivers.

Chapter 2

Older Adults in the Contemporary United States: A Snapshot

The U.S. population is aging at an unprecedented pace. The number of adults age sixty-five and older increased from just 1 million in 1870 to a staggering 48 million in 2016. The "gray tsunami," as sensationalist headlines call it, will escalate in the coming decades. By 2030, more than 74 million Americans will be age sixty-five or older. When these numbers are translated into percentages, their magnitude is even more remarkable. In 1900, just 4 percent of the U.S. population was age sixty-five and older. That proportion climbed to just under 15 percent by 2016 and is expected to reach 21 percent by 2030. Even steeper growth is expected for the oldest-old population, defined as those age eighty-five and older, and centenarians like Susannah Mushatt Jones. In 1900, just 0.2 percent of all Americans, or about 100,000 people, reached their eighty-fifth birthday. By 2016, that rate had jumped to 2 percent, and by 2030 an estimated 2.5 percent of Americans—numbering more than 20 million—will be age eighty-five and older. Relatively few Americans will survive long enough to receive a congratulatory "Happy 100th Birthday" letter from the president of the United States, yet centenarians' ranks have been increasing steadily. In 2000, just 50,000 Americans had reached their 100th birthday, while more than 72,000 did so by 2016. This number is expected to top 600,000 by 2060, although this would still constitute less than 1 percent of the sixty-five-and-older population, and less than 0.02 percent of the total U.S. population.[1]

Why has the older population grown so dramatically, and why is such steep growth projected over the next five decades? Population growth is the result of three demographic processes: fertility, mortality, and migration. Migration, or the movement of people into or out of a region or nation, cannot account for the rising number of older adults nationally because it is a rare person who emigrates from another nation into the United States in later life. Fully 90 percent of all foreign-born older adults in the United States moved here before the age of sixty-five. In-migration, or movement within the United States, helps to explain why a retirement destination like Florida is the oldest state in the nation: one in five Sunshine State residents are age sixty-five or older. However, the rising number of older adults in the nation overall is not plausibly explained by older adults migrating here.

Fertility and mortality are the two main demographic forces driving the graying of America. Fertility refers to the number and timing of babies born in a particular era, such as the high birth rates in the post–World War II years. The large baby boom cohort is now reaching old age in record numbers. The oldest of the boomers, the 1946 birth cohort, which includes Presidents Bill Clinton, George W. Bush, and Donald Trump, celebrated their sixty-fifth birthdays in 2011. Those born at the tail end of the baby boom in 1964, including former first lady Michelle Obama and entrepreneur Jeff Bezos, will make that transition in 2029. The large cohort of school-age children who made the Mickey Mouse Club and hula hoops the rage in the 1950s, who inspired the youth-centric counterculture of the 1960s, and who arguably led the charge for women's equality and LGBTQ rights in the 1970s and 1980s are now contributing to the unprecedented aging of the U.S. population.[2]

But large cohorts of infants, like the 75 million boomers born in the 1940s, 1950s, and early 1960s, are not sufficient to create a large elderly population some sixty-five years later. Those infants must survive until old age in order to contribute to the graying of society. Declining mortality rates are arguably the most powerful force influencing population aging. Life expectancy at birth in the United States jumped from forty-six years for men and forty-eight for women in 1900 to seventy-seven years for men and eighty-one for women in 2016. In the early twentieth century, rising life expectancies were due primarily to strides in conquering infectious diseases, whereas medical advances, especially those that helped reduce cardiovascular mortality, further contributed to longer life spans from the mid-twentieth century forward.[3]

In 1900, 100 out of every 1,000 babies born would die within the first year of life; by the turn of the twenty-first century, this rate had plummeted to 10 per 1,000. Improvements in nutrition and hygiene, including simple practices like regular handwashing, and major advances like water chlorination and milk pasteurization have been essential to the survival of infants and children. Late-life survival rates also have increased over the past century. In 1900, a person who had the good fortune to survive until his or her sixty-fifth birthday could expect to live another twelve years. By 2010, sixty-five-year-old men and women could anticipate living another eighteen years and twenty years, respectively.[4]

Historians and public health experts cite several reasons why life expectancies have climbed so dramatically. Infectious diseases like influenza, diarrhea, and diphtheria were the leading causes of death for young and old people alike in the early twentieth century. With the eradication of these diseases and the lengthening of life spans, other conditions that strike later in life, like cancer and heart disease, have become more prevalent.[5] Deaths from workplace accidents and injuries, which struck young men at particularly high rates in the early twentieth century, have dropped due to both improvements in occupational safety and economic transformations: workers have left the farms, factories, and coal mines for less hazardous white-collar jobs.

Scientific and medical innovations throughout the twentieth century also helped to reduce death rates and increase life expectancy. Vaccinations have virtually eliminated once-common diseases like tetanus, smallpox, and measles. Antibiotics like penicillin helped save the lives of those suffering from streptococcal and staphylococcal infections. With new treatments for cardiovascular disease, a heart attack is no longer a death sentence. In the mid-twentieth century, nearly 40 percent of heart attack victims never made it home from the hospital, dying either from the attack or from complications that followed. By 2010, fewer than 10 percent of heart attack sufferers would face a similarly bleak fate, thanks to the development of beta blockers and medical innovations like angioplasty.[6] Yet not all patients can and do take advantage of these life-saving technologies. Promising high-tech treatments often are out of reach for lower-income and African American older adults, who may lack a regular provider who refers them to specialists, as well as access to state-of-the-art health care facilities near their homes. They also tend to get care at crowded, high-volume hospitals where quality of care may be compromised.[7]

Public health initiatives also have helped to promote behaviors linked with good health and longevity, yet these campaigns are most effective in changing the practices of those who have the financial means and social supports to do so. Public health campaigns extolling the importance of wearing seat belts, quitting smoking, and cutting down on salt have raised awareness of preventive health behaviors. Reminders to get regular mammograms and colonoscopies have helped to detect and treat breast and colorectal cancers.[8] The reduction in smoking rates throughout the twentieth century is upheld as a major public health achievement. In 1955, an astounding 57 percent of men and 28 percent of women were smokers; by 2013, those numbers had dipped to 21 and 15 percent, respectively.[9]

Yet not all Americans experienced similar drops. Unhealthy behaviors that were once egalitarian or even part of a glamorous upper-middle-class lifestyle, like smoking, are increasingly concentrated in disadvantaged populations. In the 1950s, the typical American smoker might have resembled *Mad Men*'s Don Draper and his dapper advertising executive colleagues. By the 1990s, however, upper- and middle-class Americans had largely abandoned their cigarettes, heeding strong messages from the Surgeon General's office that smoking can kill. But their lower-income counterparts did not. One study found that rates of smoking among high-income Americans dropped by 62 percent between 1960 and 2000, but just 9 percent among low-income Americans.[10] That is one reason for the persistence of health and longevity disparities among older adults, despite historic advances in public health and medical technology. People with more economic resources, more education, and a higher level of literacy benefit most from public health campaigns, technological advances, and policy initiatives intended to benefit the entire population, as the examples of smoking and angioplasty reveal. This theme, which reemerges throughout the book, helps to explain an important paradox. The aging of the U.S. population is largely a good news story *in the aggregate:* average life spans, income levels, housing quality, health, and functioning have improved dramatically over the past century. Yet when we dig deeper, we see that many older adults have been left behind or have not enjoyed gains comparable to those of their wealthier peers.

Who Are Today's Older Adults? The Diverse Worlds of the Over-Sixty-Five Population

The term "older adult" is a shorthand label for people age sixty-five and older. Yet the use of this broad label can be misleading, implying that old age is a master status that tells us everything we need to know about a person. The sociologist Everett Hughes describes a "master status" as a personal characteristic that has exceptional importance for social identity, often shaping a person's entire life. One reason why this trait is so powerful is that others imbue it with meaning and treat a person as if his or her master status—whether age, race, religion, sexual orientation, or obese physique—"is more significant than any other aspect of . . . the person's background, behavior or performance."[11] Sometimes this status is bestowed importance by social institutions. For instance, upon their sixty-second birthdays, older adults may receive free or reduced bus fares and restaurant discounts, whether or not they need the financial break. At age seventy-five, they are allowed to keep their shoes on at airport security checkpoints, although some (like nonagenarian yoga master Täo Porchon-Lynch) may have better balance and lower-body strength than their grandchildren. Mandatory retirement is generally illegal in the United States, since the passage of the Age Discrimination in Employment Act (ADEA) in 1967, yet several industries still have the right to force older workers out the door—or out of the cockpit. Airline pilots must retire at age sixty-five and pilots age sixty and older on international flights must have a copilot under the age of sixty. Such policies bring into sharp focus the pervasive assumption that age is a telltale marker for health, ability, and mental acuity.[12]

The presumption that older adults constitute a monolithic category is further perpetuated by the media and confirmed by academic studies. Older adults are underrepresented in virtually all media, from television shows to movies to commercials.[13] When older adults are on TV commercials, they are almost always middle-class and impeccably dressed, with a tastefully decorated suburban home in the backdrop. A handsome older man describes how his erectile dysfunction medication gave him back his marriage, as his beaming wife looks on. A woman in her sixties working in the garden or race-walking with her friends describes how she owes her social life to her arthritis medication. Most notably, the characters are healthy and active—or at least they will be by the end of the sixty-second spot boasting the drug's efficacy. This idealized portrayal is at odds with the stereotypes that college students hold. The sociologists Anne Barrett and Laura Cantwell asked undergraduate sociology students at a large state university to draw pictures of older adults. Unlike the happy and active older adults in the final scenes of the pharmaceutical commercials, most of the students' images depicted older adults with some assistive device, like glasses or a cane. Most were frowning.[14]

All stereotypes, good or bad, contain a kernel of truth, yet they also fail to recognize the vast heterogeneity in a population. Older adults are a highly diverse group on the basis of age alone: the young-old have just celebrated their sixty-fifth birthdays, whereas the oldest-old might surpass the 116-year milepost set by Susannah Mushatt Jones. This fifty-year age span eclipses the mere eighteen-year age span that we use to define youth (age zero to eighteen), although most observers recognize that a newborn infant and a high school senior have little in common. Older adults also vary widely with respect to their physical health, cognitive capacities, wealth, social connectedness, literacy, and daily mood. Each of these dimensions of difference powerfully shapes the quality of older adults' everyday lives. A key theme of this book is that some adults will age comfortably and others will not, and that these disparities are deeply rooted in long-standing structural inequalities. To understand how and why experiences in old age vary so widely, it's important to first describe precisely who older adults are today, the economic resources they possess, and why these resources vary so widely on the basis of sex, race, marital status, education, and work history.

Demographic Characteristics

Gender A casual visit to an older adults' residential community or recreation center reveals an obvious demographic reality: older adults are overwhelmingly female, and the feminization of the over-sixty-five population increases with age. In 2015, women outnumbered men by roughly five to four among those age sixty-five and older, and by two to one among those age eighty-five and older.[15] This imbalanced sex ratio is caused by gender differences in mortality. Men die five to six years younger than women, a result of complex biological and social factors, ranging from the protective effects of estrogen to unhealthy aspects of traditional male gender roles that were central to the upbringing of many men raised in the early decades of the twentieth century. Estrogen protects against heart disease by lowering circulatory levels of harmful cholesterol. Women also have stronger immune systems, because testosterone is linked to immunosuppression.[16] Risky behaviors that are especially common among men like smoking and drinking, working in physically dangerous occupations, and refusing to take time out of work for regular checkups all contribute to the gender gap in mortality.[17] This gap has shrunk since the late twentieth century, largely because of improvements in men's health and health behaviors. For this reason, the ratio of men to women age sixty-five and older narrowed from 67 per 100 in 1990 to 79 per 100 in 2014, and it is projected to narrow even further, to 82 per 100, by 2030.[18]

The gender makeup of the older population carries important implications for social relations, living arrangements, and the kinds of support older adults can rely on. As chapters 6 and 7 will show, women are more likely than men to be widowed. Consequently, women are more likely to grow old on their own and may be especially vulnerable to social isolation. Women aging alone also are at a greater risk of poverty; that risk is amplified for women of color, who typically have spent many more years on their own than their white counterparts. Black men's relatively high rates of premature mortality, combined with relatively low rates of marriage, increase the chances that black women stay single for life or become widowed prematurely—factors that are linked to their sparser Social Security benefits in old age. Women, even those suffering from health concerns of their own, also bear a heavy burden of caregiv-

Figure 2.1 The Projected Shift in the Ethnic and Racial Composition of the U.S. Population Age Sixty-Five and Older, by Race and Hispanic Origin, 2014–2060

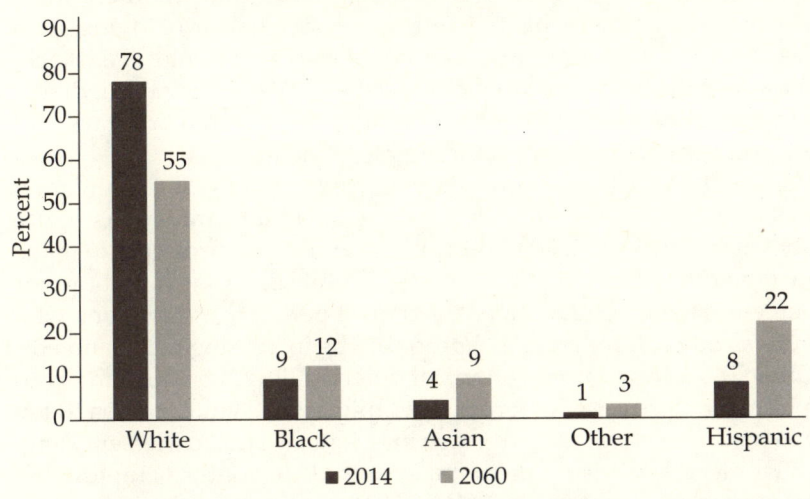

Source: U.S. Census Bureau, "Annual Estimates of the Resident Population by Sex, Age, Race, and Hispanic Origin for the United States and States: April 1, 2010, to July 1, 2014" (PEPASR6H), American FactFinder, https://factfinder.census.gov/faces/tableservices/jsf/pages/productview.xhtml (accessed September 24, 2018); U.S. Census Bureau, "Table 1. Projected Population by Single Year of Age, Sex, Race, and Hispanic Origin for the United States: 2014 to 2060" (NP2014_D1), 2014 National Population Projection Datasets, https://census.gov/data/datasets/2014/demo/popproj/2014-popproj.html (accessed September 24, 2018).
Note: White, black, Asian, and "other" refer to non-Hispanics.

ing, whether for their spouse, aging parents, or grandchildren whose parents have fallen on hard times. As subsequent chapters will show, the gender roles that men and women maintain in their younger years powerfully shape everything from their levels of financial security to their family ties in old age.

Race and Ethnicity Blacks, Latinos, and Asians may appear only rarely in popular cultural images of older adults, but they comprise a rapidly growing share of all older adults.[19] In 2014, the over-sixty-five population was disproportionately white: whites accounted for 78 percent of all older adults, blacks 9 percent, Latinos 8 percent, and Asians and persons who identified as multiracial just 5 percent (see figure 2.1). One reason why current cohorts of older adults are disproportionately white, relative to the overall U.S. population, is differential mortality. Put simply, blacks die younger than whites at every point in the life course. Despite tremendous strides in fighting infant mortality in the United States over the past century, black newborns are still more than twice as likely to die as white newborns. Among young and midlife adults, blacks (especially men) have a much greater chance of dying than whites and as a result are less likely to survive until old age. Black-white disparities in deaths due to homicide, HIV/AIDS, cancer, diabetes, and other causes that may strike fairly early in life are stark and persistent, a product of long-standing racial inequalities.

The racial and ethnic composition of the over-sixty-five population is projected to shift dramatically over the next half-century. As figure 2.1 shows, by the year 2060 non-Hispanic whites are projected to make up just over half of the older population, while blacks will account for 12 percent, Hispanics 22 percent, Asians 9 percent, and persons who identify as other or multiracial 3 percent. The increasing racial and ethnic diversity among future cohorts of older adult will be due largely to the population processes of fertility and migration. White women today are having fewer children on average than Latinas and, to a lesser extent, black women. As a result, the population of U.S. youths is rapidly becoming majority-minority. In 2015, for the first time ever, white newborns were outnumbered by infants of color. Migration patterns also matter: more than half of all older adults who were born outside the United States migrated here prior to 1970, with most hailing from Europe and Canada, whereas more recent waves of immigrants have come from Latin America, Asia, and, to a lesser extent, Africa.[20] Fast-forward these diverse cohorts fifty to sixty years and the racial composition of the older population will look very different than it does today.

Education Educational attainment, or the formal schooling one has completed, is widely considered one of the main markers of a society's well-being.[21] Education not only affects the kind of work one does and how much money one earns and saves but is considered a flexible resource that is linked to better health, healthier behaviors, effective coping skills, and other cognitive and social benefits associated with quality of life. Throughout the twentieth century, educational attainment in the United States increased dramatically for men and women, blacks and whites, and rich and poor. Nevertheless, disparities in high school and college graduation, though narrowed, still persist and contribute to late-life disparities in physical, emotional, and social well-being.

In 1950, fewer than 20 percent of adults age sixty-five and older had earned a high school diploma; by 2010, 80 percent had reached this milestone. College graduation rates also have increased dramatically. As figure 2.2 shows, college graduation rates quintupled in the latter

Figure 2.2 Educational Attainment Among U.S. Adults Age Sixty-Five and Older, by Race, 2015

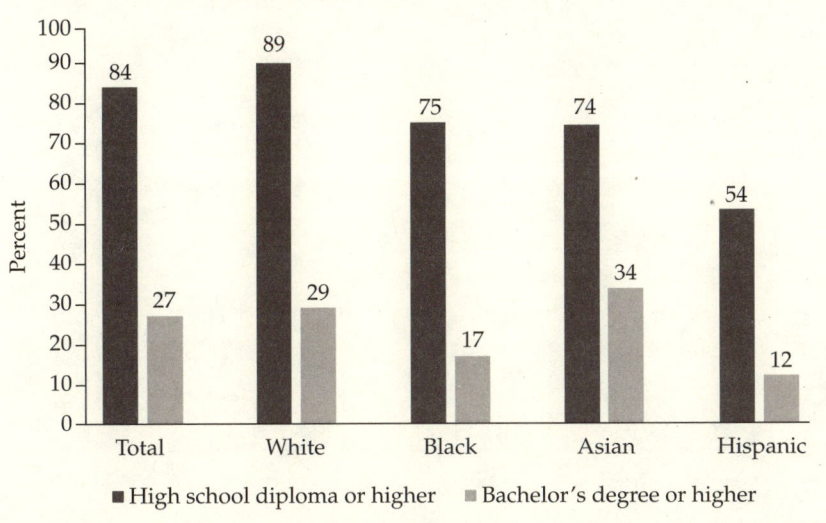

Source: Federal Interagency Forum on Aging-Related Statistics 2016.
Note: White, black, and Asian refer to non-Hispanics.

half of the twentieth century, from less than 5 percent in 1950 to more than 25 percent in 2010. Among current cohorts of older adults, men are more likely than women to have graduated from college, although this gender gap has narrowed among baby boomers and has closed and even reversed slightly among subsequent cohorts.[22] Increases in education have benefited all subgroups, yet race and ethnic disparities persist. In 2015, nearly 90 percent of white older adults had a high school diploma, compared to 75 percent of black and Asian older adults and just 54 percent of Latinos. And while one in three white and Asian older adults today have a college degree, these proportions are considerably lower for blacks and Latinos (17 and 12 percent, respectively).

These gaps matter because education is essential to healthy aging in many different ways. The most obvious is that education opens up rewarding and profitable career opportunities: college-educated young adults are more likely to enter professional occupations that provide a good salary, benefits, including pensions and health insurance, and safe work conditions.[23] Although some white-collar work is stressful, it poses fewer occupational hazards than blue-collar jobs like mining, farming, and construction.

Education also is considered one of the single best predictors of

Figure 2.3 Marital Status of U.S. Men Age Sixty-Five and Older, by Age Group, 2015

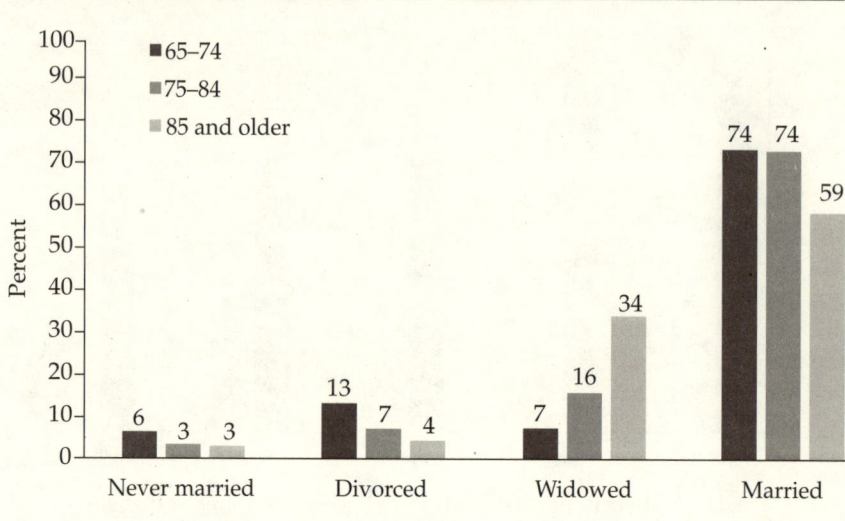

Source: Federal Interagency Forum on Aging-Related Statistics 2016.

whether a person maintains a healthy lifestyle.[24] Over the past three to four decades, more highly educated people have abandoned smoking, drinking, sedentary lifestyles, and high fat–high salt diets at much faster rates than their less-educated counterparts. They also have higher levels of health literacy, which is essential to understanding doctor's orders, following complicated instructions on prescription medication bottles, navigating the complexities of health insurance deductibles, and heeding warnings like the Surgeon General's call against smoking. As a result, highly educated people are both more likely to stay healthy and to recover quickly following a health threat. One analysis of data from the Health and Retirement Study (HRS)—a long-running survey of older adults—found that upon suffering a heart attack, college-educated older adults were more likely to quit smoking compared to those with fewer years of schooling.[25] Higher education also is linked with more ample coping resources. Educated older adults have not only the financial means to purchase those goods and services that help them age well but also the opportunity to develop effective problem-solving skills, such as self-advocacy when interacting with health care providers and health insurers, a future orientation, and a financial literacy that helps them save or invest their money strategically.

Figure 2.4 Marital Status of U.S. Women Age Sixty-Five and Older, by Age Group, 2015

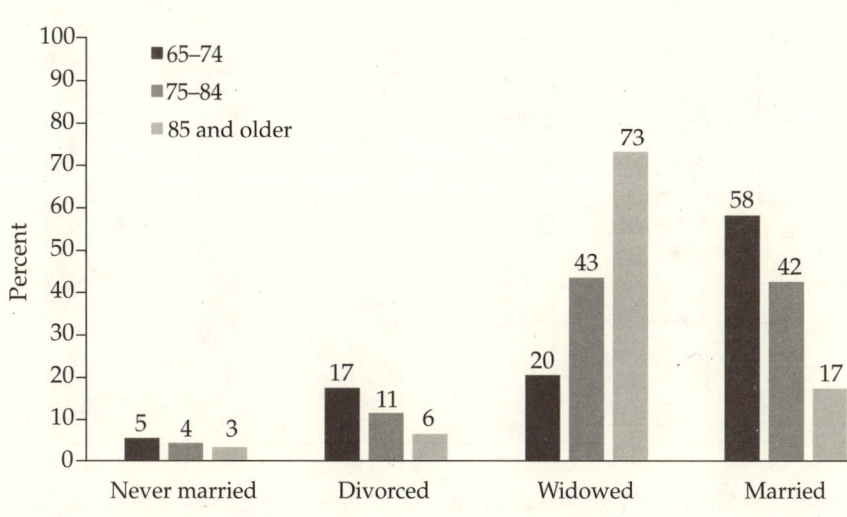

Source: Federal Interagency Forum on Aging-Related Statistics 2016.

Marital Status Older adults' health, happiness, and capacity to live safely and securely in their own homes are linked closely to whether they are married, divorced, separated, widowed, cohabiting with a romantic partner, or a lifelong single. Older men are more likely than older women to be married, and this gender gap widens with age, as figures 2.3 and 2.4 show. Today, among adults age sixty-five to seventy-four, three-quarters of men yet just 58 percent of women are married. By age eighty-five and older, fully 59 percent of men are still married, compared to just 17 percent of women. Women are more likely than men to be widowed, a gap that widens with advancing age. The widowhood gap is due to the fact that wives tend to outlive their husbands, a reality exacerbated by men's tendency to marry slightly younger women. Black women are especially likely to be unmarried, whether never married, divorced, or widowed, and the race gap in marriage has widened considerably over the past six decades.[26]

Older men also are more likely than women to remarry after spousal death or divorce. The snapshot census category of "married" includes those in long-term marriages as well as recently widowed or divorced men who have since remarried. Older women rarely remarry, due to both demographic constraints and personal preferences. Imbalanced sex

Figure 2.5 Living Arrangements of U.S. Men Age Sixty-Five and Older, by Race, 2015

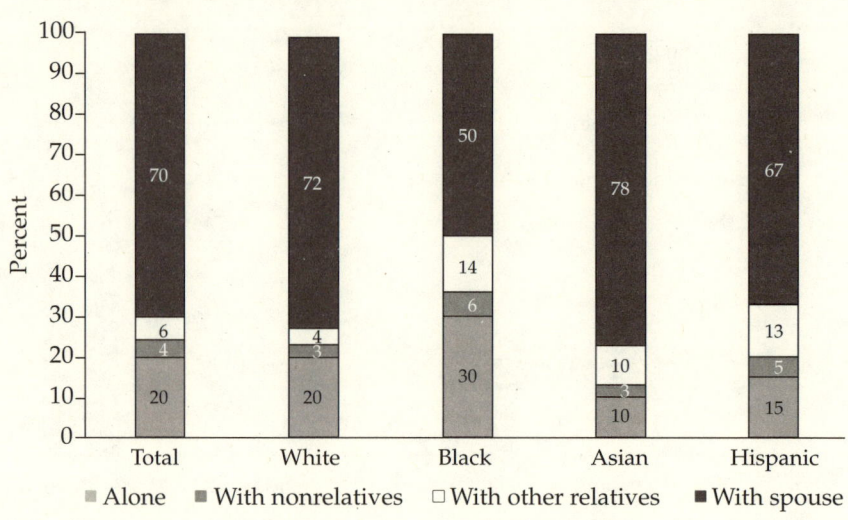

Source: Federal Interagency Forum on Aging-Related Statistics 2016.
Note: White, black, and Asian refer to non-Hispanics.

ratios, where women outnumber men, make it difficult for heterosexual older women to find a same-age male partner. Some intriguing qualitative research also shows that older women simply do not want to remarry because they know it's just a matter of time before they are providing round-the-clock care to an ailing older husband once again.[27] Divorce is relatively rare among current cohorts of older adults, yet each successive cohort is more likely than their predecessors to end their marriages. For instance, 13 percent of men and 17 percent of women age sixty-five to seventy-four are divorced, although these proportions are just 4 and 7 percent among adults age eighty-five and older. For the large cohort of baby boomers that follows, rates of "gray divorce" are rising rapidly. Experts believe that adults now in their fifties and sixties are divorcing in unprecedented numbers because they recognize that they have long lives ahead and question whether they really want to grow old with their current partner.[28]

Gender gaps in marital status make it much more likely that older women will live alone or in a nursing home or assisted living facility. Men tend to age at home, with their wife by their side. Older women, especially those who are widowed or divorced, do not have this luxury. As figures 2.5 and 2.6 show, among the 96 percent of all older adults

Figure 2.6 Living Arrangements of U.S. Women Age Sixty-Five and Older, by Race, 2015

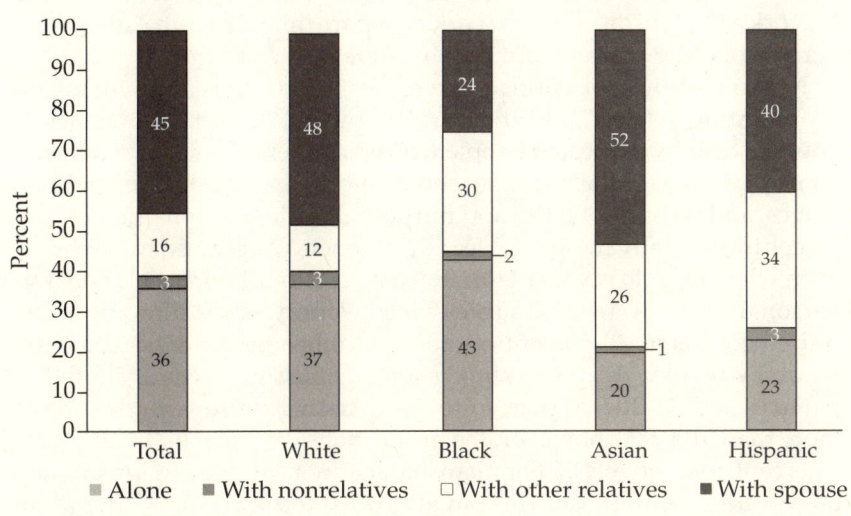

Source: Federal Interagency Forum on Aging-Related Statistics 2016.
Note: White, black, and Asian refer to non-Hispanics.

who live in their own home or apartment, women and, especially, women of color are more likely than whites and men to live alone. While just 20 percent of white men live on their own, fully 43 percent of black women do so. Just 24 percent of black women live with a spouse, whereas roughly two-thirds of men do. Chapter 7 will show how living alone can be isolating and even hazardous to frail older adults who want to stay put in their own homes ("age in place"). Older adults who live alone lack a coresident family member to help them with meals, dressing, bathing, medications, and errands. Those who are financially well off can pay for home health services, but because unmarried women and especially African American and Latino women have more limited income and savings, these services may be out of reach.

Employment and Work History A common stereotype of older adults is that they do not work for pay, with the rare exception of the genial Wal-Mart greeter. Yet census data show that the proportion of older adults who are employed has increased steadily over the past three decades and will likely continue to do so. In 2016, the number of adults age sixty-five and older working for pay topped 9 million, a record-high number accounting for roughly 19 percent of all older adults and one in three adults age sixty-five to sixty-nine. Not all of these workers have remained steadily in the workforce, however; one analysis of HRS data found that as many as 15 percent of working older adults had gone back to work after retiring. Others work on a part-time basis: an estimated 40 percent of older workers put in thirty-five or fewer hours a week.[29]

Researchers have identified two routes to later-life employment, one representing a "pull" and the other a "push."[30] Pull factors generally apply to healthy, educated people who enjoy their jobs and want to keep working for the social and interpersonal connections, intellectual challenges, and sense of identity and purpose they derive from their careers. By contrast, disadvantaged older adults tend to be pushed into working even when they do not want to, driven by economic necessity more than personal desire. A national survey asked working-age adults about their retirement plans; 40 percent of those with incomes under $40,000 said that they would "keep working as long as possible," while another 18 percent said, "I do not plan to retire." Among those with incomes of more than $100,000, however, the proportions were just half that (20 and 7 percent, respectively).[31] For many older adults, retirement is a privilege bestowed only on those who can afford to stop working. Older adults who reluctantly extend their work lives are also deprived of what sociologist Phyllis Moen calls "encore adulthood"—those years between retirement and old age that can be filled with leisure, volunteering, and other meaningful personal pursuits.[32]

Older adults' labor force participation rates have ebbed and flowed throughout the twentieth and twenty-first centuries, before reaching their current high levels. As figure 2.7 shows, more than 40 percent of men age sixty-five to sixty-nine worked for pay in 1965. At that time, paid employment was a necessity for many, given high rates of poverty and sparse public pensions. As Social Security benefits increased throughout the 1970s, older men's employment rates declined steadily, from 42 percent in 1970 to about 25 percent in 1985 for men age sixty-five to sixty-nine, and from 18 percent to 11 percent among men age seventy and older. During that same period, the average retirement age for men dipped from sixty-seven to sixty-two. Women's labor force participation rates are consistently lower than men's but started to creep up in the 1970s, owing in part to expanding occupational opportunities in the wake of the women's movement. During this period, rising divorce rates sent newly single women back into the paid labor force so that they could earn enough to support themselves and their children. Women's employment also saw an uptick in the 2000s, a pattern that some researchers attribute to the Great Recession. Because industries that employ men in large numbers, like finance, insurance, real estate, and construction, were particularly hard hit, more women had to stay in the workforce to help support their families.[33]

Figure 2.7 Labor Force Participation of U.S. Adults Age Sixty-Two and Older, by Age and Sex, 1965–2015

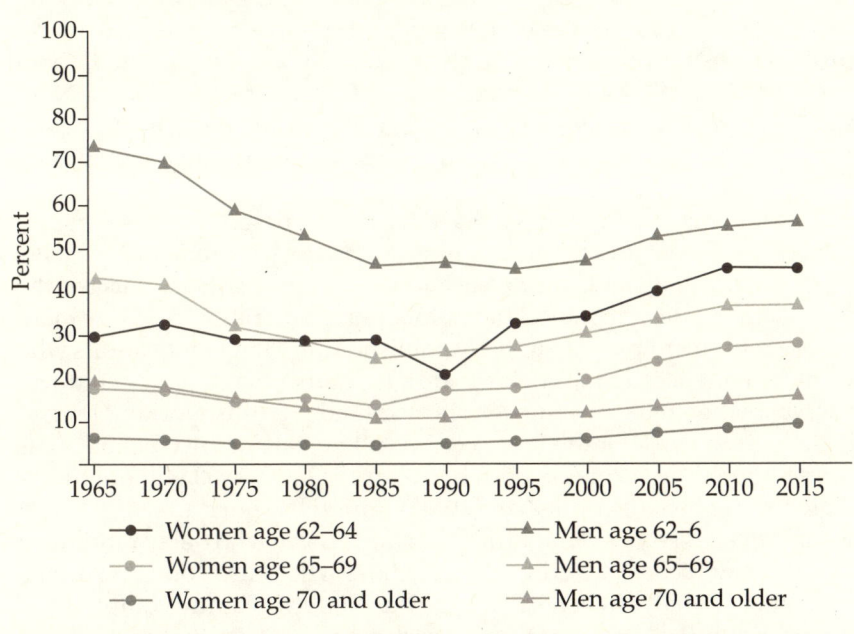

Source: U.S. Bureau of Labor Statistics 2015.

Today older men have higher labor force participation rates than they have had since the 1970s. Nearly 37 percent of men age sixty-five to sixty-nine, and 16 percent of men age seventy and older, were working in 2015. Moreover, older women's labor force participation rates have reached an all-time high, with 28 percent of women age sixty-five to sixty-nine and 9.2 percent of women age seventy and older working for pay in 2015. These high and rising employment levels in recent years are projected to persist into the future, given improvements in health and policy shifts that encourage older adults' employment. On average, older adults are healthier than ever before and can remain in the paid workforce, provided that is what they and their employers want.

Anticipated financial need also impels longer work lives. Healthy older adults recognize that if they are going to survive for another two to three decades past retirement age, they may need to extend their working lives in order to amass the salary and savings needed to finance their retirement years. Especially on the heels of the Great Recession of the late 2000s, rising numbers of older adults say that they plan to delay retirement as a hedge against possible dips in the value of their home and other unanticipated financial hits.[34] For those who had nonstandard employment like part-time work or consulting gigs in their working years, the financial need to remain in the labor force may be particularly pressing. Rising numbers of adults, especially among the baby boom and Generation X cohorts, work on a contract or freelance basis. Nonstandard workers are less likely to have steady full-time work, health benefits, and pensions and thus may need to work longer than they would otherwise prefer.[35]

Policy shifts also have encouraged (or forced, based on one's perspective) employment among older adults. Mandatory retirement ages have been largely abolished, dating back to 1967 when Congress enacted the ADEA. In the decades since, the number of industries covered by mandatory retirement provisions has diminished, allowing more adults who want to work past age sixty-five to do so. Another major policy shift will keep baby boomers and future cohorts of older adults working longer: the age at which workers can receive full Social Security benefits has been bumped up. Workers born between 1942 and 1960 will not be eligible for full benefits until age sixty-six, and those born after 1960 must wait until age sixty-seven for full eligibility. Those who delay retirement even further receive a credit, whereas those who retire younger suffer a permanent penalty in benefits. These benefit formulas are complex, but the upshot is that those who retire earlier see a substantial and permanent dip in their monthly checks, whereas those who have the physical capacity to work beyond their official retirement age reap considerable benefits.[36]

Other structural changes also are extending the working years well into old age. As we will see later in this chapter, declining numbers of older workers (especially women, ethnic minorities, and low-wage workers) receive employer-provided pensions, an important source of financial security in retirement. Yet even for those who do receive such a pension, the structure of these benefits has shifted in such a way that may keep many workers (especially lower-income workers) in the labor force, even if they would prefer to retire. Defined-benefit (DB) pension plans are increasingly giving way to defined-contribution (DC) plans, which provide an incentive (and heighten the need) to stay in the workforce longer.[37] Traditional DB plans are typically funded exclusively by employers and provide workers with lifetime annuities based on how long they were with their employer and their final salary. DC plans, by contrast, are tax-deferred savings accounts, like 401(k) plans, that provide tax and savings incentives to both employers and employees to set aside money for retirement. The payout is determined by the amount of money contributed to the plan and the rate of return on the money invested over time. The future value of DC accounts, like that of savings accounts, depends on both fluctuations in the market and the worker's savvy about investing funds wisely. A poor or misguided investment decision can strike a cruel blow to a worker's future retirement income. Moreover, not all workers have the financial wherewithal to put away money in their DCs. Lower-income workers with more immediate and pressing financial concerns may not contribute as much or as frequently as is required during their working years. That is a key reason why just 40 percent of low-income workers with DC plans, yet more than 80 percent of high-income workers with DCs, actually take advantage of them.[38]

Despite these many factors encouraging (or necessitating) paid employment in later life, staying in the workforce until one's sixties and later may be out of reach for the most disadvantaged older adults. As chapter 4 will show, lower-SES and African American adults experience earlier onset of most major health conditions, ranging from lower-body impairments to arthritis to cognitive declines. This health disadvantage is particularly troublesome because these older adults also are more likely to hold physically demanding blue-collar jobs, such as janitor or truck driver, or pink-collar jobs, such as waitress or convenience store cashier, that require standing, walking, lifting, and bending in order to carry out their tasks. In other words, those with the greatest financial need to work often are the least physically capable of doing so.

That is part of the reason why older adults' labor force participation rates vary so widely based on educational level. In 2014, 42 percent of male college graduates and 31 percent of female college graduates were working for pay after age sixty-five; comparable rates for high school dropouts were just 19 and 11 percent, respectively.[39] Thus, disadvantaged older adults have leaner pensions and savings due to their shorter work histories, they bear hefty medical expenditures years earlier than their more-advantaged counterparts, and they rely more heavily on Social Security income than on earnings to support themselves in old age, as we shall see later in this chapter.

Economic Resources

Older adults' economic standing can be captured with several different measures, including poverty status, levels and types of income, and wealth, which encompasses savings, investments, and homeownership. Each of these indicators varies based on gender, race, marital status, educational level, and work history; as such, economic resources are a crucial mechanism in explaining subgroup differences in later-life well-being.

Overall, the economic well-being of older adults has improved dramatically over the past half-century. Economists estimate that in 2015 just 10 percent of older adults lived beneath the federal poverty line, although this figure is closer to 15 percent when medical expenses are factored in.[40] This scenario is a far cry from the early 1960s, when elderly poverty was a grave national concern.[41] Roughly 30 percent of older adults lived in poverty in 1966, although this rate quickly dropped to just 15 percent by the early 1970s after substantial per capita increases in Social Security payments.[42] The Social Security Act was signed into law by President Franklin D. Roosevelt in 1935 as part of the New Deal. The program was designed to provide social insurance, or income protection, for older adults. During the program's first three decades, its benefits barely provided a minimum standard of living because monthly payments were not adjusted annually to offset inflation. The first-ever beneficiary of Social Security, retired legal secretary Ida May Fuller, received a benefit of $22.54 in January 1940, and her monthly checks remained at that amount for more than a decade. In 1950, benefits were raised for the first time. In 1972, Congress enacted a law that allowed for annual and automatic cost-of-living adjustments (COLAs).

The Social Security system is progressive, meaning that lower-wage earners receive a higher percentage benefit than higher-wage earners. In 2017, the average monthly payment was about $1,400 for a retired worker and $2,300 for a couple when both spouses were receiving benefits. Without Social Security, 40 percent of older adults, rather than the current 10 percent, would be living beneath the official poverty line.[43] Despite the undeniable success of Social Security, more than 4 million older adults still live in poverty. As many as one in three older adults have no money left at the end of the month or have to dip into their dwindling savings to pay their monthly bills.[44] And older adults accounted for more than 12 percent of all the personal bankruptcies declared in the United States between 2013 and 2016, a sad consequence of lean savings, dwindling pensions, unmanageable out-of-pocket medical expenses, and lingering debts like mortgages and their children's college loans.[45]

Poverty disproportionately strikes women and persons of color, especially those who live on their own. As figure 2.8 shows, roughly one in five Latino and black women who are householders live beneath the official poverty line, compared to fewer than 4 percent of white married couples. Across all household and family structures, whites consistently have lower rates of poverty than other ethnic and racial groups. Even among the one group consistently worst off, women living on their own, just 12 percent of white women, yet anywhere from 17 to 21 percent of women of color, live in poverty. Across all racial and ethnic groups, women on their own are one and a half to three times as likely as men to be impoverished.

These gender, race, and marital status gaps in poverty status reflect

Figure 2.8 Poverty Among U.S. Adults Age Sixty-Five and Older, by Sex, Race-Ethnicity, and Household Structure, 2014

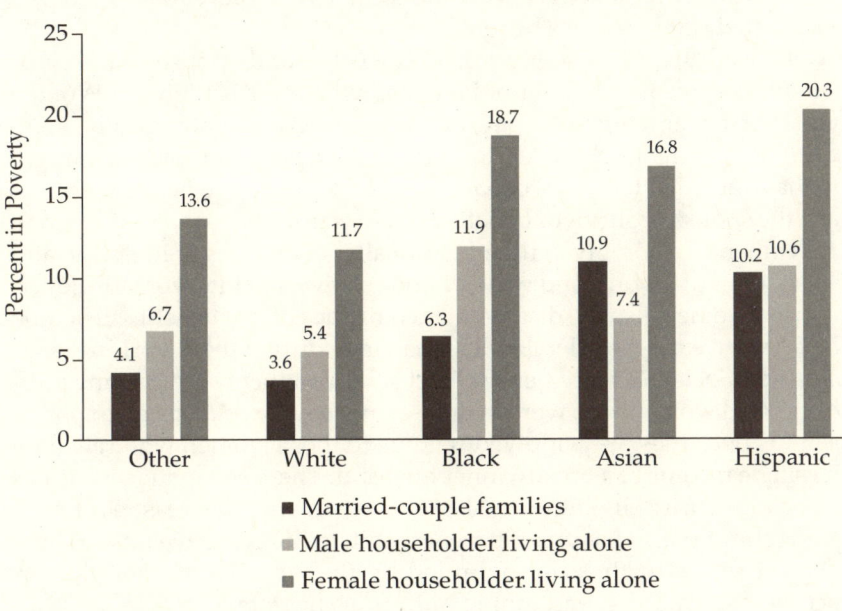

Source: U.S. Census Bureau 2014.
Note: White, black, and Asian refer to non-Hispanics.

many factors, including lower earnings and fewer savings over the life course. Yet these disparities also reflect the structure of Social Security benefits. Social Security is a complex program, yet a rudimentary understanding of the program's basic structure helps us to see why its benefits are not sufficient to eradicate race and gender disparities in poverty.[46] Social Security has a dual eligibility structure, meaning that it offers two paths to benefits. People can qualify for benefits either as a retired worker or as the spouse, ex-spouse, or widow(er) of a retired worker.[47] Yet each of these paths has additional conditions that limit their capacity to lift some out of poverty, especially women of color.

First, older adults may qualify for retired worker benefits, or Old Age Social Insurance (OASDI), if they have a minimum level of earnings over forty quarters (forty three-month periods) or a total of ten years of earnings. The benefits that retirees receive are based on the highest thirty-five years of earnings during one's working life. Second, spouse or survivor benefits are granted to those who were married to a qualified worker for at least ten years. When a married or divorced person reaches full retirement age, they are eligible for spousal benefits equal to one-half the value of their current or ex-partner's benefits. When a widow(er) reaches full retirement age, he or she receives benefits equal to 100 percent of their late spouse's benefit.

Older adults who qualify for both worker and spouse or survivor benefits receive just one set of benefits, whichever is higher.[48] Women who have never worked for pay, or who worked only sporadically, dedicating their time to child-rearing rather than paid employment, might not have accrued ten years of earnings and would have no choice but to take the spouse or survivor benefit. Social Security rules especially penalize women of color, given their historically lower rates of marriage and higher rates of divorce and widowhood relative to white women. Never-married women also are disadvantaged by the current benefits structure: they tend to earn considerably less than men during their working lives, and their Social Security benefits rest solely on their own earnings history.[49] And women who were in dual-earner couples may receive sparser benefits once they are widowed relative to those women who relied on the single income of a breadwinner husband. These economic disparities in Social Security eligibility and benefits levels are a key reason for race, gender, and marital status differences in late-life poverty status. These disparities are further compounded by the fact that women, lower-income older adults, and ethnic minorities have few sources of additional income to supplement their monthly Social Security checks.

Income Sources Older adults' retirement income has been described as a "three-legged stool," where the three legs are Social Security income, private pensions, and personal savings and investments (along with the interest generated by those investments). The stool also has a fourth leg: earnings from wages, salary, or self-employment income.[50] Although earnings historically were considered a relatively unimportant leg of the stool in an era when most older adults exited the labor force, more and more older adults are working for pay today, for reasons we saw earlier in this chapter. The types of income that older adults receive are critically important to their financial security, especially during eras in which public support for Social Security is in a state of flux or even erosion. Older adults who rely most heavily on public pensions are the most threatened by austere political shifts, whereas more financially secure older adults who rely on other income sources have a cushion against public funding cuts.

Social Security is by far the most important source of income for older adults, and especially for those with few alternative financial resources. On average, Social Security accounts for about one-third of older adults' income, although this share varies dramatically: older women, minority

Figure 2.9 Income Sources for Households Headed by U.S. Adults Age Sixty-Five and Older, by Household Income Level, 2014

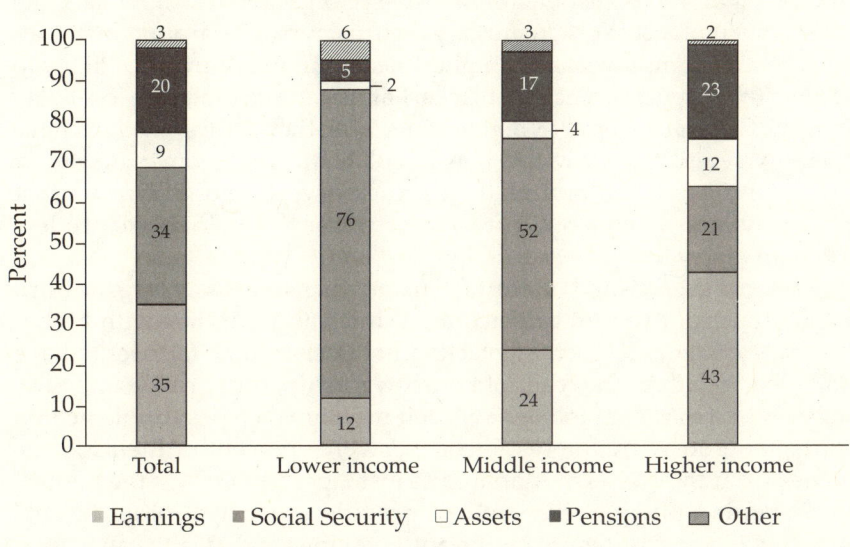

Source: U.S. Census Bureau 2015.
Note: "Lower income" includes those living at or below 200 percent of the poverty line, "middle income" includes those living between 200 and 400 percent of the poverty line, and "higher income" includes those living at or above 400 percent of the poverty line.

families, and poorer older adults are much more dependent on Social Security. Figure 2.9 shows the breakdown of older adults' income by source, based on whether they live in a lower-, middle-, or higher-income household. The lower-income category includes those living at or below 200 percent of the poverty line, and the highest are those living at or above 400 percent of the poverty line. Social Security benefits account for more than three-quarters of the monthly incomes of lower-income households, but just 52 and 21 percent of the household incomes of middle- and higher-income households, respectively.

Ethnic minority families and women are particularly dependent on Social Security as their primary or only source of income. One in five black and Latino older households survive solely on their monthly Social Security checks, compared to just 13 percent of white households. Women are more likely than men to rely on Social Security as their sole or primary income source. In 2014, Social Security accounted for 47 percent of older unmarried women's income, compared to just 34 percent among unmarried men and 29 percent among older married couples.

Employer-provided pensions are considered the second most important source of retirement income after Social Security. However, the number of employers providing these plans has dropped dramatically since the late 1990s; just half of private-sector employees now have access to such plans. Workers for larger firms, typically around one hundred or more employees, and higher-income workers are most likely to receive these benefits. Because blacks, Latinos, and women are less likely to work for large firms or in higher-wage jobs, they are less likely to have their own employer-provided pension plan. Married women may have access to such a plan through their spouse's work—another factor that puts private pensions out of reach for women of color, who are less likely to marry and stay married.[51]

Personal savings and interest from one's personal assets are the third major source of retirement income. Whites and families with higher incomes are more likely than blacks and lower-income families to have amassed wealth in the form of homeownership, other real estate, savings, and investments and to have their monthly incomes supplemented more generously by interest income. Twelve percent of their income comes from their assets, compared to just 2 percent among the poorest households.[52] Interest income can provide a boost to older adults' monthly income, but more importantly, savings and wealth can help to sustain a family's standard of living when a crisis such as job loss, retirement, death of a spouse, or illness strikes. Race and ethnic gaps in wealth (and consequently interest income) are vast, reflecting the persistence of economic obstacles and racism facing blacks and Latinos over the life course.

Blacks have lower levels of education, more sporadic work histories, and lower earnings over the life course relative to whites. As a result, blacks are less likely than whites to have a solid savings account, to own a home, to invest in stocks and bonds, or to acquire other interest-generating assets. These discrepancies reflect long-standing patterns of race-based discrimination in the labor market, institutional discrimination like bank lending practices, and public policies that disadvantage blacks, like the GI Bill.[53] Blacks may also have more difficulty saving any money at the end of the month because they are more vulnerable to educational, medical, and housing debt, often accruing high monthly interest charges through high-cost loans.[54] As a result, the black-white gap in assets widens dramatically over the life course. One recent analysis of Survey of Consumer Finance (SCF) data found that, in their thirties, whites have an average of $147,000 more in wealth than blacks (three times as much). By their sixties, whites have over $1.1 million more in average wealth than blacks (seven times as much).[55]

Finally, earnings are an increasingly important income source for older adults, especially those age sixty-five to seventy-four who are healthy enough to work and who hold white-collar jobs that are compatible with aging bodies. As figure 2.9 shows, the proportion of monthly income coming from earnings is 43 percent among the highest-income households, yet just 12 percent among the lowest-income households. This pattern reflects the facts that higher-income households tend be younger and that poorer adults experience the earlier onset of major illnesses and physical impairments, which shorten their work careers. Physical impairments are especially likely to cut short the work lives of those who are on their feet all day, like waitresses and cashiers, or workers who do heavy lifting and bending, like stockroom or construction workers. Higher-income older adults, by contrast, are more likely than their lower-income counterparts to have held white-collar jobs with benefits, so it is not surprising that they receive a larger share of late-life income from private pension sources (23 versus 5 percent).

In sum, despite the many benefits of Social Security, it is not sufficient to overcome the cumulative disadvantages that women and ethnic minorities experience over the life course. Social Security replaces about 40 percent of an average worker's income when they retire, although financial advisers typically caution retirees that they will need at least 70 percent of their pre-retirement income to live comfortably.[56] Money cannot buy happiness, according to the time-worn adage, yet economic stability is powerfully linked to physical and mental health, provides a cushion when unexpected expenses arise, and allows older adults to purchase the goods and services they need to feel safe and secure in their homes and neighborhoods. Economic resources are an important engine that can either buffer against or exacerbate the challenges of old age, widening the divide between those who enjoy their golden years and those who do not.

Chapter 3

Life-Course Perspectives on Social Inequalities in Later Life: A Brief Overview

A popular saying among life-course sociologists is that "aging starts at birth." This claim succinctly captures a core theme of life-course perspectives in sociology: our experiences in old age are tightly linked to the social advantages and disadvantages that we have experienced throughout life, dating back as early as infancy or even in utero.[1] Social scientists seeking to understand inequalities in later life, such as why one person dies at age sixty-five and another at ninety-five, or why one person has a lively social life and another is a recluse, recognize the importance of present-day influences, like the comfort and security of our home and neighborhood, whether we have enough money to live on, and whether we are happily married or have children living nearby. Yet life-course approaches recognize that each of these immediate conditions is at least partly shaped by earlier experiences such as childhood nutrition, the quality of the schools we attended, the jobs we held during our working years, or the coping skills we developed over time. Yet our early experiences do not cast our destinies in stone. Life-course researchers also debate the extent to which advantages like supportive role models, a college education, a loving marriage, a healthy lifestyle, or a warm and gregarious personality can diminish, offset, or even undo the harmful impact of some early-life adversities.

This long-term view is not unique to sociology. Physicians and medical researchers also recognize that older adults' health and longevity reflect the advantages they have enjoyed and the struggles they have encountered from "cradle to grave" (or the less dignified "sperm to worm" or "lust to dust"). Biomedically oriented researchers tend to emphasize the long-term impacts of early biological influences, such as genetics or fetal development. Social scientists, by contrast, consider a wider array of influences, from highly personal experiences, like encouragement and nurturance from parents or teachers, to sweeping social conditions, like economic booms or public policy initiatives like the GI Bill, which provided life-changing benefits to many World War II veterans in the 1940s and 1950s. One subset of life-course theories, cumulative inequality perspectives, argue further that it is not simply that early experiences directly shape later-life outcomes. Rather, accumulation perspectives emphasize that small advantages (or adversities) early in life beget subsequent advantages (or adversities) over time, such that relatively small differences early in life can become large and highly consequential decades later. This recognition that late-life disparities unfold and even intensify over many years underscores the importance of social programs, policies, and interventions that can help to level the playing field years earlier than one's sixty-fifth birthday. Despite the importance of Social Security and Medicare in providing older adults with an income floor and access to health care, they are not a panacea against late-life poverty and poor health.

The general focus of life-course perspectives on explaining differences rather than similarities in how individuals age departs from classic developmental theories, which emphasize universal aspects of aging. To provide a historical context for understanding the pathbreaking contributions of life-course perspectives, I briefly describe the core themes of classic developmental theories of aging. I then describe the general themes of life-course and cumulative inequality perspectives and underscore how these themes help to explain social inequalities in later life and set a foundation for developing policies or programs to mitigate against these disparities.

Developmental Theories of Late-Life Well-being: A Brief History

The notion that inequalities in late-life health, wealth, and happiness are a product of accumulated life experiences, large and small, may seem obvious today, but this long-term perspective is a quite contemporary advance in how social scientists think about aging. Through much of the early and mid-twentieth century, psychologists and gerontologists relied on developmental models of aging that focused on contemporaneous influences and universal processes. As such, these perspectives paid relatively little attention to differences rooted in persistent inequalities, like the opportunities bestowed or denied on the basis of a person's gender, race, or socioeconomic background. Four of the most influential perspectives—disengagement, activity, continuity, and successful aging theories—provide important foundational insights into how we age, yet these perspectives also are limited in that they pay scant attention to how social inequalities shape the opportunities we have to age well.

Disengagement Theory

Disengagement theory, a prominent perspective in the mid-twentieth century, argued that paring down and ultimately withdrawing from one's social roles and responsibilities is the path to a salubrious and satisfying old age.[2] Drawing heavily on biological views of aging, this framework asserted that it is best for aging minds and bodies to recede from the demands of everyday life and to instead focus on our inner needs as we prepare psychologically and spiritually for death. Elaine Cumming and William Henry argued that such disengagement was beneficial to society as well as to older adults themselves: their withdrawal from work and family roles would open up those opportunities to the younger generation.[3] This perspective is out of step with contemporary views of old age, which promote vigor and engagement until very old age and recognize the many meaningful ways in which older adults can contribute to their families, communities, and society.[4] Presuming that chronological age is a reasonable marker for the biological and cognitive declines that may necessitate withdrawal from social responsibilities, disengagement theory failed to recognize that the timing and severity of age-related health declines vary based on an individual's social location. Some workers may have no choice but to leave their jobs while still in their fifties or early sixties.[5] Those with early onset of health problems may struggle to keep up with work tasks, especially those working in manual jobs that require physical strength and stamina. By contrast, adults working in professional jobs with health benefits, comfortable working conditions, and flexible schedules may have the capacity to remain active, engaged, and vital even into extreme old age.[6]

Activity Theory

Activity theory challenged the core assumptions of disengagement theory. Rather than envisioning late life as a time of solitude and introspection, activity theory argued that staying busy and engaged is essential to well-being.[7] Proponents of this view argued that the voids created by later-life transitions like retirement and widowhood should be filled with pleasant substitutions. Activities were viewed as more or less interchangeable: any manner of keeping busy could provide social and cognitive engagement, a boost to self-esteem, and a sense of purpose, independence, and autonomy. Activity theory was influential in shaping social programs for older adults in the 1960s and 1970s, when senior centers with group activities like bingo and singalongs flourished; even more stimulating activities were organized in the decades that followed, including senior volunteer corps and lifelong education programs like Elderhostel (since renamed Road Scholar), which began in 1975.[8] The underlying assumption of activity theory is strongly supported by research. Social activity and engagement, whether volunteering, visits with friends and family, attending religious services, or participating in activities like travel, sports, and the arts, are linked with older adults' well-being. For instance, volunteering just two or three hours a week is linked with fewer depressive symptoms, better health, and longer lives for older adults.[9]

Yet activity theory presumed that the same activities are equally valuable or desirable to all, failing to consider older adults' personal preferences, capabilities, and access to resources that facilitate participation in these activities. Like disengagement theory, activity theory neglected the social and economic factors that may hinder gainful activity. Poor health may prevent older adults from volunteering, visiting with friends, or attending religious services, while those living in poverty may not have the means to travel or enjoy other pricey leisure activities.[10] The perspective also presumed causation—that is, that activities enhance well-being, rather than the equally plausible possibility that being healthy, happy, and mentally sharp enables and inspires older adults to remain active. More generally, activity theory conceptualized well-being as a result of personal choices and initiative, failing to consider that the goal of staying active and engaged is out of reach for the most physically vulnerable and socially isolated older adults.

Continuity Theory

Like activity theory, continuity theory held that activity and engagement are essential to older adults' well-being.[11] Yet it also recognized that merely staying busy is not sufficient; rather, older adults should engage in activities similar to those that they carried out during their younger years. A retired schoolteacher might volunteer in an elementary school classroom, a professional musician who has left the concert circuit might give afternoon recitals in local nursing homes, or a former construction worker might help build homes for Habitat for Humanity. Continuity theory also emphasized the importance of stability in one's living space, recommending that older adults who move into long-term care facilities arrange their rooms in ways that resemble their longtime homes. Such continuity and stability, the theory proposed, provides a sense of comfort and predictability that is integral to well-being. Yet critics note that this emphasis on continuity neglected the fact that some older adults might not have chosen or enjoyed the jobs, relationships, activities, and places that filled their younger years. Older adults who had limited economic resources or who faced discrimination on the basis of their race, gender, sexual orientation, or other personal traits might not have willingly selected their jobs, neighborhoods, and homes, but instead defaulted to whatever options were available to them. Still others may want desperately to leave behind the conditions of their earlier years, such as an unpleasant workplace, demanding caregiving responsibilities, or a run-down home. The underlying assumption was that our experiences in early and midlife are positive and should be continued, although this assumption is questionable for those whose earlier lives were marked by constrained or few opportunities.

Successful Aging Theories

Successful aging models, proposed by the physician Jack Rowe and the psychologist Robert Kahn, are probably the most widely cited perspective in social gerontology today.[12] The underlying premise is optimistic and consistent with current cultural and social messages that old age can be a time of vigor, vitality, and social engagement, provided we put in the effort and make healthy lifestyle choices. In their original formulation, Rowe and Kahn proposed that successful aging encompasses high levels of cognitive and physical functioning, minimal risk of disease and illness, and active engagement with life. The main pathways to successful aging are leading a healthy lifestyle and remaining socially active and engaged. Despite its popularity, this model drew extensive critiques on the grounds that it used a very narrow definition of "success," such that successful aging may be out of reach for those with early onset health conditions, disabilities, or cognitive impairments.[13] Perhaps a more serious concern about the original model, at least in the eyes of sociologists, is its emphasis on choice rather than structure. Sociological perspectives on aging build on successful aging models by recognizing the social patterning of good health, opportunities for social engagement, and access to the goods, services, and environments that facilitate healthy lifestyles. Sociologists' focus on opportunity structures rather than personal agency underscores that individual choice and personal initiative are not enough to ensure that all adults will have the opportunity to age well.

Sociological Perspectives on Aging and the Life Course

Sociological perspectives on aging rest heavily on the life-course paradigm, a framework credited primarily to the sociologist Glen Elder. While developmental models conceptualize aging as a function of biological influences and behavioral adaptations to these biological changes, sociological approaches emphasize the influence of historical contexts, social structures, and public policies on older adults' lives. Life-course researchers are particularly interested in documenting the links connecting early and later-life experiences, paying careful attention to race, gender, and socioeconomic differences in these experiences. Given this attention to diversity, scholars working in the life-course tradition often rely on large longitudinal data sets that track thousands of people over long periods of time, spanning as many as five or six decades. Data collected at multiple time points help to identify the pathways through which early experiences shape life-course trajectories of health, wealth, and well-being, while large sample sizes enable researchers to explore the ways in which gender, race, and other factors may contribute to divergent life-course experiences.[14]

Life-course research rests on four assumptions: (1) human lives are embedded in and shaped by historical contexts; (2) the meaning and impact of a life experience is contingent on a person's age at which it occurs; (3) human lives are linked through social relationships; and (4) individuals construct their own lives through their choices and actions, yet within the constraints of historical and social circumstances. Each of these themes provides a framework for understanding why and how social disparities in later-life experiences emerge, why these processes may unfold differently based on the larger social, political, and economic context, and the extent to which disparities might be mitigated by fortuitous historical circumstances, personal ingenuity, supportive social relationships, or inventive public policies.

The Importance of Historical Context

The first theme guiding life-course research is that our lives are shaped by the historical eras in which we live. Social and historical changes, including cultural shifts in attitudes toward old age, public policies related to pension and health benefits, and biomedical and technological advances that may extend the human life span, powerfully influence the lives of older adults. Recognizing the importance of historical context also helps us to understand why the experiences of older adults in the early or mid-twentieth century were very different from those projected for the large cohort of baby boomers entering old age in the late twentieth and early twenty-first centuries. The careers we pursue, whether we can afford to buy a home, whether our education is interrupted by war or a recession, and the medications and medical technologies available to us are tightly tied to sweeping macroeconomic, social, and political factors.[15] Even our most private and intimate choices are shaped by cultural and historical contexts: when (and whether) to marry and have children, how spouses choose to divide up household chores, and our expectations for caring for or living with aging relatives vary across time periods.

The notion that our lives are shaped by historical contexts dates back to the classic writings of C. Wright Mills. In *The Sociological Imagination*, Mills observed that to understand human lives, scholars must consider both their "biography" and their "history."[16] For instance, current cohorts of older adults born in the 1920s and thereafter have longer life expectancies than the generations that came before them, thanks in part to the medical advances that were introduced shortly before they were born. An infant born in 1930 is more likely than an infant born in 1900 to survive until old age, given pathbreaking advances in sanitation, medicine, and public health that were introduced in the early twentieth century. School and work opportunities also are powerfully shaped by historical and policy contexts. The Supreme Court's *Brown v. Board of Education of Topeka* decision in 1954 ruled it unconstitutional for states to maintain separate public schools for black and white students. This ruling helped to chip away at racial disparities in the quality of schooling that children received. Equal employment opportunity and equal pay laws passed in the 1960s opened up new career doors for women and African Americans and helped to diminish long-standing wage gaps.

Racial disparities in the quality of education, and gender and race disparities in employment and earnings persist today. Still, legislation targeting structural inequalities helped to open up opportunities for young adults in the late twentieth century that their parents and grandparents never could have dreamed of. For instance, U.S. census data show that as recently as 1950, 43 percent of all employed black women in the United States were working in "private service" occupations such as maids, cooks, or caregivers to others' children, as Susannah Mushatt Jones did. In sharp contrast, nearly 70 percent of black women who graduate from high school today enroll in college the following autumn.[17] Given the strong links among education, high-quality employment, and late-life well-being, progressive social changes throughout the late twentieth century created a context in which future cohorts of older adults, especially women and persons of color, may fare better than those who came before them.

Timing Matters

The second guiding principle of the life-course perspective is that timing matters, such that the long-term impact of a personal experience or historical event is contingent on one's age when it occurred. For instance, the long-term consequences of parenthood (and grandparenthood) depend on whether individuals had their first child at age fourteen or forty. A recession may have a more serious impact on a twenty-two-year-old looking for her first job and apartment, relative to a seventy-year-old retiree who has already paid off her mortgage.

In general, a personal transition made earlier than is typical among one's peers and before one is considered ready emotionally, financially, or socially is described as an "off-time" transition.[18] Off-time transitions, such as dropping out of high school in order to work and support one's family, or exiting the labor force before retirement age, whether to be the primary caretaker of one's grandchild or to take disability leave when still relatively young, are considered particularly harmful to a person's well-being in the longer term. Off-time transitions are especially likely to befall people from disadvantaged backgrounds and are a mechanism linking early-life disadvantage with later-life difficulties. Entering the workforce at age seventeen after dropping out of high school may relegate a young person to a lifetime of low-wage work. Exiting the labor market at age fifty because of disability or to meet caregiving demands may result in fewer savings, lower pensions, and less accumulated wealth in the long term. Off-time work and family transitions also put people out of step with their peers socially, depriving them of the social support that could help them adapt to the transition. Losing a spouse at thirty-five makes one an anomaly, whereas those widowed at age seventy-five can draw support and advice from empathetic peers going through a similar experience.

The personal impacts of historical contexts and public policies also depend on an individual's age when those events occurred. These processes are brought to life in Glen Elder's book *Children of the Great Depression*. Elder discovered that World War II affected soldiers very differently, depending on their age during the war years.[19] Young enlistees had few family or work responsibilities when they shipped off to Japan or Europe, whereas older soldiers were leaving behind jobs, homes, and marriages. The young soldiers returned home to promising new educational and career opportunities. The Servicemen's Readjustment Act of 1944, widely referred to as the GI Bill, provided tuition benefits and stipends for living expenses to help these young men earn college or trade school degrees. They also could receive low-interest, zero-down-payment home loans, which enticed young men to purchase homes in newly emerging suburbs. The older soldiers, however, were more established when they shipped overseas; many were married, had jobs, and owned homes. The perks provided by the GI Bill were simply less relevant to men in their thirties. Not only did they not benefit from the bill, but many soldiers came home to find their marriages strained and their former jobs no longer available. These divergent experiences carried long-term consequences for the careers, finances, and well-being of the soldiers, such that younger men benefited from their military service in ways that the older men did not.[20] Elder's work underscores that the value and impact of public policies depend on one's capacity to take advantage of the benefits conferred.

Linked Lives

"Linked lives" refers to the embeddedness of our lives in networks of social relationships—with parents, children, siblings, friends, coworkers, in-laws, romantic partners, and others. This concept is especially helpful in understanding how and why childhood and adolescent conditions can affect a person's physical, emotional, social, and financial well-being even five or six decades later. One pathway through which lives are "linked" is intergenerational transmission, or the ways in which parents' characteristics or behaviors get passed down to their offspring. These processes can happen directly or indirectly. Early-origins theories of health, proposed by the epidemiologist David Barker, argue that a mother's health can have direct long-term effects on the health of her child, with these influences taking hold as early as in utero.[21] Poor maternal nutrition, a problem particularly common among low-income women, may affect a fetus's development such that prenatal conditions directly increase the offspring's risk of diabetes, heart disease, and other illnesses even seventy years later.[22]

Sociological perspectives shed further light on indirect pathways linking parent experiences and traits to child outcomes. Socioeconomic disadvantage during childhood, typically captured by early-life poverty, low household income, or low paternal or maternal education, is associated with a greater risk of functional limitations, cancer, heart disease, high blood pressure, and even early death among midlife and older adults.[23] The main explanation offered is that children from disadvantaged backgrounds are especially likely to experience subsequent adversities, including more problems in school, slimmer chances of going on to college and getting a good job, more relationships problems, more risk-taking and unhealthy behaviors like drinking and smoking at a young age, more strenuous or dangerous jobs, and financial problems of their own in adulthood that directly affect their health and well-being.[24]

The sociologists William Sewell and Robert Hauser have used data from the long-running Wisconsin Longitudinal Study (WLS) to explore the ways in which a child's socioeconomic background affects his or her education, career, and financial success in adulthood.[25] Focusing on men and women who were born in the late 1930s and graduated from high school in 1957, the researchers found that sons and daughters of fathers with higher levels of education and with professional occupations were more likely than the children of less-advantaged fathers to graduate from college, obtain more prestigious jobs, and earn higher salaries by the time they reached their thirties. These advantages were due in part to having the financial means to afford college, but they also reflected the higher levels of support and encouragement from parents, teachers, and classmates. By contrast, the teens from less-advantaged backgrounds tended to befriend classmates who also had no plans to attend college and were less likely to receive encouragement from their teachers.

Nearly forty years later, the sociologist John Robert Warren revisited the WLS data to explore how these early experiences mattered for the later-life health of the study participants, now in their seventies.[26] He found strong and consistent patterns: the now-retirement-age adults from less-advantaged backgrounds had poorer mental health, poorer self-rated health, and worse musculoskeletal health than their more-privileged classmates, and these patterns were largely explained by the study participants' own socioeconomic resources.

Like the impacts of life transitions and historical events, the impact of early economic adversity on individuals depends on their age when their family experienced hardship. The sensitive period model proposes that the long-term impact of early disadvantage depends on a child's age when the experience happened.[27] For instance, a parent's job loss might derail a child's life chances if the layoff strikes precisely when the child is heading off to college. If the family cannot pay tuition bills, the child might be forced to forgo college, with long-term implications for the child's own career, relationships, and health. By contrast, a parent's job loss when the child is a toddler may have less bearing on his or her college prospects. In fact, some studies have suggested (somewhat counterintuitively) that having an unemployed parent at home during the day helps a young child's development, provided that the unemployment spell is short-lived.[28] The long-term impact of early life conditions also depends on their duration—longer spells of child poverty, family strife, or parental mistreatment may have more profound and long-lasting effects than shorter periods of disadvantage.[29]

Agency Within Constraints

Sociologists' heavy emphasis on historical, economic, and intergenerational influences might appear deterministic, allowing little room for innovation, resilience, or creative adaptation in how people respond to the opportunities and obstacles before them. Yet life-course approaches do explicitly consider the role of personal agency, recognizing that individuals shape their own lives through their choices, actions, and ingenuity—yet within the constraints of historical and social circumstances. Those who are from disadvantaged backgrounds or who face obstacles on the basis of their race or gender may have fewer opportunities to seek out and pursue their goals, especially during those historical periods when obstacles are many and opportunities few. To revisit an earlier example, the GI Bill was designed as "race-neutral" legislation, intended to help World War II veterans purchase homes and go to college.[30] Yet in practice, these benefits were enjoyed largely by whites. The Federal Housing Administration (FHA) prevented black veterans from taking advantage of the zero-interest loans because few banks were willing to issue mortgages for homes in black neighborhoods, while racism kept blacks from buying homes in largely white suburbs.[31] Consequently, young black veterans who aspired to college degrees and homeownership would be less likely than their white peers to have attained that dream.

Yet life-course scholars recognize that restrictive policies and structures, though daunting, are not sufficient to dictate one's life experiences. Personal characteristics like motivation, psychological resilience, persistence, and supportive social ties, like having a mentor or advocate, may help some to overcome obstacles where others do not. The psychologists Edith Chen and Greg Miller identified coping strategies they dubbed "shift and persist"—an intriguing combination of strategies that weakens the link between childhood economic disadvantage and poor health outcomes in late life.[32] This model proposes that even in the face of severe adversity, some young people manage to find adults who teach them to trust others and to focus on the future. Over time they learn how to solve their problems by "shifting"—accepting stress and adapting to it—while at the same time "persisting" or trying to find meaning and optimism, despite their challenges.

"Shift and persist" is just one of myriad coping tactics that help people to manage and even overcome adversity. Life-course sociologists' emphasis on agency and personal choice does not diminish the fact that structural obstacles are pervasive and daunting, yet it does reveal the power of resilience, initiative, and human connectedness. As we will see throughout this book (and especially when focusing on mental health and social relationships), some older adults have lived lives marked by unimaginable adversity yet still enjoy happiness, rewarding social ties, and wisdom in their later years.

Cumulative Inequality Perspectives

Cumulative inequality perspectives build on life-course principles by proposing that disparities in health, wealth, and well-being widen over the life course. The main argument is that advantage begets further advantage, and disadvantage begets further disadvantage, such that relatively modest inequities in early life amplify over time.[33] Cumulative inequality perspectives have their conceptual roots in the sociologist Robert Merton's "Matthew effect" principle. Merton was studying the productivity of research scientists, not the lives of older adults, although his model is particularly appropriate for understanding aging.[34] Merton discovered that some scientists who enjoyed small advantages or special opportunities early in their careers would parlay these perks into ever more opportunities. Over time the gap in researchers' productivity levels would widen dramatically as those who were anointed as "stars" early in their careers became more productive and those without the early career advantages grew less productive. Merton named this process the Matthew effect after the biblical verse: "For everyone who has will be given more, and he will have abundance. Whoever does not have, even what he has will be taken from him" (Matthew 25:29).

It is easy to understand how disparities between the haves and have-nots could widen over time. Imagine that two elementary school classmates, Don and John, differ in one fundamental way: Don is born into a poor family, and John is born into a middle-class family. Don drops out of high school to help support his family, settling for the menial or physically hazardous jobs available to a young high school dropout. His backbreaking work poses minor threats to his health in the short term. Over the longer term, however, Don's aches and pain worsen, and he self-medicates each night by having a few beers. After showing up for work hungover, he loses his job and health insurance; unable to afford the medical treatments that he needs, he experiences worsening health problems. This process whereby one adversity begets another may create an increasingly vast chasm between Don and John, his middle-class schoolmate who went on to graduate from high school and college, took a well-paying professional job, and had few financial worries in later life. While the differences between the two classmates might have been fairly small in early life, over time these differences escalated such that Don experienced poor health and financial insecurity during his retirement years, while John enjoyed good health and a comfortable life.

Cumulative inequality perspectives are not without their critics. Some researchers have proposed a countermodel called the "age as leveler" effect (although a more apt name may be the "*old* age as leveler" effect). This perspective holds that with advancing age, disparities between the haves and have-nots narrow or level off, for two main reasons. The first is selective mortality; people facing the most severe economic, interpersonal, and social hardships early in life, like Don, are most likely to die prematurely. Those who are hardy and resilient enough to overcome early-life obstacles and survive until old age may have important genetic, psychological, or interpersonal attributes that protect them in later life. In short, those who manage to withstand multiple adversities in early life and survive until old age may be healthier, happier, and more socially integrated than their counterparts who do not survive. Thus, the gap between the haves and have-nots looks narrower in later life because the most vulnerable have died off, to put it coarsely.

The second reason is that social policies provide an important buffer for older adults. Social Security provides a source of monthly income, while Medicare provides health insurance benefits to older adults. Taken together, these programs help to chip away at economic and health gaps that might have been particularly large at midlife—a time before people are eligible for these benefits. Yet, as we shall see throughout this book, Social Security and Medicare cannot fully eradicate persistent disparities in health and well-being and may be too little too late for the most disadvantaged.

Cumulative inequality perspectives are especially useful for understanding disparities in later-life physical health and economic security.[35] In general, people who enjoy social and economic privilege early in life are better positioned to acquire additional resources and benefits than those who have fewer early advantages and opportunities.[36] Higher education is an especially important resource, as it carries far-ranging benefits for a person's health, well-being, and financial stability. Yet, in the early and mid-twentieth century, college was out of reach to many low-income persons, women, and blacks, who were often discouraged subtly or outright from attending college. A 1946 *Newsweek* magazine article told women that "books and babies" didn't mix.[37] Several years later, in 1962, James Meredith became the first black student to enroll at the University of Mississippi. Although this was an inspiring historical turning point for blacks, many Southern whites did not see it that way. Violence and riots erupted, causing President John F. Kennedy to send five thousand federal troops to calm the campus. The years that followed ushered in federal programs to help low-income youth attend college, like the Pell Grants program created by the Higher Education Act of 1965. While the 1965 act played a pivotal role in the lives of many baby boomers born in the 1940s and 1950s, it was too late for those born in the 1920s and 1930s, who already had jobs and family responsibilities by the mid-1960s.

Work histories also contribute to cumulative inequalities. Many older adults today abided by a gender-typed division of work and family roles during their younger years, with long-term consequences for men's and women's divergent economic prospects. Young married women in the mid-twentieth century tended to cut back on paid work or stopped working altogether during their child-bearing and child-rearing years. Women who did pursue careers often were discouraged from pursuing lucrative careers in business, medicine, law, and engineering and instead opted for lower-paying jobs deemed more appropriate for women, like teaching, social work, and nursing.[38] Racial discrimination in the workforce contributed to black men's more sporadic work histories, lower earnings, and greater likelihood of working in jobs without health or pension benefits, relative to their white peers. Discrimination in hiring, firing, and promotion and the well-established fact that during economic downturns blacks are more likely than whites to be laid off have all contributed to blacks' lower earnings in the short term and sparser pensions and leaner savings in the long term.[39]

Cumulative disadvantage processes also apply to experiences of stress exposure. Stress, or the difficult events and persistent strains one encounters over the life course, can snowball in such a way as to threaten one's physical and emotional health and personal relationships. This snowballing process is a powerful mechanism through which health disparities are perpetuated and amplified in later life. As chapters 4 and 5 will show, stress is socially patterned such that less-advantaged people tend to experience both a greater number of and more severe stressors. They also have fewer material and social resources to help them cope with or overcome these stressors. The late sociologist and eminent stress researcher Leonard Pearlin described this process as stress proliferation, whereby "people exposed to a serious adversity [are] at risk for later exposure to additional adversities."[40] For example, an event like a spouse's job loss may trigger a chain of new and chronic strains, like financial worries, more frequent marital spats, and the added stress of the unemployed spouse's depression and drinking. Conversely, chronic strains may precede and even give rise to a stress-inducing event. A decades-long marriage to a partner who is abusive or has substance use problems is inherently stressful, and it also may lead to divorce, creating a new cycle of financial and personal challenges.

In sum, late-life experiences are powerfully shaped by long-term, persistent, and accumulating inequalities over the life course. The next five chapters will show how these processes contribute to race, gender, and socioeconomic disparities in late-life physical and mental health, social relations, living conditions, and quality of dying experiences, and why social programs targeting older adults are not sufficient to eradicate these persistent disparities.

= Chapter 4 =

The Fit and the Frail: Physical Health Among Older Adults

When Americans are asked to name their biggest worry about getting old, two answers consistently top the list: health and the loss of independence that accompanies illness and disability. It is not surprising that fears about declining health are so common. Aphorisms tell us that "when you have your health, you have everything," while the best-selling memoirist Augusten Burroughs offers the corollary: "When you do not have your health, nothing else matters at all."[1] Survey data from AARP affirm these words by showing that good health beats out a dozen other candidates like family relationships and money as the strongest predictor of life satisfaction among older adults.

Poor health can cast a shadow over nearly every aspect of life. Getting out of bed in the morning is a chore for the 54 percent of older adults with arthritis.[2] Getting a good night's sleep is a struggle for the 50 percent who have trouble falling asleep or staying asleep because of medication side effects, breathing problems, gastrointestinal symptoms, and other health issues.[3] Older adults with functional or sensory impairments often must rely on friends and family to carry out once-simple tasks like preparing meals and getting dressed, a source of particular frustration for members of the Greatest Generation cohort, who pride themselves on being self-sufficient.[4] Whether and how often older adults leave their home, visit with friends and family, go to religious services, volunteer, or participate in activities that give life meaning are dictated by physical health and functioning.[5]

Senescence happens. It is a fact of life that with old age, physiological changes bring on illness and disability. Blood vessels lose elasticity, and this hardening of the arteries can increase the risk of heart disease. Weakening immune systems leave older adults vulnerable to infection. Diminishing lung capacity means that a once-effortless skip up a flight of stairs leaves some older adults breathless. But biology is only part of the story. Social factors powerfully shape the symptoms and diseases a person experiences, the timing of when health starts to decline, and one's capacity to manage symptoms, seek effective medical care, and adapt the physical environment so that symptoms are a nuisance rather than an insurmountable obstacle to living an engaged and independent life. That is why physical aging, while universal, starts younger for those who have experienced the most substantial social and economic hardships. Early onset of physical and cognitive declines, in turn, may set in motion other difficulties, like prematurely exiting the workforce (and losing earnings and pension wealth in the process), abandoning the activities that were once a source of enjoyment, and suffering from social isolation and depression.

Health disparities, or gaps in the health enjoyed by more- versus less-advantaged people, are evident at every stage in the life course, and old age is no exception.[6] Adults of lower socioeconomic status die younger and experience earlier onset of nearly every major health condition relative to their more-advantaged counterparts.[7] These disparities are so persistent across time and consistent across diverse health outcomes that the sociologists Bruce Link and Jo Phelan have argued that socioeconomic resources are a "fundamental cause" of health.[8] Higher SES encompasses benefits like money, knowledge, power, and helpful social connections that can protect one's health no matter what the specific disease or the specific mechanisms contributing to it.

But health disparities are not limited to socioeconomic hierarchies: race and, to a lesser degree, gender matter. Blacks uniformly fare worse than whites when it comes to physical health, and while much of this gap is accounted for by blacks' sparser socioeconomic resources in both childhood and adulthood, disparities persist even when SES is controlled.[9] One reason why is that socioeconomic resources bring fewer health benefits for older blacks relative to whites. Each additional year of schooling or dollar of income accrues fewer health and longevity benefits for blacks relative to whites, underscoring the powerful ways in which racial discrimination can undermine older blacks' health.[10] Gender gaps in older adults' health also are well documented, such that women generally have poorer health than men, although men die younger.

Medicare plays an important role in providing older adults access to health care, but it is not sufficient to erase health disparities because they are the end product of (dis)advantages that have been accumulating over decades. An influential editorial in the *New England Journal of Medicine* argues that access to health care explains just 10 percent of premature death in the United States (see figure 4.1). In stark contrast, social factors like daily stress, habitual smoking or drinking, and exposure to

Figure 4.1 Estimated Share of Contribution to Premature Death in the United States, 2007

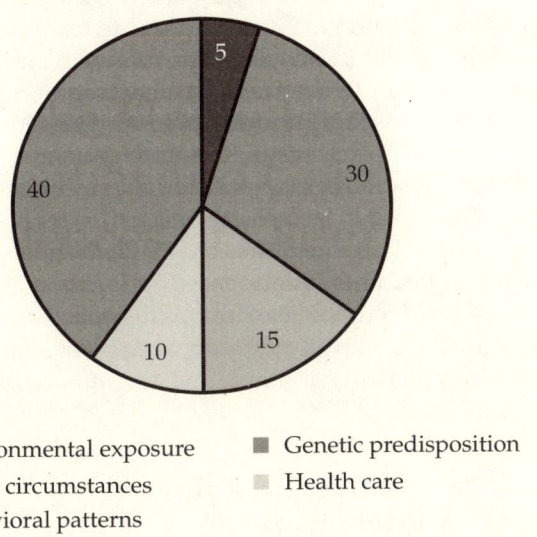

- Environmental exposure
- Social circumstances
- Behavioral patterns
- Genetic predisposition
- Health care

Source: Schroeder 2007.

environmental hazards like pollution account for 60 percent; genetics account for the final 30 percent.[11] As the eminent sociologist James S. House has observed, "the major determinants of health lie not in medical care but rather in the conditions of life and work."[12]

This chapter shows how unequal life and work conditions lead to vast disparities in the physical health of older adults, and why these disparities persist despite major medical advances throughout the twentieth and twenty-first centuries. I begin with a brief overview of biological theories of aging and disease, underscoring how social factors may speed up or slow down the physical declines that are inevitable in old age. I then describe the concepts, data, and measures that social scientists use to study health and provide a snapshot of death, disease, and disability patterns in the late twentieth and early twenty-first centuries.

At first blush, a simple snapshot of older adults' health reveals a good news story. For much of the past century, life expectancies have increased while rates of disability and disease have decreased. Scientific advances like new medications, innovative surgical procedures, and state-of-the art hearing aids and pacemakers are helping older adults to thrive, even when new health conditions erupt. Yet a simple snapshot conceals stark disparities in health, life span, and quality of life. I describe why and how key aspects of social stratification—including race, gender, and both early life and adult socioeconomic resources—affect older adults' health and survival. I elaborate on three main pathways through which social disadvantages affect health and longevity: stress, health behaviors, and, to a lesser extent, access to medical care, and I show how each of these risk factors can be minimized by public policies that prioritize social welfare and population health.

This chapter just scratches the surface of later-life disparities in physical health and longevity.[13] Subsequent chapters dig deeper into the specific social factors that contribute to or compound these disparities: mental health conditions like depression (chapter 5); problematic or deficient social ties, including isolation, elder mistreatment, and difficult caregiving burdens (chapter 6); living conditions, neighborhoods, and physical environments (chapter 7); and the quality of care received at the end of life (chapter 8).

Biological Perspectives on Aging and Health: A Brief Overview

Graying temples, wrinkled skin, fuzzy vision and hearing, aches and pains, and declining memory are inevitabilities of aging. Many biological theories of aging seek to explain why disease and disability strike older adults, ranging from perspectives that emphasize "wear and tear" on the body over time to cellular aging theories that focus on the progressive weakening of cells' capacities to divide and replicate over time. Each of these perspectives recognizes, whether explicitly or implicitly, that social and environmental factors can speed up or slow down the physiological changes that accompany old age.[14] The main force behind these speed-ups is stress: the persistent threats like poverty, sporadic employment, discrimination, neighborhood crime, and strained relationships that "get under our skin" and undermine the functioning of our major organ systems. A full discussion of biological models of aging is beyond the scope of this book, yet I highlight just a few examples to reveal how universal processes of biological aging are intensified and sped up for those exposed to stress and adversity.[15]

Cellular Aging Approaches

Research on cellular aging demonstrates that telomere length shortens with age. Telomeres are the caps at the end of each strand of DNA that affect how our cells age. We can liken them to the plastic cap that protects the end of a shoelace. Without the protection of telomeres, our cells will gradually age and die. This progressive shortening of telomeres with age is linked with increasing rates of poor health and disease for all adults, and this general process of telomere aging is intensified by social stress and adversity.[16] Researchers analyzing data from the National Health and Nutrition Examination Survey (NHANES) found that older adults with lower levels of education had shorter telomere lengths, compared to their better-educated peers.[17] And emerging research shows that this shortening process starts as early as childhood. School-age children whose parents did not attend college have shorter telomeres than children of college graduates, a difference that equaled roughly six years of additional cellular aging for those from less-advantaged backgrounds.[18]

Oxidative Stress Approaches

Free radical and mitochondrial theories emphasize the role of oxidative stress in biological aging. These are complex theories, but the crux is that age-related disease results when the body's balance of pro-oxidants and anti-oxidants tilts to favor pro-oxidants, which can damage healthy cells. Anti-oxidants, by contrast, are chemical compounds that bind to free radicals and prevent cell damage. (That is why nutritionists urge us to eat blueberries, beans, and other anti-oxidant-rich foods.) These imbalances are linked with neurodegenerative diseases such as Parkinson's and Alzheimer's disease, cancers, heart and blood vessel disorders, atherosclerosis, heart failure, heart attack, and inflammatory diseases.[19]

Oxidative stress is linked to social factors, most notably SES. Studies focused on both young and older adults find that those with fewer years of education, lower income, and greater exposure to environmental hazards have higher levels of oxidative damage, measured with biological markers such as gamma-glutamyltransferase.[20] These socioeconomic disparities hold even when health behaviors like smoking and drinking are controlled; smoking is linked with higher levels of oxidative stress and heavy drinking increases free radical concentrations. Researchers also attribute disparities to other behavioral and social factors, like environmental toxins in poor neighborhoods and some dangerous work sites. Emotional reactions to persistent stressors like caregiving or marital strife also pose risks; depression can increase oxidative stress levels directly by activating physiological stress axes.

Immune System Approaches

Immunosenescence perspectives argue that immune functions decline with advancing age. Our T cells, which fight antigens, gradually lose their efficiency with each passing year. This diminishing capacity to fight off viruses, bacteria, and other threats renders older adults more susceptible to disease and infection, slower recovery, and poorer responses to medications and vaccinations meant to fight infection. These universal processes are amplified by stress. One analysis of NHANES data demonstrated the strong protective effects of education and income on older adults' immune function.[21] These results suggested that doubling older adults' family income could result in eight fewer years of age-related antibody response.

Genetic Perspectives

Gene-environment interaction studies reveal that while a genetic predisposition toward a particular disease increases one's risk of that condition, the magnitude of this risk diminishes over the life course and in response to protective social factors. Genes shape key aspects of who we are—our eye color, hair texture, height, and risk of some diseases, especially those that strike early in life like juvenile (type I) diabetes and early-onset Alzheimer's disease.[22] Yet most diseases that strike older adults have only modest heritability (the proportion of risk for a particular trait or disease derived from our genes).[23] Although juvenile diabetes has an estimated 88 percent heritability factor (and eye color is 98 percent heritable), diseases that strike in middle age or later life have much lower heritability. Heritability is estimated at roughly 30 to 50 percent for heart disease, hypertension, stroke, and prostate cancer, meaning that 50 to 70 percent is explained by nongenetic factors.[24]

The simplest explanation for this diminishing power of genes is that with each passing year, adults are exposed to more and more social and environmental influences that might intensify or dampen their genetic predisposition to a particular condition. Decades of smoking two packs of Marlboros a day can put one at high risk for lung cancer, even without a genetic risk. Years of healthy living, by contrast, can mute or even turn around a genetic predisposition. For instance, one study of more than fifty-five thousand older adults found that those with a genetic predisposition to heart disease had double the risk of the condition compared to those who did not share that predisposition. Yet when researchers examined the combined effects of genetic risk and lifestyle, they found that the risk of heart disease for older adults who had a high genetic risk but also exercised regularly, did not smoke, ate a healthy diet, and maintained a healthy body weight was only half that of their counterparts who had a high genetic risk and followed an unhealthy lifestyle.[25] Gene-environment research provides a powerful example of how social and behavioral factors can shape older adults' health and even erase what some may think of as their genetic destiny.

Bridging the Biological and the Social: Early-Origins Models

Cellular aging, oxidative stress, immune system, and genetic perspectives help us understand the underlying biological processes through which health declines, but they do not pinpoint the specific social or environmental factors that hasten decline. The British physician and epidemiologist David Barker developed a pathbreaking framework for understanding how social factors leave their imprint on biology. Noting the importance of intrauterine conditions, Barker discovered that adults who had been low-birth-weight or preterm infants had an elevated risk of ischemic heart disease, diabetes, lung disease, liver disease, high blood pressure, and other chronic diseases as many as seventy years later.[26] He developed Fetal Origins of Adult Disease (FOAD), a theory to explain how poor maternal nutrition could "program" or permanently change the structure of the fetus's organs while still in utero. Delayed lung development as a premature baby could give rise to lung disease in old age, while abnormal pancreas development in utero could make a person vulnerable to diabetes decades later.

Barker expanded FOAD and renamed it the Developmental Origins of Health and Disease (DOHaD) model to more explicitly acknowledge the role of social factors linked to maternal nutrition and, consequently, fetal development. His revised model recognizes that mothers who have poor nutrition and receive insufficient prenatal care—both common problems among economically disadvantaged young women—are more likely to have preterm or low-birth-weight babies. These babies, often born into the multiple disadvantages of poverty, low birth weight, and prenatal and neonatal health problems, are more likely to suffer from childhood illnesses and consequently to perform more poorly in school. Their poor school performance and their parents' limited economic resources, in turn, make them less likely to attend college and then to find well-paying professional jobs. These accumulating biological and social disadvantages conspire to undermine health in midlife and later life and hasten mortality.[27] Early-origins theories exemplify the core theme of cumulative disadvantage theories: relatively small social and biological differences early in life, such as birth weight, can set off a chain of experiences that lead to ever-growing health disparities over time.

Measuring Later-Life Health and Mortality

Identifying the complex ways in which biological and social factors affect older adults' health requires extensive data over long time periods. Social and biomedical scientists use a range of measures and methods to study older adults' health, each with its own distinctive meanings and limitations. Although black-white and socioeconomic disparities follow generally similar patterns across most measures of physical health and functioning, the magnitude and sources of these gaps can differ across outcomes. Identifying the specific mechanisms that account for particular disparities is necessary to develop potential interventions and protections.

For instance, socioeconomic disparities in rates of diseases that develop slowly over time may reflect long-term exposure to hazardous work or environmental conditions. The median latency period for mesothelioma (a cancer that affects the lining of the lungs and chest wall) is thirty to forty-five years, so several decades typically pass between the time a worker is first exposed to asbestos and the time that a doctor diagnoses the disease. Workers in construction or demolition jobs may become aware of their condition in their sixties and seventies when their persistent cough or breathing troubles become debilitating.[28] Other diseases, like diabetes or emphysema, are more closely tied to long-term health behaviors like decades of unhealthy eating and smoking.[29]

By contrast, disparities in rates of diseases that are highly amenable to treatment are explained in part by differential access to care. Racial disparities in breast cancer survival—white women have an 83 percent chance of surviving five years post-diagnosis yet black women have just a 68 percent chance—are partly explained by the fact that black women are less likely to get follow-up care after an irregular mammogram. As a result, their cancer is detected and treated at a later and more serious stage.[30] One recent *Journal of the American Medical Association* study found that 20 percent of black women (but just 11 percent of white women) with breast cancer do not learn of their disease until it has advanced to stage 3 or 4. And once diagnosed, black women are less likely to have access to state-of-the art care and experimental drug treatments, either because there are no top-notch hospitals nearby or because they lack insurance to access that care.[31]

Because different health conditions have different risk factors, researchers consider a range of outcomes. Three of the most commonly used measures are official records of mortality status, like death certificates; self-reported data in large population-based surveys; and biological or behavioral measures obtained during face-to-face interviews or medical encounters.

Mortality Data

The most commonly studied and presumably most incontrovertible health outcome is mortality: whether an individual died and if so, at what age and of what cause. This information can be obtained from death certificates, which researchers then link to survey data through the National Death Index (NDI); these matched data allow researchers to explore social factors related to mortality. For instance, Joe Feinglass and his colleagues used linked data from the NDI and HRS to examine whether socioeconomic characteristics at midlife, like education, income, and wealth predicted whether a study participant would die over the subsequent ten-year observation period. They found a strong gradient in survival, even after health behaviors were controlled.[32]

An alternative approach for measuring an older adult's vital status is through a proxy interview conducted as part of a survey. For long-running surveys of health and aging like the HRS, researchers often learn that a study participant has died when they contact the participant's home for an interview. A proxy, typically a bereaved spouse or adult child who lives at the decedent's address, will inform the researcher about the older adult's death and also answer a series of questions that ascertain the date, cause, and place of the death. These proxy reports are more susceptible to error than death certificate measures, which are completed by a physician, coroner, or medical examiner at the time of death. A grieving spouse might not accurately recall the death date, might not know exactly how their loved one died, or might be reluctant to report the cause of death if it was a suicide or the outcome of a stigmatized condition like cirrhosis or HIV/AIDS.[33]

Yet death certificate data are not perfect when it comes to measuring the social factors that may contribute to late-life mortality, like socioeconomic status or race. Death certificates indicate the decedent's occupation, ideally identifying the main job that the decedent held during his or her working life. These data enable researchers to document whether coal miners die younger than college professors, how many fewer years they live, and the main causes of death for each occupation. The demographic data on a death certificate, like occupation and race, are typically filled in by a funeral director. The funeral director is likely to ask the decedent's family members for this information, who might respond "he's retired," or they might mention the last job the decedent held, which may not provide an accurate snapshot of the health risks he experienced throughout his work life. A coal miner who developed lung disease after twenty-five years of exposure to hazardous dust might have moved into a less taxing job in his fifties, so his death certificate might say "store clerk," even though he held that job only at the very end of his life.

Studies that contrast occupational data as reported on the death certificate with self-reported occupational data from linked surveys show that the specific job titles (such as coal miner or sociology professor) match only about 50 to 60 percent of the time, although the match rate is closer to 90 percent when broad occupational groups such as construction or professional occupations are used.[34] Consequently, some researchers have suggested that occupational disparities in mortality rates might be understated, requiring parallel analyses that also explore educational or wealth disparities.[35]

Death certificate indicators of race also are susceptible to misreporting. The funeral director (or occasionally the coroner) responsible for the death certificate's demographic data offers his or her best guess as to the decedent's race based on physical appearance or cues from the family members. Researchers have found that racial death certificate data are excellent for blacks and whites: they match survey data about 99 percent of the time. Match rates are considerably lower, however for Asian, Native American, and Latino decedents, ranging from 60 to 80 percent; these errors of classification are attributed to their more ethnically ambiguous facial features.[36]

One fascinating study further suggests that some misclassifications may reflect biases on the part of the funeral director or professional filling in the death certificate data. The sociologists Andrew Noymer, Andrew Penner, and Aliya Saperstein found that the race designations on death certificates are biased by cause of death: some funeral directors are more likely to assign a race that is consistent with stereotypical notions regarding the people who might die of the condition named on the certificate.[37] For instance, those who died of cirrhosis, a disease often precipitated by heavy alcohol use, are disproportionately classified as Native American, and homicide victims are disproportionately classified as black. Overall, researchers conclude that these different types of misclassifications may lead to an underestimation in deaths to Native Americans, but with negligible consequences for understanding mortality disparities among other ethnic groups. However, these misclassifications may become more prevalent as Latino, Asian, and multiracial populations increase among future cohorts of older adults.

Self-Reported Measures

Most population surveys of aging collect extensive self-reported measures of physical health and health care use. Survey participants are asked to describe how good their overall health is, which conditions they have, how much their health affects their daily functioning, when they last saw a doctor, and whether they have been recently hospitalized. The most widely used measure is a single indicator of self-rated health, which asks, "In general, would you say that your health is excellent, very good, good, fair, or poor?" Despite its widespread use, researchers debate its value as a snapshot of health. Some consider it a "gold standard" indicator, noting that it is a better predictor of subsequent mortality than a doctor's assessment of the respondent's health.[38] However, critics say that it is a better predictor of mortality for younger rather than older adults, and that other snapshots of health may be more appropriate when studying older adults.[39] Older adults' health self-assessments may be excessively positive, whereas younger adults may offer more accurate appraisals, reflecting age differences in the thought processes that guide such appraisals. Older adults might compare themselves to their least healthy and frailest peers. Some may find their social circles being diminished by recent deaths of family members and friends. As a result, even a quite unhealthy older adult might think, *I'm in pretty good shape. I'm still alive, aren't I?* For this reason, studies of older adults' self-rated health might also use a comparative measure such as "compared to people your age, would you say your health is excellent, very good, good, fair or poor?"[40] This helps to ensure that older adults appraise their health relative to a reasonable standard.

Self-reported measures of illnesses and symptoms also are commonly used. The illness checklist approach asks respondents to indicate which of a dozen or so chronic illnesses they have been diagnosed with, such as cancer, heart disease, hypertension, or arthritis. Some researchers find these measures problematic, because the phrase "that you have been diagnosed with" might lead those who do not have a regular health care provider, and consequently would not have received a diagnosis, to reply "none." Symptom checklists, by contrast, capture the number of times in the past week (or past month) a person experienced health symptoms such as headaches, back pain, sleep troubles, nausea, or excessive sweating. No diagnosis is needed; respondents simply need to feel and experience these symptoms. Self-reported disease and symptom measures can be used in several ways. Some researchers are interested in respondents' specific conditions, whereas others are interested in summing up the total number of respondents' conditions or frequency of symptoms in order to capture the intensity, number, or variety of their health problems. Multimorbidity, or having two or more simultaneous chronic illnesses, is a serious concern for two-thirds of older adults.[41]

Disability, or difficulty in navigating everyday life due to health conditions, also is measured with self-report instruments, such as the activities of daily living (ADLs) which capture the capacity to dress, bath, toilet, and perform other basic daily activities, and instrumental activities of daily living (IADLs) scales, which assess the capacity to carry out more complex activities like doing housework or managing medications.[42] Researchers are interested in disability as an outcome in its own right, as it reveals how functional limitations affect the quality of older adults' daily lives. ADL and IADL measures also can be used in tandem with mortality data to construct an indicator of active life expectancy (ALE) or disability-free life expectancy. This measure indicates the proportion of an older adult's final years that are relatively healthy versus the proportion marked by impairment and chronic disability.[43] Of particular interest to policymakers and practitioners is whether morbidity is compressed (packed into a short time period at the very end of life) or whether years are spent suffering with disability that requires services and supports for long durations. Most evidence suggests that more-advantaged older adults experience compressed morbidity, whereas less-advantaged older adults experience longer periods of disablement that compromises their independence and quality of life.[44]

Health care use—such as the number of hospitalizations in the past year, whether the respondent has a regular provider, and whether the respondent had a bone density scan in the past year—is regularly measured in surveys. Health behaviors also are a key component of most large surveys; these questions capture the frequency with which respondents smoke and drink, their body weight, and how often they engage in light versus vigorous exercise. Researchers recognize the importance of taking lifetime histories of these behaviors, like the total number of years a respondent smoked, or the period in a respondent's life when he or she drank most heavily. These lifetime measures are particularly important when assessing the consequnces of smoking and drinking for older adults' health; abstinence today may be a consequence of problematic health behaviors in decades past. Older nonsmokers include both longtime smokers who quit when they learned they had emphysema and those who never lit up a cigarette. Teetotalers include those who never had a drink as well as once-heavy drinkers who entered recovery, perhaps following a frightening diagnosis of liver disease. Health disparities researchers require these lifetime data so as not to over- or understate the importance of health behaviors relative to other explanatory mechanisms.

Biomarker Data

Over the past two decades, population-based surveys of aging have started collecting biomarkers, or biological indicators of health, in addition to self-reported measures. Research team members who administer a survey may draw blood, take a saliva or hair sample, or do a blood pressure reading on their study participants. These biological data can be used to generate indicators of cardiovascular and metabolic risk factors, as well as markers of inflammation like C-reactive protein (CRP) and interleukin-6 (IL-6). Inflammation markers are especially important for understanding older adults' health because they signal problems with the immune system. Researchers also collect blood and saliva samples to create genetic markers to carry out genome-wide association studies (GWAS), which explore links between genetic markers and psychosocial, behavioral, and health outcomes. Some investigators are also starting to collect stool samples, which can be used to assess microbes associated with inflammation and other biological risks for late-life illness. Performance measures are a second type of biomarker that researchers collect—for example, tests of balance, walking speed, grip strength, and the capacity to get up out of a chair. Although these performance measures are not indicators of health per se, they do reveal the impact of health on older adults' functioning. For instance, gait speed, or the time it usually takes an older adult to walk a distance of about twenty feet, is one of the best predictors of a person's risk of mortality.[45]

Just as survey measures of health can be used to understand specific outcomes or a composite indicator of health, researchers using biomarker data may focus on either specific or aggregated outcomes. For example, several studies based on the Midlife in the United States (MIDUS) study have found that low-income older adults have higher levels of the specific inflammation markers CRP and IL-6.[46] Meanwhile, other researchers have used multiple biomarker measures to create a composite measure of health, such as allostatic load (AL). The neurophysiologist Bruce McEwen developed the concept and measure of AL, which refers to a collection of symptoms and conditions that indicate accumulated wear and tear on the body. People who score high on the AL index have a heightened risk of early mortality and illnesses such as heart disease and diabetes.[47] Biomarkers have become very popular in recent years, as they help researchers to understand the physiological processes through which cumulative social inequalities affect older adults' health. While behavioral measures like exercise, diet, smoking, and health care–seeking partially explain why disadvantaged older adults have more illness, disability, and early mortality, they do not tell the whole story. Biological markers can reveal the surprising ways in which bodies respond to cumulative stress—ways that often are invisible until too late.

Later-Life Health and Mortality: Patterns and Disparities

Historical and Global Contexts

Studies tracking older adults' health throughout the late twentieth and early twenty-first century tell a largely uplifting story. Life expectancy at birth has increased steadily over the past century, despite a slight

Figure 4.2 Death Rates for U.S. Adults Age Sixty-Five and Older, by Disease, 1981–2014

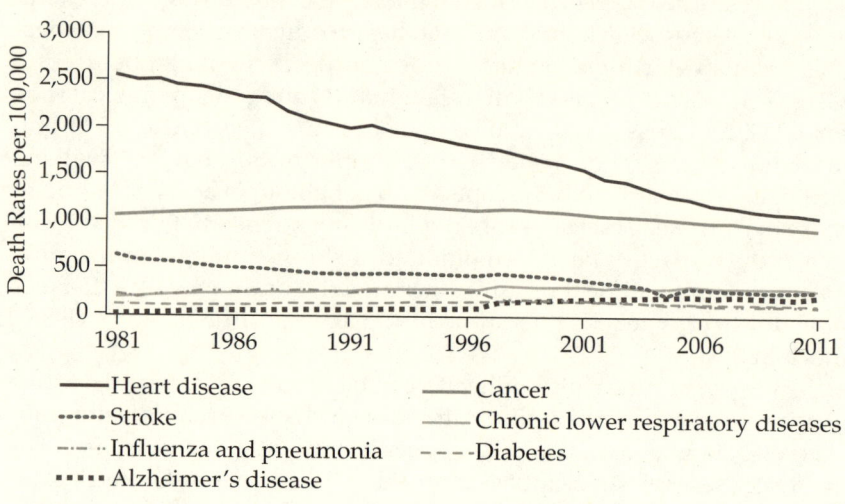

Source: Federal Interagency Forum on Aging-Related Statistics 2016.
Note: Rates are deaths per 100,000 population. ICD-9 codes were used prior to 1999; ICD-10 classifications were used thereafter.

downward dip starting in 2015.[48] Death rates for heart disease, stroke, diabetes, and other diseases have declined or leveled off, as shown in figure 4.2. Declines have been steepest for heart disease: the death rate from heart disease declined by 50 percent between 1981 and 2014, from 2,500 to 1,250 per 100,000. Disability levels are inching downward, and many older adults can function on their own until well into their eighties and nineties.

Yet this good news is tempered by some jarring realities. These aggregate trends conceal stark disparities along nearly all health outcomes. Although rates of most diseases and disability have declined steadily or leveled off over the past century, these declines have been much steeper for the advantaged and much flatter for the disadvantaged. For instance, Robert Schoeni and his colleagues tracked rates of ADLs and IADLs between 1982 and 2002 using National Health Interview Survey (NHIS) data and found that older adults in the lowest income quartile and those with less than a ninth-grade education showed virtually no improvement in ADLs over the twenty-year period, while their more-advantaged peers experienced significant improvements.[49] As a result, the socioeconomic gap in disability widened even further between the 1980s and 2000s, despite the coarse aggregate trends showing improvement.

The relatively poor health among the most-disadvantaged Americans is part of the reason why life expectancies in the United States lag behind other wealthy industrial nations by as many as eight to ten years. A 2017 study in *The Lancet* showed that South Korea tops the list of thirty-five nations, with life expectancies of ninety-one and eighty-four for women and men, respectively, while the United States is mired in the bottom tier alongside eastern European nations, like Poland and the Czech Republic, which are not as wealthy.[50] The study investigators attribute the relatively poor standing of the United States to factors like high obesity rates and lack of universal health insurance, both of which disproportionately affect older adults from poorer economic backgrounds and racial minorities.

Fundamental cause theory helps us to understand why stubborn health disparities persist in the United States despite major advances in medical technologies over the past century and medical spending that far outpaces that of other wealthy nations.[51] Link and Phelan argue that even if new scientific knowledge or promising medical interventions are developed, it is the most highly educated, wealthiest, and most well-connected individuals who are best equipped to take advantage of these advances.[52] Major medical breakthroughs over the past century, such as effective cancer screenings and surgical techniques like angioplasty, disproportionately benefit those with access to doctors working in top-notch hospitals and using cutting-edge technologies. Public health campaigns against risky behaviors like smoking and a sedentary lifestyle are most likely to benefit those who are literate and have the means and support to kick unhealthy habits and adopt healthy new behaviors. In short, if only the most advantaged benefit from these health-enhancing advances, then the gap between the haves and have-nots will persist.

Changes in breast cancer rates illustrate this point vividly. In 2002, the Women's Health Initiative made the startling discovery that hormone replacement therapy (HCT) was linked to heightened risk of breast cancer, shattering the widely held belief at the time that it would help women lower their risk of breast cancer and heart disease. News media blasted the findings far and wide, establishing a "new normal" for women's health. In the years that followed, breast cancer incidence among older white women in high-income U.S. counties dropped dramatically, although similar decreases were not detected among less-well-off women and women of color.[53] Breast cancer is just one example; late-life health disparities are far-reaching and intransigent, despite medical advances and older adults' access to health care through Medicare benefits.

Later-Life Health and Mortality: A Statistical Snapshot

It seems painfully obvious to state that age is the biggest risk factor for mortality and illness. As figure 4.3 shows, death rates follow a clear age gradient: each age group is more likely to die than the next-younger age group—with the exception of school-age children, who have lower death rates than infants and preschool-age children. These patterns largely reflect the mortality transition that occurred throughout the twentieth century; the leading causes of death shifted from infectious diseases that can strike at any age, like pneumonia, to chronic illnesses like cancer and heart disease that disproportionately afflict older adults.[54] Gender and race gaps also persist. Women outlive men by roughly five years. In 2017, women's life expectancy was eighty-two and men's just seventy-seven. And among both men and women, blacks lag behind whites and Latinos.[55] In 2014, the life expectancies of black women and men were seventy-eight and seventy-three, respectively, compared to eighty-one and seventy-seven for white women and men (figure 4.4). For Hispanic women and men, life expectancies were eighty-four and seventy-nine, respectively (not shown).

It is important to recognize that it is not old age per se that causes death. Rather, it is the onset of age-dependent diseases like cancer, heart disease, osteoporosis, and dementia that can hasten death.[56] Of the 2.7 million Americans who died in 2016, roughly 75 percent were age sixty-five or older. The five leading causes of death to older adults are heart disease (27 percent), cancer (22 percent), chronic lower respiratory diseases like emphysema and bronchitis (7 percent), stroke (6 percent), and Alzheimer's disease (5 percent); these five conditions alone account for three-quarters of all deaths to persons age sixty-five and older. Cancer edges out heart disease (32 to 21 percent) as the leading cause of death to midlife adults age forty-five to sixty-four. Accidents rather than illness are the leading cause of death for young people: unintentional injuries account for 38 percent of all deaths to people under age twenty-five and for one-quarter of deaths to those age twenty-five to forty-four.[57]

Black and lower-SES older adults fare worse than white and higher-SES adults on nearly all health outcomes, evidencing higher rates of disease, earlier age of onset, and poorer survival rates once diagnosed. Given how systematic these disparities are, it would be tedious and redundant to report each and every one. Suffice it to say that their consistency is remarkable. These disparities are all the more disheartening in light of the possibility that selective mortality actually mutes late-life health disparities. Selective mortality refers to the fact that those with the fewest economic and social resources tend to have the poorest health at every stage of the life course and, as such, are less likely to survive

Figure 4.3 Male and Female Age-Adjusted Death Rates, by Age, 1955–2014

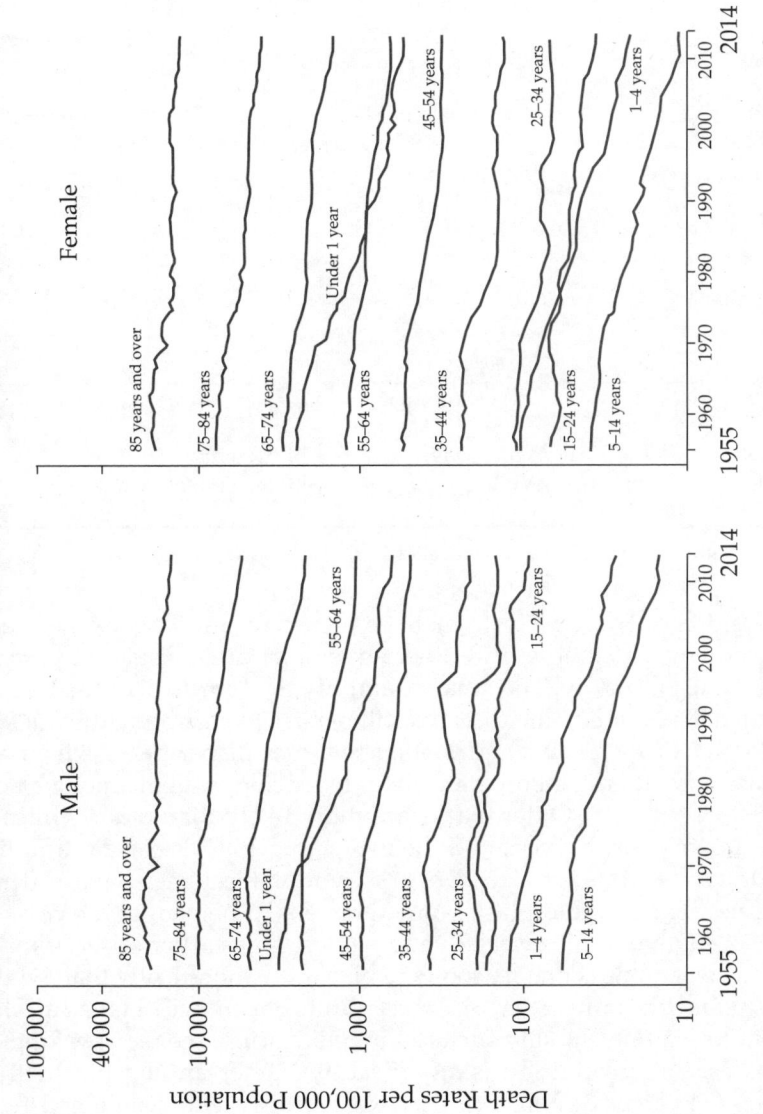

Source: National Center for Health Statistics 2016.

Figure 4.4 Life Expectancy at Birth, by Race and Sex, 1970–2015

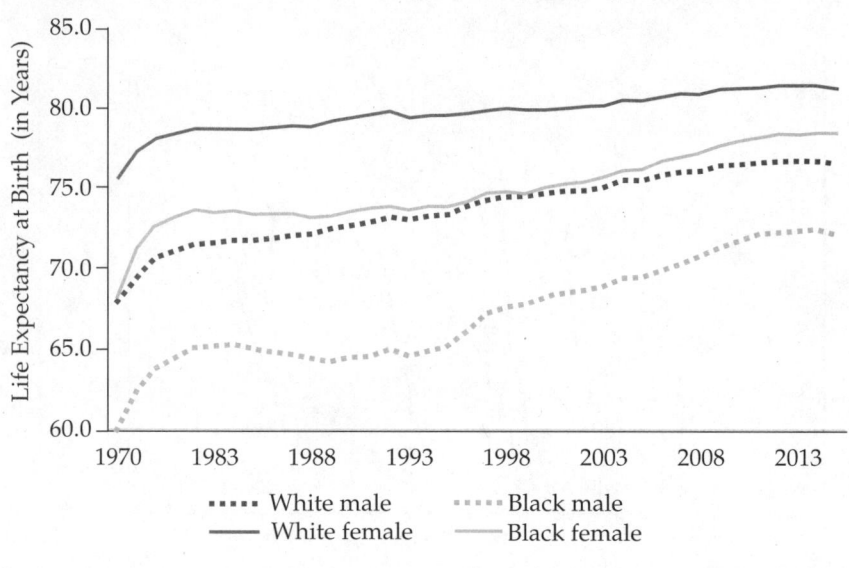

Source: National Center for Health Statistics 2016.

until old age. Those who do manage to survive until age sixty-five in spite of poverty, illness, and other adversities are considered particularly robust or hardy. They may exemplify the "survival of the fittest," yet disparities in late-life diseases still persist, even among the fittest.

To give just a few examples of current race disparities, Alzheimer's disease and other dementias are about twice as prevalent among blacks as among whites.[58] Older blacks are more likely than older whites to suffer from heart disease, and the race gap begins as early as midlife. Among Americans age forty-five to sixty-four, black men have a 70 percent elevated risk and black women have a 50 percent greater risk of developing heart failure relative to whites. This earlier onset of major health conditions is one reason why blacks are more likely than whites to have health-limiting impairments. While one in five older adults has a health-related disability such as limited hearing, seeing, speaking, or walking, this proportion is significantly higher among blacks than whites (26 versus 21 percent). These disparities are not explained away even when socioeconomic resources are controlled.

Socioeconomic differences are just as consistent. Regardless of whether socioeconomic status is measured by parental education or one's own education or wealth in later life, disparities exist along nearly every imaginable health outcome, including mortality risk, cardiovascular disease, diabetes, arthritis, asthma, and most forms of cancer as well as earlier onset of dementia and disability. To revisit the case of dementia risk, one recent analysis of HRS data found that dementia rates decrease steadily with each additional year of education.[59] This link partly reflects biological processes: more schooling helps to build a cognitive reserve that enables older adults to better compensate for changes in the brain that could result in dementia. Geriatricians have suggested that education increases connections between neurons in the brain and helps the brain to compensate for early neurological changes by using alternate routes of neuron-to-neuron communication to complete cognitive tasks. Social scientists also have identified behavioral pathways. Highly educated older adults get more physical exercise, which protects against dementia by forestalling illnesses linked to brain disease, such as diabetes, hypertension, heart disease, and inflammation.[60]

Studies consistently detect a clear gradient where health improves with more years of schooling or as the tier in the occupational hierarchy increases—a phenomenon that the epidemiologist Sir Michael Marmot refers to as the "status syndrome."[61] The association between income and health is more complex, however, with important implications for policy, as we will see later in this chapter. Higher levels of income are linked with better health, but only up to a point. The health gains reaped with each additional year of income are steepest for those at the lower rungs of the income distribution; they level off thereafter. For the poor and near-poor, each additional dollar of income may boost health, but for those with a middle-class or higher income, each additional dollar does not bring further health benefits.[62]

Explaining Late-Life Health Disparities: Three Mechanisms

Late-life health disparities are difficult to eradicate because they are a consequence of long-standing social, economic, and behavioral factors. There is no pill to cure or surgical intervention to excise economic deprivation, loneliness, exhausting caregiving duties, or persistent discrimination. Several biological and methodological arguments attempt to challenge the notion that social inequalities drive health disparities, yet empirical analyses generally show that the explanatory power of these competing perspectives is modest—holding only for particular health outcomes, subpopulations, or life-course stages.

First, some scientists attribute black-white health disparities to biological differences. It's true that a handful of diseases like sickle cell anemia have a clear genetic basis, but they are far outnumbered by disparities that are better explained by social and economic factors.[63] Hypertension provides a case in point. Blacks are more likely than whites to suffer from hypertension: 71 percent of older blacks but just 54 percent of older whites have high blood pressure. Some historians and cardiologists have attributed this gap to genetic vulnerabilities.[64] The controversial (and largely unsupported) "slavery hypertension hypothesis" argues that blacks' higher rates of hypertension trace back to slaves' greater capacity to conserve salt, which protected them from disease and death when they sailed the rocky passage across the Atlantic from Africa. The capacity to retain salt would be a helpful hedge against diarrhea and vomiting-induced weakness at that time. This same capacity today can intensify one's risk of high blood pressure, because salty foods are a staple of U.S. diets and especially the "Southern diet," which is popular among many African Americans.[65]

Social scientists offer a much more compelling (and empirically supported) explanation, pointing to enduring systems of inequality in the United States as the primary source of black-white health disparities. From this vantage point, race is conceptualized as a social construct that may limit individuals' access to economic opportunities in particular contexts; it is not a biological reality.[66] If biology were the primary explanatory mechanism, then race disparities in health and mortality would be generally similar across geographic, social, and historic contexts. One particularly compelling study shows that older blacks in the United States fare worse than blacks in both the Caribbean (also a slave-receiving location) and West Africa across multiple health conditions, including hypertension—a pattern that some have attributed to uniquely high levels of discrimination against blacks in the United States.[67] Even within the United States, black-white health disparities vary widely by state: blacks generally fare worse in states with less generous social welfare programs, like Mississippi, and fare better in states with a more protective safety net, like Massachusetts.[68]

Similarly, some biomedically oriented researchers attribute women's life expectancy advantage to biological factors like the protective effects of estrogen and the disadvantageous effects of testosterone, which impel men (especially young men) to risky or potentially deadly aggressive behaviors. The Darwin Award, a project developed in a Usenet group twenty-five years ago, is an annual tongue-in-cheek award presented to the individual who died in the most reckless or foolish way in the past year. Without fail, these distinctions are bestowed upon young men whose deaths resulted from actions like jumping into a lion's cage at the zoo (after having chugged a six-pack of beer) or from ostentatious feats of strength gone awry, like the young man who plunged to his death after triumphantly "planking" on a high-rise balcony railing.[69] These sensationalist catastrophes aside, biology does play a small role in men's mortality disadvantage over the life course. An estimated 107 baby boys are born per every 100 girls, but those numbers quickly even out due to boys' higher infant mortality rates, a function of weaker cardiopulmonary systems and greater genetic susceptibility to illness.[70]

If gender gaps were due to biological factors alone, then health and mortality disparities would be relatively constant over time. Yet that is not the case. The gender gap in mortality has narrowed considerably over the past several decades, largely because men (especially middle-class men) have abandoned unhealthy behaviors like smoking, and left dangerous manual jobs for white-collar work, while women's rates of unhealthy behaviors (especially smoking) have increased.[71] Some evidence also suggests that liberalizing gender ideologies throughout the late twentieth century have freed men from the cultural expectations consistent with hegemonic masculinity, a view of masculinity that privileges being strong, silent, and invincible. The desire to appear invulnerable, combined with the need to support one's family financially, has been linked with men's unhealthy behaviors like ignoring painful symptoms until it's too late, going to work when sick, avoiding regular checkups, and not divulging symptoms that might be viewed as a sign of weakness (like depressive symptoms) when they do go for checkups.[72]

The gender gap in late-life health and mortality may continue to narrow even further in the coming decades, especially for white working-class baby boomers, but for the wrong reasons. New data documents rising mortality rates among lower-SES middle-aged women—a function of obesity, smoking, opioid use, the stress associated with being a family's main breadwinner, and other problems to which poor women are particularly vulnerable.[73]

Some researchers also challenge the notion that social inequalities cause poor health, drawing on methodological concerns. Adherents of the social selection (or "downward drift") hypothesis counter that poor health is a cause rather than a consequence of low socioeconomic status. A sickly child or a young adult fighting major depression and substance use may have bleak chances of earning a college degree or finding steady work, both of which provide health-enhancing benefits. A middle-aged worker in poor health may need to quit his or her job, cut back to part-time hours, or go on disability—actions that would reduce earnings in the short term and savings and pension payments in the longer run. Empirical studies show some evidence of social selection, especially among middle-aged workers, but on the whole causation arguments are supported more strongly by the data.[74]

The three most convincing social explanations for health disparities are stress exposure, health behaviors, and, to a lesser extent, access to care. Social and economic disadvantage is linked with higher levels of stress, fewer healthy and more unhealthy behaviors, and less access to preventative care and treatment over the life course; each of these disparities in turn compromises physical health in old age. Although these three pathways may, at first blush, appear to reflect individual-level choices, they are closely intertwined with macrosocial conditions and public policies. For instance, older adults residing in states with more generous social welfare programs and policies that prioritize population health fare better along multiple indicators of health and well-being, in part because these policies can help to minimize some stressors, promote positive health behaviors, and enhance access to care.[75]

Stress Exposure

Stress makes us sick and kills us slowly. As biological models of aging and disease show, stress undermines our health gradually, often taking years for the harmful effects of early assaults to come to fruition. Years of exposure to social, interpersonal, psychological, and environmental slights can undermine one's cardiovascular, immune, and central nervous systems and bring about disease and premature death. Hollywood dramas would have us believe that stress can kill older adults instantaneously, but that is rarely the case. Classic film buffs may recall the scene in *Now, Voyager* when Charlotte Vale, a mousy spinster who blossoms into a worldly sophisticate, has a heated argument with her disapproving mother, who promptly dies of a heart attack. A similar fate strikes Horace Giddens in *Little Foxes*. A frail and mild-mannered man with a serious heart condition, Horace dies of a heart attack following a vicious spat with his contemptuous wife, Regina. The actual ways in which stress hastens death are less dramatic, but more pernicious because they unfold slowly, increasing one's risk of multiple conditions over the life course.

How Stress Hurts Us Physiological responses to stress involve the direct stimulation of the central nervous system (CNS) and a hormonal relay system among three organs: the adrenal glands, located at the top of each kidney, and the hypothalamus and pituitary gland, located in the brain. Both the CNS and the hypothalamic-pituitary-adrenal (HPA) axis play a critical role in linking stress with physical health. A key mechanism is cortisol, also referred to as the "stress hormone." When faced with an immediate and short-term stressor, such as an intense argument, a near-miss traffic accident, or the sound of footsteps close behind us as we walk down a deserted street, our cortisol levels rise. Small increases in cortisol levels can be good for us in the short term: increased cortisol boosts our memory and immune function and gives us the adrenaline rush we need to escape from imminent danger. This release serves as an anti-inflammatory hormone and increases levels of circulating glucose and energy storage. However, when we live under conditions of constant stress, such as persistent worries about paying the monthly bills, the prolonged high levels of cortisol in our bloodstream elevate our risk of suppressed thyroid function, blood sugar imbalances, high blood pressure, lowered immune responses, slower wound healing, and decreased bone density. Consistently high levels of stress-induced cortisol also are linked with abdominal adiposity, or belly fat, which heightens the risk of heart attack, stroke, and metabolic syndrome.

Stress exposure also affects vascular inflammation, which leads to atherosclerosis, a buildup of plaque in the arteries. When arteries are clogged with plaque buildup, blood flows less freely and increases the risk of myocardial infarction and stroke. Stress also increases the production of platelets, a type of blood cell whose main purpose is to prevent bleeding. Platelet activation releases substances into the bloodstream that stick to arteries, leading to plaque buildup and possibly increasing the risk of heart disease. Stress also has powerful effects on mental health symptoms like depression and anxiety, which can be particularly overwhelming for older adults; chapter 5 delves into these linkages and shows how mental health problems can undermine physical health. Biological models of stress exemplify the key premise of cumulative disadvantage theories: repeated exposure over long periods of time accumulate to take a toll on older adults' health.

Differential Exposure to Stress It is a rare person who is blessed with a stress-free life. Even the most privileged individuals are subject to stress. Wall Street moguls worry about hostile takeovers, Hollywood celebrities suffer the relentless surveillance of aggressive paparazzi, and highly paid athletes and coaches might fear job loss after a crushing Super Bowl defeat. However, the frequency, intensity, variety, and duration of stress is especially high for those occupying the lower tiers of the social hierarchy, where the tiers are defined by one's economic and social power in a particular context.[76] Dozens of studies show that persons of color and of lower SES have higher levels of stress exposure at every point in the life course.[77] Low SES increases a person's risk of stressful life events ranging from divorce to job loss to early onset of health problems, as well as chronic stressors such as overcrowded or dilapidated living conditions, marital strife, and discrimination.

Many of the stressors affecting African Americans have their roots in persistent economic disadvantage, but economic factors do not tell the whole story. Some scholars have suggested that blacks, regardless of

SES, face an entirely separate set of stressors from which European Americans are spared. Minority stress, as the psychiatric epidemiologist Ilan Meyer calls it, includes long-term exposure to racial discrimination, prejudice, tokenism, interpersonal mistreatment, and struggles to balance one's own cultural practices with those of the majority-white society.[78] These stressors, which may be compounded by persistent economic strain, dangerous neighborhoods, limited access to high-quality health care, heightened risk of death to family members, and problems that befall loved ones (like a grandchild's imprisonment or unemployment), conspire to put blacks at a heightened risk of health problems in later life.[79]

The epidemiologist Arline Geronimus argues that this accumulation of both personal and macrosocial stressors like economic adversity and political marginalization leads to a process she calls "weathering."[80] Weathering describes the physiological deterioration that blacks disproportionately experience over the life course, leading to earlier onset of morbidity, disease, and mortality. She and her collaborators find stark racial gaps in later life that range widely across biological outcomes—including allostatic load—increase with age, and are not explained by racial differences in poverty. These disparities persist because they result from "living in a race-conscious society that stigmatizes and disadvantages Blacks"; such lives require sustained and high-effort coping, which takes a further toll on minds and bodies.[81]

Differential Coping Resources   It is not just differential exposure to stress that contributes to health disparities, but differences in the resources we possess to ward off or cope with those stressors. Older adults who have suffered long-term deprivation may lack some essential coping resources that help them to thrive in the face of stress. That is not to suggest that they lack resiliency or problem-solving savvy. In fact, experts increasingly recognize that modest amounts of adversity can be protective, enabling us to learn how to effectively cope with and overcome difficult obstacles. But disadvantaged older adults have had fewer tangible and structural resources over the life course to help them manage or circumvent stressful situations, such as having enough savings for a down payment for a home in a safe neighborhood, or to pay for a quality education that will open career doors and provide flexible problem-solving skills, or to hire a home health aide to assist with daily tasks that exceed one's physical capacities.[82]

Older adults whose lives have been marked by cumulative adversity also tend to lack the one coping resource that stress researchers deem most important: social support. Of course, neither race nor social class affects a person's capacity to love or be loved. But it does affect the availability of family members and friends to provide assistance in times of need. Adult children who face struggles of their own or who live paycheck to paycheck might not be able to take time off work to care for an ailing parent.[83] Older adults who live in poor neighborhoods may find that their neighbors come and go, renting for a few months and then moving out. That "churning" or rapid turnover of social ties leads to a less consistent and dependable base of support and assistance.[84] Chapter 6 will say much more about how social support and isolation can either intensify or buffer against the effect of stress in older adults' lives.

Our thought processes also affect how we cope. Some evidence suggests that people with lower levels of education feel a greater sense of hopelessness and fatalism and as a result may resign themselves to a stressful situation rather than try to fix it. This acquiescence may be a completely rational and realistic reaction to insurmountable stressors; still, it prevents people from extricating themselves from the very situations that may gradually erode their health.[85] For instance, the "poverty-cancer spiral" derives from the observation that people with low levels of education are especially likely to view cancer as an inevitable death sentence and to consequently see screening and treatment as exercises in futility.[86] Conversely, some blacks may react not with hopelessness but with a fervor to overcome whatever obstacles are placed in their path. Yet this persistence, which the epidemiologist Sherman James has dubbed "John Henryism," may ultimately harm their cardiovascular health.[87]

Named after the American folklore hero who worked himself to death while building a railroad tunnel, John Henryism refers to the process whereby some blacks expend very high levels of effort to succeed against all odds in a majority-white society. Survey questions measure John Henryism by asking respondents to indicate their level of agreement with statements like "When things don't go the way I want them to, that just makes me work even harder." This coping approach may help people overcome daily challenges, yet it also exacts a physical toll in the long term, in the ways that Arline Geronimus's weathering hypothesis describes. James and his colleagues have found that older blacks with high scores on John Henryism scales have an elevated risk of physiological symptoms, including high blood pressure. Just as John Henry died clutching his hammer, some African Americans may slowly suffer by working tirelessly to succeed in untenable and high-pressure situations, ultimately hastening their deaths.

John Henryism also partially helps to explain the "diminishing returns" phenomenon, whereby each extra year of education or extra dollar of income brings fewer health benefits to older blacks than it does to whites. One particularly disheartening study compared a cohort of older white physicians who graduated from Johns Hopkins University Medical School in the 1950s and 1960s and black physicians who graduated from Meharry Medical College during the same era. The doctors were tracked for several decades, and by their sixties and seventies the black doctors had double the rates of diabetes and hypertension relative to the white doctors.[88] Why didn't the critical coping resources of education and income benefit blacks and whites in the same way? One plausible explanation is that upward social mobility may lead African Americans to largely white neighborhoods and workplaces, where they experience the strains of tokenism and discrimination. Efforts to overcome these obstacles, by working as hard as one possibly can in the spirit of John Henry, may engender frustration and ultimately compromised health.[89] Others have observed that blacks' more modest health gains reflect factors like racial discrimination, unequal employment opportunities, differences in educational quality, and other stressors associated with being a visible minority in the United States.[90]

Public policies can play an important role in mitigating against stress, albeit indirectly. Of course, some stressors simply are not amenable to policy interventions; the pain of losing a spouse or child is just as devastating for rich and poor, black and white. But many stressors can be muted, and many coping resources strengthened, via policies such as affirmative action programs to improve blacks' access to higher education and employment, antidiscrimination legislation, and antipoverty or income support programs. Financial insecurity is consistently named by most Americans as the single biggest stressor in their lives.[91] This insecurity can be alleviated somewhat by income support programs like the Earned Income Tax Credit (EITC) for working-age adults and Supplemental Security Income (SSI) benefits for older adults. Importantly, these programs target poor and near-poor adults, which may be particularly effective in narrowing health disparities, given that the health benefits linked to income are largest at the lowest levels of income and taper off thereafter.

EITC, one of the largest federal antipoverty programs in the United States, began in 1975 and provides a refundable tax credit for low-income working adults. In addition to the federal credits, twenty-six states and the District of Columbia offer state credits.[92] The state credits, combined with the federal EITC, help working adults avoid poverty and the hardships it could impose on them and their families. EITCs also have demonstrated long-term effects on health and well-being, which they achieve in part by minimizing health-depleting financial strain and freeing up money for things like healthy foods or apartments in less hazardous neighborhoods. Recent studies show that older adults living in states with a long history of offering EITC are less likely to have functional impairments.[93] Relatively few older adults are currently working and thus may not be direct and immediate beneficiaries of these credits, yet the physical health benefits may accrue in the much longer term. Additionally, the benefits of living in a state with EITC may extend to older adults' network members, including friends, family, and community members, enabling them to provide support to older adults in need.[94]

The effects of income programs directly targeting low-income older adults also have been proven to improve health. Pamela Herd, Robert Schoeni, and James House focused their analysis on SSI, a means-tested income supplement program established in 1972 for older adults, blind, and disabled persons.[95] Like EITC, these cash supplements can be used to meet basic needs like food, housing, and clothing. About 6 percent of older adults receive SSI. Although benefit levels vary by state, the minimum benefit brings older adults' monthly income up to three-quarters of the federal poverty line. The research team found that a $100 monthly increase above and beyond that minimum was linked with a significant drop in functional limitations. Income transfer programs targeting low-income working-age and older adults may be a particularly cost-effective way to help reduce late-life health disparities, as they may help to reduce stress, enhance coping, and facilitate the adoption of healthy behaviors.

Health Behaviors

Health behaviors, including smoking, diet, exercise, alcohol and drug use, and sleep patterns, are among the most powerful explanations for race and socioeconomic disparities in health and gender differences in mortality risk. As noted earlier, an influential *New England Journal of Medicine* article concluded that health behaviors account for as much as 40 percent of premature deaths.[96] The direct effects of health behaviors on disease and mortality risks are substantial, although the magnitude of these effects may diminish with age.[97] For instance, the harmful impact of being overweight and obesity on mortality is smaller among older adults relative to younger and midlife adults because caloric reserves can bring some protection in old age.[98] Still, changes in health behaviors even at advanced ages are linked with better health. A study of smoking cessation in the Coronary Artery Surgery Study (CASS) found that quitting smoking reduced the mortality risk of older adults with coronary artery disease (CAD), while those who continued to smoke had higher risks of both heart attack and death over a six-year follow-up period.⁹⁹ These studies clearly challenge the misperception of some older smokers that "it's too late to quit," or that quitting will not make a difference.

Besides having direct harmful effects on health and mortality, unhealthy behaviors also have multiplicative effects—that is, one unhealthy behavior begets more health-depleting stress and additional unhealthy behaviors. Heavy drinkers may have more frequent marital feuds, legal run-ins, and shakier employment prospects than nondrinkers or abstainers, and these additional stressors may drive them to drink even more. Obesity increases one's risk of stressors like weight-related discrimination, relationship strains, and lower body impairments, which in turn may trigger more stress-related eating and less exercise.¹⁰⁰ While some mood-enhancing behaviors, like drinking, smoking, and eating comfort foods, may feel good in the short term, their longer-term health consequences can be dire. These unhealthy behaviors can snowball to take a major toll on older adults' health. The researchers Benjamin Shaw and Neda Agahi examined heath profiles of older adults in the HRS and found that smokers who were also heavy drinkers had a significantly higher mortality risk compared to those who engaged in just one of the two behaviors.¹⁰¹ And studies based on the Whitehall data in the United Kingdom similarly found that older adults who were smokers and heavy drinkers had a much steeper decline in cognitive functioning over a ten-year period relative to nonsmoking moderate drinkers.¹⁰²

Health behaviors are a popular target of public health campaigns. It's easy to tell someone to "just say no" to drugs, that "smoking kills," or to "just do it" and start an exercise regimen. The message is that if we just put our mind to it, we too can be as fit and flexible as Tāo Porchon-Lynch, the world's oldest yoga master, or Jacinto Bonilla, a prostate cancer survivor and the oldest man to compete in the 2017 Crossfit Games. But studies repeatedly show that people cannot simply will themselves to engage in healthy behavior. It requires money to buy healthy food, time to prepare it, and safe neighborhoods to facilitate exercise. For those who experience chronic stress day in and day out, a cold beer or two might help to take the edge off, especially for those who either cannot afford professional mental health care or fear the stigma of seeking such care. Addictions in all forms, whether food, drugs, alcohol, or nicotine, are extraordinarily difficult to overcome. The Centers for Disease Control and Prevention (CDC) reports that roughly half of all smokers try to quit each year, but only about 6 percent succeed.¹⁰³ Most make several attempts and start smoking again after an initial quit in response to withdrawal symptoms.

Health behaviors play a powerful role in later-life health disparities because the behaviors themselves are highly stratified.[104] To revisit the example of smoking, just 9 percent of older adults currently smoke, yet the rate is twice as high among those living beneath the federal poverty line than among those living at 200 percent or more of the poverty threshold (7 versus 14 percent). Obesity, a function of a high-fat, high-calorie diet and sedentary lifestyle, follows a steep gradient over the life course. Blacks, and especially black girls and women, have the highest obesity rates of any demographic group. Although obesity rates have been rising steadily over the past three decades for all groups, rich and poor, black and white, these increases have been steepest for those with the least education and lowest income.[105]

Most sociological approaches emphasize that structural inequalities underlie these patterns.[106] Low levels of education are linked with poorer health literacy: those from disadvantaged backgrounds are less able to fully comprehend the long-term consequences of unhealthy behaviors. Poor older adults living in crowded low-income neighborhoods cannot easily access healthy and affordable foods at their local grocery stores. Access issues are compounded by the fact that purveyors of unhealthy behaviors, including fast-food corporations, soda and snack food companies, cigarette manufacturers, and alcohol distributors, explicitly target blacks, inner-city communities, and low-income populations in their marketing campaigns.[107] Older adults living in rundown or crowded neighborhoods also may lack safe places to walk and get basic exercise, and they may struggle to fall asleep at night, given high levels of noise in the neighborhood, as we will see in chapter 7.

That's not to say that personal choices do not matter, but choice is constrained by social contexts. Foods that are high in salt and fat taste good and meet our natural cravings.[108] Yet these natural (albeit unhealthy) cravings are easier to satisfy when one lives in a poor neighborhood where fast-food restaurants with dollar menus outnumber farmers' markets. It also takes money to develop a palate for healthy foods, and a palate developed in childhood often stays with us for life, especially if we do not have the means to explore more varied food choices. The sociologist Caitlin Daniel found that middle-class parents introduce their children to healthy fruits and vegetables slowly and gradually, encouraging them to develop a taste for foods that will help them stay healthy and slender. It may take as many as eight to fifteen tries on average, but eventually many middle-class children come around to embracing Brussels sprouts. In stark contrast, Daniel found that lower-income parents might try once or twice to convince their child of the benefits of broccoli, but they cannot afford to waste money on food their children will spit out. Money spent on white bread and boxed macaroni and cheese is seen as a much surer bet that their children will be filled up, albeit with fewer nutrients.[109] Not surprisingly, studies of adults find that higher SES is linked with greater consumption of whole grains, lean meats, fish, low-fat dairy products, and fresh vegetables and fruit, whereas lower SES is linked with eating less nutritious foods like white bread and fried foods.[110]

Public policies can help bring affordable healthy foods to economically disadvantaged populations, with long-term implications for health and survival. The Supplemental Nutrition Assistance Program (SNAP) (formerly the Food Stamp Program, which began in 1961) provides low-income Americans of all ages with monthly benefits that they can use to purchase healthy foods and drinks, whether at grocery stores or farmers' markets. In 2015, 11 percent of all SNAP recipients were older adults, three-quarters of whom lived alone.[111] These programs are highly effective in promoting nutrition and health; SNAP reduces poor families' chances of being "food insecure" by anywhere from 10 to 30 percent; food insecurity means either skipping meals or eating too little because food is unaffordable. Federal and state investment in programs like food stamps and SNAP have demonstrated long-term benefits for health that can linger through old age. One assessment found that access to food stamps in the 1960s was linked with older adults' better self-rated health and lower odds of metabolic symptoms more than five decades later.[112] The program also has direct impacts: in 2015, SNAP households with an older adult received $128 in monthly benefits, boosting their annual income by 15 percent. These dollars can go directly to improving nutrition and reducing anxiety about food bills.

Just as public policies can promote healthy behaviors, they can help to reduce unhealthy ones. Rates of smoking (and consequently smoking-related diseases like lung cancer) and overall mortality rates tend to be lowest in states that invest most heavily in programs like antismoking ad campaigns, smoking bans in public places, antismoking curricula in schools, laws restricting tobacco companies from marketing, raising the legal smoking age from eighteen to twenty-one, and increasing cigarette taxes. The last is a particularly effective strategy. Residents of all fifty U.S. states currently pay a $1.00 federal excise tax per pack of cigarettes, yet additional state-level taxes range from as low as 17 cents per pack in Mississippi to $4.35 a pack in New York. "Red" states that historically are under Republican-controlled governments, like Alabama, Mississippi, South Carolina, and Tennessee, tax less than a dollar per pack, while traditionally blue states like Connecticut, Minnesota, Rhode Island, and Vermont tax well over $3 per pack.

Although taxes are always political hot buttons, they are also extremely effective, revealing a principle that economists refer to as "price elasticity." In short, the higher the tax, the fewer cigarettes are bought and smoked. This pattern is strongest for those with the least income to spend, including teenagers, low-income smokers, and racial and ethnic minorities. One recent study showed that for each 10 percent increase in the price of cigarettes, rates of teen smoking dropped by 7 percent.[113] Given that smoking habits form early in life, tax policies that affect young people's behaviors have implications for their health and well-being many decades later.

But public health initiatives to quash poor health behaviors and promote positive ones are not sufficient to erase health disparities. As fundamental cause theory has argued and multiple empirical studies have demonstrated, public health initiatives like antismoking campaigns are much more effective in promoting healthy behaviors among those with more ample socioeconomic resources, given their higher levels of health literacy, financial means to purchase healthier foods, greater receptiveness to health-promoting messages, and access to more effective stress-reducing techniques than smoking cigarettes.[114]

Access to Care

Most health researchers and policymakers believe that access to care is critical to health over the life course, although it makes only a modest dent in eradicating health disparities. Recall the *New England Journal of Medicine* editorial arguing that health care access explains just 10 percent of premature mortality in the United States.[115] More than three decades before that, the seminal 1982 *Black Report* revealed the then-stunning finding that social class disparities in sickness and mortality actually widened in the United Kingdom after it introduced universal health care through the National Health Service.[116] Produced by the United Kingdom's Department of Health and Social Security, the *Black Report* revolutionized conversations about health disparities by showing the far-reaching ways in which social class shapes health, citing pathways like work conditions, diet, housing quality, and substance use.[117]

Unlike the United Kingdom, the United States does not have national health care. Health insurance historically has been provided by employers, meaning that health benefits have been a privilege afforded to full-time workers or those married to full-time workers. In 2010, shortly before the implementation of the Affordable Care Act (ACA), roughly 70 percent of working-age Americans received health insurance through their employers. Those who were too young to work, too old to work, or out of work often relied on public insurance programs. Low-income adults were eligible to receive health insurance through Medicaid, older adults through Medicare, and children through state-based Children's

Health Insurance Programs (CHIP) if their parents earned too much to qualify for Medicaid. Roughly one in five older adults who were Medicare beneficiaries had income low enough to also be eligible for Medicaid, a status referred to as dual-eligible.

Yet this piecemeal system left 45 million adults, mostly working-poor and lower-middle-class persons, uninsured in 2010—a number that dropped to 28.5 million by the end of 2015, thanks to the implementation of the ACA. According to the Kaiser Commission on Medicaid and the Uninsured, low-income families, especially blacks and Latinos, have been most likely to remain uninsured since the implementation of the ACA, because even under the ACA the costs of coverage are prohibitive.[118] As of June 2018, the future of the ACA and its subcomponents was uncertain; the Congressional Budget Office (CBO) projected that, if the ACA is repealed, the number of uninsured Americans would jump from 28 million to at least 50 million by the year 2026.

Despite the importance of health insurance to the well-being of a society, it does not guarantee that all Americans will receive care, especially high-quality care. That is one major reason why health insurance alone is not sufficient to eradicate health disparities, consistent with the core argument of fundamental cause theory.[119] Medicaid recipients may have difficulty finding a physician who will take them as a patient; many doctors refuse to see them because the Medicaid reimbursement rates are too low. An estimated 70 percent of doctors in the United States will accept a Medicaid recipient as a new patient, yet this rate ranges from just 40 percent in New Jersey to 99 percent in Wyoming. New Jersey ranks dead last because of the low reimbursement rates.[120] According to some estimates, New Jersey family physicians were reimbursed an average of just $23.50 in 2014 for an office visit from a Medicaid-covered patient, although that same visit would be reimbursed for as much as $111 in other states.[121] Even when doctors do accept Medicaid patients, those patients often fall to the end of the queue, waiting longer to get appointments and referrals because private pay and employer-insured patients take top priority. Sometimes Medicaid recipients will eventually find a provider who will take them on as new patients, only to find that they cannot easily travel to the faraway office or medical center. As a result, Medicaid patients who must travel long distances to their providers have later-onset diagnoses and delayed treatment for diseases like breast cancer.

Physical distance is not the only obstacle; some researchers argue that social distance also matters. Lower-income patients may feel uncomfortable with doctors, fearing that they will be looked down upon or judged for being on public assistance.[122] African Americans also have a long history of mistrust toward the medical system, rooted in travesties like the Tuskegee study conducted for forty years in the mid-twentieth century, in which physicians allowed black men to die from untreated syphilis, all in the name of science. That is one reason why black and Latino patients report greater trust, comfort, and willingness to seek out care when their doctor shares their ethnic or racial background.[123] But racial concordance between doctor and patient is elusive: although blacks make up 13 percent of the U.S. population, they account for less than 5 percent of practicing physicians.[124]

And despite the great success of Medicare over the past half-century, it is not a guarantee that older patients will receive all the treatments and medical services they need. Health care providers are more willing to take Medicare patients than Medicaid patients because of the higher Medicare reimbursement rates. Still, an estimated 20 percent of doctors refuse to accept new Medicare patients.[125] Even Medicare patients with a regular doctor may find that many treatments and services are excluded under the program's standard benefits. For instance, the infamous Medicare "donut hole" refers to the gap in coverage for prescription medications that prevents some low-income older adults from being able to pay for the pricey drugs they desperately need. Drugs like Cognex and Aricept, prescribed to Alzheimer's patients, can run from $180 to $400 per month, so partial coverage may put these drugs out of reach for older adults who have a limited income and few savings.

Medicare also provides no hearing, vision, or dental benefits, each of which is a serious concern for older adults' functioning and social engagement. For example, just half of all older adults and 25 percent of low-income older adults have seen a dentist in the past year. This might not have been considered a serious concern decades ago, when most older adults had lost their natural teeth and wore dentures. But as more and more older adults are keeping their teeth, thanks to improved hygiene and fluoridation, dental care is increasingly important to their physical health and social engagement. Older adults who struggle to eat solid food are at risk of nutritional deficits, while embarrassment about missing teeth and bad breath may keep some older adults from socializing with friends and families, compounding their social isolation.[126]

Medicare also excludes some long-term care benefits that older adults need, such as home health care or payments for residential long-term care, as we shall see in the following chapters. Because of these gaps in coverage, older adults with several illnesses or serious functional limitations often must bear out-of-pocket costs that can top thousands of dollars a year. Moreover, Medicare does not place a cap on the out-of-pocket costs that patients bear, so the burden can be prohibitive for older adults living on modest incomes. According to recent estimates, more than one-quarter of all Medicare beneficiaries and nearly 40 percent of those with incomes below 200 percent of the federal poverty line spent at least one-fifth of their income on health care and insurance premiums in 2016.[127] Older adults can purchase additional coverage such as Medicare Supplement Insurance (Medigap), to help pay for services, like vision and hearing care, that are not covered by traditional Medicare benefits, but insurance premiums average $2,000 a year. Premiums for Medicare Part D, which helps cover prescription medications, average more than $400 a year.[128] Yet the costs of and access to these plans vary widely, such that they may be out of reach for some Americans. For instance, Medicare Advantage is a supplemental insurance offered by private insurance companies that are approved by Medicare. One-third of all Medicare beneficiaries were enrolled in a Medicare Advantage plan in 2017, yet because these plans often operate under a health maintenance organization (HMO), older adults living in rural or poor areas may lack access to them and to participating providers.[129]

Given these many limitations of Medicare, substantial race and socioeconomic gaps in treatment-seeking and treatment receipt persist, even among Medicare beneficiaries. For instance, one analysis of Medicare Current Beneficiary Survey (MCBS) data found that older blacks were less likely than whites to get flu shots (67 versus 43 percent), a pattern that the researchers attributed to whites' more positive attitudes toward and willingness to seek out the flu shot.[130] Other studies document significant race gaps in treatments ranging from chiropractic services to colorectal cancer screening, to hip replacements and coronary artery bypass grafting (CABG).[131]

These limitations of public insurance programs should not minimize the fact that access to timely high-quality preventive care and treatment does matter for older adults' health and longevity, especially because most diseases that kill older adults have their initial onset years before they are eligible for Medicare benefits. Early access to preventive care like colonoscopies for colorectal cancer and mammograms for breast cancer is essential so that older adults can learn whether they are sick before their tumor progresses to dangerous levels. For many cancers, patients start to notice symptoms only when the disease has progressed to a point where the prognosis is dire.

Some older adults, like super-centenarian Susannah Mushatt Jones, have the good genes, healthy behaviors, and meaningful work and family ties that promote long and healthy lives. But how long one lives, the illnesses one suffers from, and one's likelihood of surviving an illness once diagnosed are highly stratified by socioeconomic status and race. Medicare is not sufficient to erase these vast and persistent gaps, heightening the need for what the sociologist James House refers to as "nonhealth policies—especially those involving socioeconomic position, race-ethnicity, or gender—that shape the conditions of life and work, especially among the half or so of our population who live and work in disadvantaged conditions and whose health is consequently affected."[132] As the next three chapters will show, these "conditions of life and work," including social isolation, elder abuse, unsafe neighborhood conditions, and even natural disaster, can undermine older adults' physical and mental health, rendering them even more vulnerable to other social, interpersonal, and economic adversities.

… Chapter 5 ═

The Satisfied and the Sorrowful: The Mental Health of Older Adults

The emotional lives of older adults have been described both as the best of times and the worst of times. Confucius observed that "old age . . . is a good and pleasant thing," a time of happiness and contentment, while the French military and political leader Charles de Gaulle declared that "old age is a shipwreck," implying that our later years are plagued by misery and sorrow. Similar contradictions are detected in the scientific literature. Researchers have documented a U-shaped curve in happiness: older and younger adults report greater happiness than the middle-aged.[1] Epidemiologic studies consistently report that common mental health problems like depression, anxiety, and substance use decline steadily with age.[2] Yet these largely upbeat portrayals are challenged by data revealing a bleaker side of older adults' mental health. White men over age sixty-five have suicide rates nearly three times higher than the U.S. average.[3] And with advancing age, men and women from all walks of life become vulnerable to stressful experiences that may threaten their emotional well-being. The loss of meaningful social roles like worker and spouse, the deaths of friends and loved ones, chronic health conditions, and ageism are stressors that older adults inevitably encounter. The emotional toll of these stressors is all the more profound for those also struggling with financial insecurity, social isolation, and health problems of their own, exemplifying the life-course theme of cumulative disadvantage.

To revisit the competing proclamations of Confucius and de Gaulle, is old age the best of times or the worst of times when it comes to psychological health? The answer, in short, is that it depends. Whether later life is marked by joy or sorrow depends heavily on the advantages or adversities experienced over the life course, the presence of resources to cope with those adversities, access to mental health treatment, and genetic and psychological factors that may protect against or intensify the emotional ups and downs that are an unavoidable part of life. Although population-level statistics tell us that older adults generally fare better than younger people with respect to mental health symptoms ranging from happiness to depression to anxiety, these snapshots conceal important disparities among older adults.

Race, socioeconomic status, and gender powerfully shape the number and types of stressors faced by older adults, their financial and social resources to cope with stressors, the cognitive capacities that help them creatively adapt to stress, their willingness (or reluctance) to acknowledge symptoms like depression, and their capacity to access treatment for those symptoms. Late-life mental health disparities also reflect advantages or disadvantages that have accumulated over time; lifelong exposure to stressors like poverty, illness, and discrimination erode not only one's emotional health but undermine one's capacity to access important coping resources. Yet a lifetime of disadvantage does not predestine anyone to an old age marked by sorrow, just as lives of advantage are no guarantee of emotional bliss. Many older adults manage to thrive emotionally and are resilient, drawing strength from strong social ties, affirming religious beliefs, well-honed coping skills, and formal support systems.

This chapter begins by describing the main components of emotional health in later life, focusing primarily on depression but touching on other common problems such as anxiety, anger, substance use, and one of the most serious indicators of mental health: suicide and suicidal ideation.[4] I describe trends and differentials in each of these facets of mental health and point out reasons why standard survey and diagnostic measures may offer an unrealistically optimistic portrayal of older adults' mental health and understate or mask important gender and race disparities. I then describe several stressors that are common among older adults, yet particularly so among those already facing persistent economic, social, or physical disadvantages. I delve into the question of why some older adults are particularly vulnerable to stress while others are resilient even in the face of significant challenge. I also underscore that poor mental health is not inevitable late in life, even for the most disadvantaged older adults, and I highlight personal resources, public policies, and practical interventions that may mitigate against the long-term mental health consequences of cumulative adversity.

Late Life Mental Health: Definitions, Components, and Trends

Mental health is a very broad concept. Many scholars and practitioners rely on the World Health Organization's definition: mental health, according to WHO, is more than "the absence of mental disorders or disabilities." Rather, it is "a state of well-being in which an individual realizes his or her own abilities, can cope with the normal stresses of life . . . and is able to make a contribution to his or her community."[5] Consistent with this expansive view, social science and clinical studies of mental health focus on diverse indicators because each provides a slightly different perspective on emotional health. Focusing on a single aspect of mental health could conceal important disparities given that men and women, blacks and whites, and older versus younger adults experience, describe, and have their mental health problems diagnosed and treated in very different ways.

Depression: Trends and Disparities

Depression is the most widely studied mental health condition, a consequence of its high prevalence. As many as one in six U.S. adults have been diagnosed with depression at some point in their lives.[6] Scholars and practitioners dating back to Sigmund Freud have observed that depression is a reaction to loss or "exit events" that are especially common in later life, such as retirement, widowhood, a reluctant move out of a longtime home, or the loss of independence that accompanies failing vision, hearing, and cognitive functioning. Depression is commonly studied because it is measured in most major surveys of health and can be screened fairly easily by health care providers. As such, researchers can readily obtain data to identify its social patterning and causes.[7]

One of the most commonly used instruments for measuring depressive symptoms in population-based studies is the Center for Epidemiologic Studies Depression Scale (CES-D).[8] This twenty-item checklist captures how often in the past week the respondent experienced symptoms like sadness, hopelessness, and loneliness; however, the measure is not designed to gauge whether the respondent has the more serious clinical diagnosis of major depressive disorder, which occurs when a person experiences severe depressive symptoms for two weeks or more. These severe symptoms interfere with the ability to work, sleep, eat, and enjoy activities that were once pleasurable. Major depressive disorder can be assessed with instruments like the Composite International Diagnostic Interview (CIDI) and Diagnostic Interview Schedule (DIS). Regardless of the measure used, studies consistently show that older adults have depressive symptoms levels and rates of major depressive disorder that are comparable to or lower than those of younger persons.[9]

Depression is an especially important outcome when studying late-life disparities because it is both a product of cumulative disadvantage and an engine perpetuating it. Rates of depression are consistently highest among those who have experienced lives of economic disadvantage and personal hardship. Yet depression, in turn, increases a person's risk of subsequent adversities. It elevates older adults' risk of disease, disability, and death, renders them vulnerable to self-neglect, social isolation, mistreatment, and exploitation, and makes them less receptive to the well-intended efforts of potential caregivers.[10] Researchers have found that depression is linked with reductions in life span of anywhere from seven to ten years, and that older adults with frequent depressive symptoms are twice as likely as their peers without symptoms to experience elder abuse and neglect.[11]

Although depression is often thought of as a singular experience, marked by persistent sadness, it actually has four distinctive components: emotional, cognitive, motivational, and somatic symptoms. Emotional symptoms are the sadness and diminished pleasure that almost always accompany depression. The cognitive component refers to the changes in our thought processes when we are depressed: we may feel hopeless about the future, believe that we are worthless, or think that others dislike us. The motivational component refers to lethargy and a diminished ability to "get up and go" with everyday activities. Finally, somatic symptoms include physical conditions like fatigue, headaches, or sleeping too much or too little.[12] These distinctions are especially important for studying, diagnosing, and treating the mental health of older adults, who are particularly susceptible to somatic symptoms like fatigue and who may be reluctant to report cognitive or emotional symptoms; as a result, their depression may go undetected.

Some experts suggest that current generations of older adults are especially reluctant to report their feelings of sadness and depression—whether on a survey or to their health care provider—because of embarrassment, fear of stigma, or the belief that sadness is just a normal part of getting old. This potential source of bias reflects what demographers call a "cohort effect": generations are socialized differently and carry certain generation-specific beliefs throughout their lives. Older adults today, many of whom grew up during the Depression and World War II, were raised in a culture in which complaining and showing negative emotions were frowned upon. They were taught to keep a stiff upper lip even in troubled times, and in continuing to do so, they may hide their symptoms from physicians, family members, and care providers.[13] Depressed older patients may admit to somatic symptoms like sleep troubles and poor appetite or motivational symptoms such as low energy or lethargy, yet if they do not report feelings of sadness, their doctors may (incorrectly) attribute their symptoms to physical illness and "normal aging" rather than depression and may not offer proper treatment.[14] Older adults who believe that depression is a normal and expected response to aging are only 25 percent as likely as those who acknowledge their symptoms to talk about their mental health concerns with a physician.[15]

Studies of depression consistently show clear gendered patterns, such that older women are more likely than men to be diagnosed with depression, whether by a health care provider or based on their responses to standard survey items like the CES-D. Current data show that 15 percent of women but just 10 percent of men age sixty-five and older report clinically significant depressive symptoms. The magnitude of the gender gap diminishes in very old age (eighty and older), yet women are more likely than men to evidence both depressive symptoms and major depression at every age, as shown in figure 5.1.[16]

These persistent gender gaps do not mean that older men are spared of depression; rather, they experience and report their symptoms differently. Men are more likely to report somatic or cognitive symptoms and less likely to acknowledge feelings of sadness, whether on a symptom checklist or when visiting their health care providers.[17] Especially for men who were raised in an era when being strong, silent, and invincible was the cultural norm, acknowledging feelings of vulnerability and reporting symptoms like crying may be seen as a sign of weakness. Yet older men's reluctance to acknowledge or report these symptoms may lead to misdiagnoses and undertreatment by health care providers, who may view somatic symptoms like fatigue as simply a "normal" part of aging.[18] That is one critical reason why older men have such high rates of suicide: their underlying depression has gone unacknowledged or untreated.[19]

The gender gap in depression is well documented, but racial differences are less clear-cut. The data generally show that blacks and Hispanics report lower rates of depressive symptoms and major depression than whites. This mental health advantage has been described as a paradox, because ethnic minorities are exposed to more persistent stress and strain over the life course than whites.[20] Researchers offer different explanations for this paradox. Some believe that blacks' and Latinos' lower rates of depression reflect their rich coping resources like religion, strong family networks, and the personal resilience that comes from surviving a lifetime of stressors like racism. Others view the gap as a methodological artifact that conceals the reality of blacks' and Latinos' experiences. Proponents of this perspective point out that a pervasive mental illness

Figure 5.1 U.S. Adults Age Fifty-One and Older with Clinically Relevant Depressive Symptoms, by Sex and Age Group, 2014

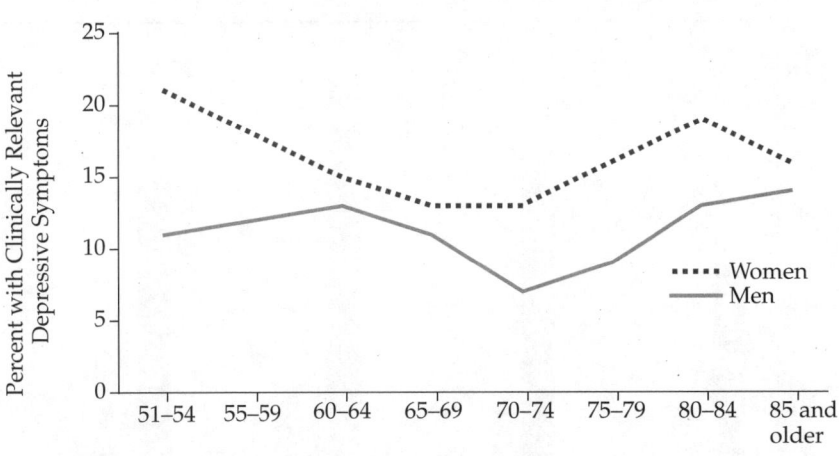

Source: Federal Interagency Forum on Aging-Related Statistics 2016.
Note: Clinically relevant depressive symptoms indicate the presence of four or more of eight depressive symptoms from an abbreviated version of the CES-D among participants in the 2014 Health and Retirement Study.

stigma among African Americans and, to a lesser extent, Latinos makes ethnic minorities less likely to report mental health symptoms on a survey checklist, to admit their symptoms to a health care provider, or to seek professional help for depression.[21] As a result of this reluctance, combined with less regular access to health care over the life course and (for some) a distrust of mental health providers, their depressive symptoms may go undetected and untreated.[22]

Compelling evidence shows that older blacks are less likely than whites to receive timely and effective treatment for their depression. When black older adults do seek treatment for their depression, they tend to go to primary care offices or emergency departments, where providers may be less adept at diagnosing their depression because older blacks (like men) tend to exhibit somatic symptoms that are viewed as just a part of normal aging rather than a mental health problem requiring treatment.[23] As a result, black older adults with depression are only one-half to one-third as likely as their white counterparts to take antidepressants and are less likely to receive what practitioners call "adequate treatment" for depression.[24] Adequate care means that the patient had a sufficient number of visits with a specialty or general health provider in the past year or received adequate antidepressant medication.

Figure 5.2 Quality of Treatment Received by Persons with a Depressive Disorder in the Past Twelve Months, by Race-Ethnicity, 2001–2003

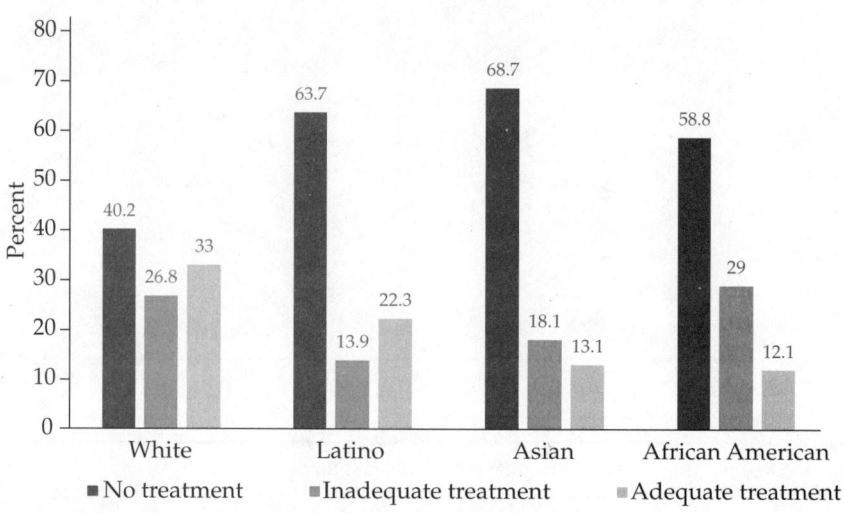

Source: Alegría et al. 2008. Reprinted with permission from Psychiatric Services (copyright ©2008). American Psychiatric Association. All Rights Reserved.

Across samples and methods, studies consistently find that among depressed older adults, blacks and Hispanics are significantly less likely than whites to receive adequate treatment.[25] For example, data from the nationally representative National Institute of Mental Health (NIMH) Collaborative Psychiatric Epidemiology Surveys (CPES) finds that while one-third of whites with a depressive disorder received adequate treatment within the past year, this proportion was just 22 percent among Latinos and a mere 12 percent among African Americans (see figure 5.2).

Disparities in depression also reflect economic inequalities. It seems painfully obvious to say that older adults who grew up in economically disadvantaged homes, have less education and income, hold poorer-quality jobs, and live in dilapidated homes in unsafe neighborhoods may be more susceptible to symptoms of sadness and demoralization. Statistics bear out this assumption. One of the most consistent findings in epidemiologic research is the strong inverse association between socioeconomic status and depression. Across samples and regardless of whether SES is measured in terms of income, education, assets, or a composite measure, studies consistently show that those of lower SES have roughly twice the rates of depression as their better-off counterparts.[26]

Just as race and gender disparities in depression reflect both the reality of humans' lives and the intricacies of how scientists measure and study depression, socioeconomic disparities do as well. Researchers attribute SES disparities in depression to two distinct factors: social causation and selection. Social causation means that experiences of socioeconomic adversity negatively affect mental health by exposing people to higher levels of stress, undermining their coping resources, and rendering them vulnerable to depression. Social selection, conversely, means that depressive symptoms are a cause rather than a consequence of economic adversity. People suffering from depression are less likely to graduate from high school, attend college, obtain and hold down rewarding jobs, and earn adequate earnings, in part because of symptoms that may undermine their performance and concentration.[27]

Moving Beyond Depression: Other Mental Health Concerns Most of the research described in this chapter focuses on depression, yet mental health encompasses other conditions, including anxiety, substance use, suicidal ideation, and suicide. Focusing only on depression creates a potentially misleading portrait of mental health disparities among older adults, so researchers now cast a wider net. Anxiety includes unsettling feelings, worry, and nervousness, as well as physical symptoms associated with nervousness like heart palpitations, difficulty breathing, heightened blood pressure, and sweating. Older women are more susceptible to anxiety than men are, although the gender gap narrows with age. Among people in their sixties and seventies, women are twice as likely to suffer an anxiety disorder, but by age eighty-five this gap disappears.[28] Anxiety and depressive symptoms tend to be comorbid, meaning that they often co-occur because the stressful experiences that trigger anxiety also may bring on sadness (and vice versa). When a spouse dies, a widow(er) may feel deep sadness over the loss of their beloved, yet may also worry about new challenges like living alone or taking on new responsibilities that their late spouse once managed, like finances, home repair, or cooking. Likewise, a serious illness and accompanying disability may bring on sadness about the loss of independence and anxiety about activities like climbing stairs or getting in and out of the shower.

An estimated 10 percent of older adults experienced an anxiety disorder in the previous year—a rate considerably lower than the 18 percent rate for the overall U.S. population.[29] However, this rate varies widely by gender and socioeconomic status. Anxiety rates are roughly twice as high among high school dropouts and women as they are among college graduates and men.[30] These gaps largely reflect stressful experiences that are particularly common among women and those with more limited socioeconomic resources, including worry about managing illness, fear of falling either at home or while navigating daily errands, and concern regarding neighborhood crime.[31]

Anger and frustration are less frequently studied emotions among older adults, perhaps a consequence of stereotypical beliefs that we mellow with age. Frustration is an emotional reaction to obstacles that block or derail one's pursuit of personal goals, whereas anger is a response to a perceived threat, injustice, or provocation. In fact, both are common emotions among older adults; studies using survey and daily diary methods find that as many as 40 percent of older adults report regular feelings of frustration, often in response to physical limitations and challenges in maneuvering their environment.[32]

It is easy to understand why these unhealthy emotions are more common among those who have faced the most daunting obstacles and injustices over the life course, especially African Americans and those with bleak prospects for economic advancement. However, it is not simply the feeling of anger that varies by social location, but the expression of those feelings: disadvantaged groups tend to silence or suppress their anger, a reaction that has long-term implications for physical and emotional health. Social scientists have found that the license to express anger outwardly and freely (dubbed "anger-out" or expressed anger) is a privilege afforded to those with social power, whereas groups with less social or economic power are more vulnerable to "anger-in"—suppressed feelings that are bottled up and experienced silently—for fear of retribution or retaliation.[33] A fast-food worker who is berated daily by his boss may suppress his feelings of rage because shouting or lunging at the boss could get him fired, if not worse. Suppressed anger has even more powerful and far-reaching effects on cardiovascular health and mortality risk than expressed anger, underscoring yet another pathway through which cumulative disadvantages contribute to later-life disparities in well-being.[34]

Alcohol use or excessive drinking is considered an important indicator of mental health, especially for older men. When men are under stress, they tend to externalize their symptoms by drinking alcohol or acting out toward others, whereas women tend to internalize their feelings, showing symptoms like sadness or worry.[35] The gender gap in alcohol use is much narrower among older adults than younger adults, yet this disparity is still stark. About 40 percent of older adults drink alcohol, although fewer than 10 percent are classified as unhealthy drinkers. However, men are four times as likely as women (16 percent versus 4 percent) to be classified as such. Unhealthy older drinkers are defined as having more than two drinks a day for men and more than one drink per day for women, or more than four drinks on a single day during the past month.[36] It is rare for someone to start drinking heavily

Figure 5.3 Suicide Rates over the Life Course, by Race and Sex, 2010

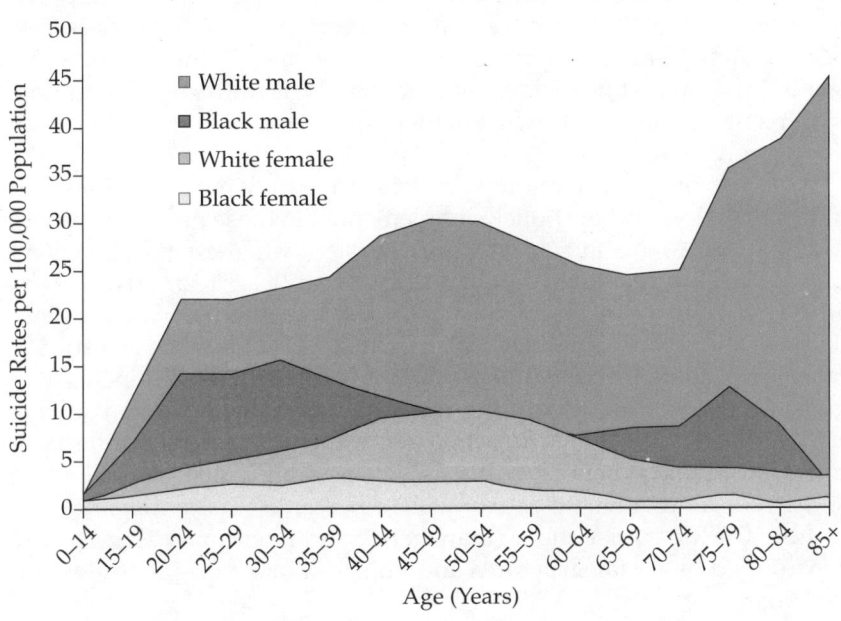

Source: Crosby, Ortega, and Stevens 2013.
Note: Suicide rate refers to number of suicides per 100,000 persons in the United States in 2010.

for the first time in later life. Only one-third of older problem drinkers started this behavior recently; most have long histories of heavy drinking. However, stress can trigger new and short-term bouts of heavy drinking, especially among older men when they experience a life-altering transition, like widowhood or retirement, or as they cope with chronic strains like social isolation.[37]

Two of the most dire indicators of late-life mental illness are suicidal ideation (thinking about killing oneself) and suicide. Suicide is often thought of as a tragedy of youth rather than old age. After all, fewer than 1 percent of all deaths of older adults are due to suicide, making it the seventeenth most common cause of death among those age sixty-five and older.[38] In sharp contrast, suicide is the second most common cause of death among young people age fifteen to thirty-four, accounting for roughly one in five deaths in this age group.[39] Yet these aggregate-level statistics conceal the fact that the one group most likely to commit suicide is older white men. As figure 5.3 shows, suicide rates are relatively low but peak in midlife for white and black women, and in young adulthood and young-old age (sixties and seventies) among black men.[40] Suicide rates are consistently highest for white men at every age and spike up after age seventy-five, a trend that experts attribute to the dark side of masculinity and autonomy, as we will see later in this chapter. The leading risk factor for suicide, not surprisingly, is untreated depression: 85 percent of older adults who kill themselves had been struggling with depression.[41]

Access to means also matters, underscoring how the places in which older adults live and the policies implemented in those places contribute to disparities. Men's suicide rates are consistently highest in states where gun ownership rates are highest and gun laws least restrictive.[42] Even after researchers control for other risk factors like income, education, divorce, and crime rates, they find that state-level male firearm suicide rates increase by roughly 3 per 100,000 for each 10 percent increase in gun ownership rates. Wyoming leads the nation in male gun suicide rates (26 per 100,000) and firearms ownership (73 percent), while Massachusetts trails far behind, with a gun suicide rate of just 4.2 per 100,000 and a firearm ownership rate of just 14 percent.[43] These disparities illustrate the life-course theme that agency and intentions can be highly constrained by social structures and policies that prioritize health and personal safety.

Later-Life Stress and Mental Health

At every stage in the life course, one of the most powerful risk factors for mental health problems is stress. Older adults' mental health is closely tied to immediate or recent stressors, as well as persistent long-term stressors that may date back years or even decades. Stressors fall into three broad categories, with each affecting older adults' mental health in slightly different ways: life events, chronic strains, and daily hassles. Life events are acute changes or occurrences such as the death of a spouse or having major surgery. Life events are generally thought of as single point-in-time transitions, whereas chronic strains are ongoing demands that require adaptation over longer periods of time. Chronic strains such as managing serious health problems, caring for an ailing spouse, worrying about the costs of prescription medications, feeling anxious walking through an unsafe neighborhood, or being the target of racism or ageism can persist over weeks, months, or even years. That is why chronic strains are considered more hurtful than acute life events: they are persistent and often reflect situations that cannot be easily changed or escaped.[44] Stress also takes a less obvious form: daily hassles. Daily hassles are minor and seemingly insignificant occurrences that get on our nerves throughout the day, such as difficulty maneuvering a new walker through a small kitchen, overhearing a neighbor's daily arguments, or being put on hold when phoning a health insurer with an urgent question.

Although life events, chronic strains, and daily hassles often are described as separate and discrete experiences, they are closely intertwined and often co-occur. Leonard Pearlin and his colleagues described this process as stress proliferation, where "people exposed to a serious adversity [are] at risk for later exposure to additional adversities."[45] A life event like midlife job loss may trigger a chain of new chronic strains, such as financial worries, loss of health insurance, and exposure to age discrimination while trying to find a new job after age sixty. Conversely, chronic strains may precede and even give rise to a stressful life event. Caring for a spouse who is dying from cancer is inherently stressful and will likely precede the eventual death of the spouse, which then creates a new cycle of stressors like settling the estate and managing life alone.

The extent to which a particular stressor harms a person's mental health depends, in part, on its magnitude (how serious?), desirability (was the change desired or not?), expectedness (was it anticipated or was it a surprise?), and timing (at what age did it occur?). In general, life transitions that are unexpected or premature are particularly distressing. For those who lose their job suddenly and without warning, the loss can be a jarring blow, and they may be ill prepared to find another position. Stressors that happen "off-time"—earlier or later than is typical—also are particularly difficult. Men who retire younger than the typical age of sixty-five experience more depression than those who retire "on time," even when physical health symptoms are controlled.[46]

A life transition that we experience at an age earlier than our peers do is often unexpected (or unwanted), so we are not adequately prepared to manage our new role or status. Consistent with the "timing matters" theme of the life-course paradigm, early-onset stressors—whether premature retirement, health problems, loss of a family member, or even a physical appearance considerably older than our biological age—puts us out of step with our peers, depriving us of the social networks and support we may need. An eighty-five-year-old woman may find support from her many widowed peers when her husband dies, whereas a fifty-year-old woman who is the first among her friends to lose a spouse may feel adrift and alone as her peers struggle with what to say and do for her. People who experience early-onset health problems and other life transitions may be subjected to unkind or demeaning treatment from others. Workers in their early fifties who retire due to debilitating arthritis, or a relatively healthy-looking person who uses a handicapped parking space because of an invisible health condition like lupus may be maligned by others as lazy, dishonest, or "faking" their symptoms.[47]

The number, severity, and timing of stressors vary by social class and race. Women and men tend to experience different types of stressors, with older men typically having more work-related stressors and women more family-related stressors over the life course, yet there is little evidence that one gender is exposed to either a greater number of stressors or more intense stressors. However, the evidence is incontrovertible that racial minorities face more stressors than whites, and that those with fewer economic resources face more daunting stressors than their better-off counterparts.

Blacks are more likely than whites to experience racial discrimination, lower income and earnings, material deprivation, and early onset of health problems; to have a greater number of network events such as a child's or grandchild's incarceration; to live in an unsafe neighborhood; and to be confronted with other stressors related to being a minority in the United States.[48] Latinos, on average, experience many stressors similar to those encountered by blacks, and Latinos who migrated to the United States experience additional stressors related to immigration and linguistic isolation and challenges with understanding or speaking fluent English.[49] The number and magnitude of stressors is also much greater for those who have experienced lives of economic disadvantage, relative to their peers who grew up more comfortably. Stressful life events like job loss or the premature death of family members, chronic strains like living in an unsafe neighborhood or working in a physically dangerous job, network events like a sibling's bout of unemployment, and daily hassles like family squabbles or noisy neighbors are more numerous and long-lasting among those whose lives are marked by financial precarity, especially because they lack the economic wherewithal to remove themselves from these situations.[50]

Inevitable Stressors of Later Life

Stress is an inescapable part of life. Teenagers fret about their high school grades, fitting in with peers, and getting into college. College students stress out over graduate school applications and finding jobs after earning their degrees. Employees worry about meeting work deadlines or, worse yet, losing their jobs during economic downturns. The stressors of parenthood keep nervous mothers and fathers awake at night. Older adults struggle with the deaths of friends and family, physical health problems, financial worries, and ageism or mistreatment on the basis of their age. Here I focus on two specific stressors that are ubiquitous experiences in later life—ageism and chronic health problems—and show

how a person's vulnerability to and capacity to withstand these stressors is all the more difficult for those with the sparsest social and economic resources.

Ageism "Old fart." "Geezer." "Gramps." "Little old lady." Each of these phrases commonly used to describe older adults can be hurtful and a trigger for sadness, an undermined sense of competence, and even a weakened desire to live. "Humorous" birthday cards remind us that with each passing year we grow more wrinkled, saggy, and forgetful. Widely ridiculed characters like the frail older woman who cries "Help! I've fallen and I can't get up!" in a medical alert system advertisement perpetuate negative stereotypes of older adults as irritable, dependent, and addle-minded. Just as toxic as inappropriate jokes and greeting cards are the daily interpersonal slights that older adults experience. Family members, neighbors, store clerks, and even health care providers often slip into "elderspeak" or the infantilizing language and tone that people may use when speaking to older adults. Speaking unnecessarily loudly or slowly and using overly simplistic language, a singsong voice, and seemingly benign greetings like "How are you today, young lady?" are viewed as condescending and disingenuous by older adults and gerontologists alike.[51]

Although offensive cartoon images and the occasional "sweetie" dropped into conversation may seem innocuous, these subtle yet pervasive slights are part of the larger social problem of ageism, a term coined by the visionary geriatrician Robert Butler. Ageism refers to "systematic stereotyping of and discrimination against people because they are old, just as racism and sexism accomplish this with skin color and gender."[52] What makes ageism different from racism or sexism is that all of us who survive long enough will eventually be old and thus susceptible to the slings of ageism. Butler argued that ageism is rampant because it is rooted in a deeply embedded fear and dread in modern societies: "a personal revulsion to and distaste for growing old, disease, disability, and fear of powerlessness, uselessness, and death."[53] Other scholars have described ageism as the widespread "prejudice against our feared future self."[54]

Statistics bear out the insidiousness of ageism. National surveys of older adults show that more than 80 percent say they have been the target of ageism—ranging from being subject to insensitive jokes or treated as if incompetent to being passed over for a workplace promotion, losing out to a younger and less experienced colleague.[55] And onethird have received greeting cards that poke fun at their age, with images like the fictional "Seven Dwarves of Old Age" ("Nappy, Wrinkly, Squinty, Rocky, Saggy, Farty, and Leaky"). Qualitative studies, blogs, and casual conversations with older adults are replete with personal anecdotes of ageist treatment. The septuagenarian scholar and aging activist Martha Holstein shares the following encounter in her latest book, *Women in Late Life:* "The ticket agent at the Amtrak counter slowly and deliberately told me not to lose the ticket that she just handed me because, if I do, I'll have to buy another one. Humiliation is among the most painful of social wrongs."[56]

It is not just callous young people who believe that older people are out of touch and incompetent: even older adults themselves hold these views. Psychological studies consistently show that people do not "age out" of holding stereotypical views of older adults. One way in which researchers evaluate prejudicial attitudes is through the use of Implicit Attitude Tests (IATs), which are less susceptible to social desirability effects than more direct measures of personal attitudes. Even the most callous person knows not to tell a researcher that he or she thinks of older people as "fogies." The IAT projects a screen image such as a photo of an older adult or a teenager or words such as "Old" and Young." Participants then must very quickly click their computer mouse on either the positive word or negative word presented side by side on the screen. For instance, they might see a portrait of an older woman and then have the option to quickly click on a positive word like "strong" or a negative word such as "weak." After proceeding through this task for several images associated with old age versus youth, the study participant receives a score indicating whether he or she holds implicitly positive or negative views toward older adults. The IAT can capture our subconscious stereotypical beliefs about age, gender, race, sexual orientation, and so on. Multiple studies conclude that when both older and younger adults are administered the IAT, their responses are remarkably similar: both groups more often associate images of old age with negative words and images of youth with positive words.[57]

Older adults who hold negative beliefs about old age are particularly susceptible to mental health symptoms, such as hopelessness and depression, and feelings of neediness, worthlessness, and dependence. The psychologist Becca Levy has discovered that simply exposing older adults to words and messages associated with negative stereotypes of aging, such as the words "forgetful" or "feeble," raises older adults' stress levels while also impairing their memory skills, as measured through a standard memory test. Conversely, those who are exposed to positive images of aging show increases in happiness, self-esteem, and even the will to live.

Likewise, ageism and ageist encounters perpetuated by others—whether condescending words from the pharmacist or having a driver's license taken away unnecessarily by an overly controlling adult child—may undermine an older adult's mental health.[58] Exposure to ageism, as with racism, sexism, or any other "ism," is a chronic strain that undermines a person's sense of worth and compromises mental health.[59] Studies of nursing home patients show that older adults have depleted self-esteem and behave in a more dependent manner when the nursing staff treat them as if they were children.[60] And older adults are less likely than younger people to be referred for the psychiatric or neurological treatments they need because doctors view their symptoms of sadness as part of normal aging rather than as a medical condition that requires treatment.[61]

Besides its direct toll on older adults' emotional health, ageism can also undermine mental health indirectly by derailing or stalling an older adult's prospects for employment, triggering financial insecurities and anxiety. For instance, in 2015, job-seekers over age fifty-five took thirty-six weeks on average to find a new job, compared to just twenty-six weeks for younger workers, a gap that analysts attribute in part to ageism. These obstacles are worse for women than men, casting light on the complex ways in which the indignities of ageism and sexism are intertwined. One experimental study of more than forty thousand mock job applicants found that while men and women in their sixties were less likely than younger job applicants to be hired for jobs ranging from janitor to office administrator, the age gap in hiring was much larger among women than men.[62] Experts attribute this gendered pattern to the high premium placed on youthful beauty among women (especially in jobs, like sales, which require high levels of customer contact); this premium makes age a greater liability for older women than men when searching for a job.[63] Given older women's greater financial precariousness in the first place, especially among those who may need to reenter the labor market after widowhood or divorce, this added threat to financial stability is a particularly cruel source of anxiety and emotional strain.

Some intriguing research further suggests that ageism may be especially inescapable for those of lower socioeconomic status because they tend to "look old" for their age.[64] Wrinkled skin, age spots, thin lips, gray hair, and tooth loss render people prime targets for ageism, although these physical signs of maturity tend to appear earlier for those who have experienced cumulative disadvantages such as economic strain, poor health behaviors like smoking, and physical exhaustion.[65] Cosmetic treatments that can turn back the clock, like regular hair highlights, facials, Botox, and cosmetic peels, are luxuries that may be out of financial reach (or deemed superficial priorities) for older adults struggling with more pressing financial concerns.[66]

Physical Health Problems Senescence, or biological aging, is inevitable. Our clear vision, sharp hearing, taut muscle tone, cognitive acuity, and cardiopulmonary strength will wane as we reach old age, although these transitions typically happen at younger ages for those who faced more social and economic disadvantage earlier in life, as we saw in chapter 4. According to a Johns Hopkins University analysis of Medical Expenditure Panel Survey (MEPS) data, fully 88 percent of people age sixty-five to seventy-four and 93 percent of those age seventy-five and older have at least one chronic illness. Serious health conditions are one of the most powerful influences on later-life mental health. While just 1 to 5 percent of older adults overall have major depression, rates are as high as 10 to 12 percent among those with major physical health problems.[67] "Comorbidity between medical and mental conditions is the rule rather than the exception," according to the Robert Wood Johnson Foundation, the largest foundation in the United States dedicated to promoting health research.[68]

Studies based on surveys, clinical data, and medical claims data uniformly show that physical and mental health are tightly intertwined. Older adults with cancer, dementias, diabetes, heart disease, lung disease, musculoskeletal conditions, and vision impairments are more likely than those without these conditions to suffer from mental health symptoms, most notably depression and anxiety. Complex biological and social processes underlie these associations, yet researchers are reluctant to conclude that physical conditions necessarily "cause" mental health problems, because two-way linkages are equally plausible for many health conditions. People with long-standing mental health conditions often have experienced challenges and adversities that also have eroded their physical health, such as disrupted education, a sporadic work history, fractured interpersonal relationships, and higher rates of smoking, drinking, and obesity. All of these experiences, in turn, elevate one's risk of subsequent physical health problems, as well as continued symptoms of mental health troubles, in later life.[69]

Biological pathways also may account for associations between physical and mental health problems. Cardiovascular disease damages the brain's prefrontal white matter. When this damage occurs, older adults have fewer cognitive control mechanisms to regulate their emotions, making them more vulnerable to depression and sadness.[70] Medications for physical health conditions, such as antihypertension drugs, beta blockers, corticosteroids, hormones, anti-Parkinson's agents, respiratory or gastrointestinal medications, and some cancer medications, also have side effects that may increase an older adult's risk of depressive symptoms. Insomnia, a common ailment among older adults, also is strongly linked with depression.[71]

The links between the physical and mental health of older adults reflect two additional pathways: symptom management (daily efforts to manage illness and medications) and functional impairment (the extent to which health problems limit the capacity to lead a full and independent life). Moreover, how these processes unfold reflects persistent race, class, and gender inequities.

Symptom management provides a vivid example of how fairly "normal" and expected everyday hassles may be particularly distressing for disadvantaged older adults. Managing health problems can entail a time- and energy-depleting set of activities that detract from more personally satisfying pursuits, and the amount of time and energy these activities sap reflects access to resources like convenient and predictable transportation, a regular health care provider, and short wait times at the pharmacy or doctor's office. Data from the American Time Use Study (ATUS), a daily diary study of how Americans spend their time, show that persons in ill health spend an average of two hours per day on self-care, including activities like taking medications, self-administering insulin shots, and testing blood sugar levels.[72] They also spend an average of two and a half hours seeking medical care outside the home on those days when they need to see a health care provider. That time encompasses traveling to and from the visit (thirty-five minutes), waiting in the doctor's office or ER (forty-seven minutes), and time spent in the clinic receiving care (seventy-two minutes).

Yet the ATUS data also reveal stark race and socioeconomic differences, reflecting the added obstacles that ethnic minorities and lower-income patients face when navigating complex health care systems. Blacks and Latinos spend roughly 50 percent more time than whites seeking care, with much of this time spent traveling to health care facilities far from their homes (and often using unreliable public transportation) and waiting for long periods in overcrowded health care settings.[73] Patients living in lower-income neighborhoods spend about 10 percent more time on their visits compared to those from higher-income neighborhoods.[74] Although a ten-minute difference in travel time or twenty-minute difference in waiting time may seem inconsequential, these differences add up—especially for older adults with multiple health problems. The stress and time involved in seeking care can undermine older adults' emotional health by creating daily stress and hassles, threatening their sense of control, reducing the time they can spend in leisure or family activities, and providing a constant reminder of their physical declines.[75]

Functional limitations and disability are a second pathway through which chronic illnesses undermine older adults' mental health. Disability refers to the difficulties of carrying out everyday tasks and activities due to a "lack of fit between individuals and their environments."[76] Disability not only limits older adults' ability to socialize, engage in activities that they used to enjoy, and navigate their physical environment with ease but also threatens their sense of autonomy, competence, and independence.[77] Disability may trigger secondary stressors, such as living in fear of falling, moving to an assisted living facility, scraping together money to pay for a home health aide, or trying to set up a schedule of informal care among family members and friends who may be reluctant to do so or who may disagree about their duties.[78] These stressors are all the more common among those who lack the money to pay for assistance or who have no nearby family members to offer a hand. Disability-related stress, compounded by the stress of underlying illness, can take a powerful toll on older adults' emotional health.

The Importance of Coping Resources

The extent to which stressors like ageism and health declines undermine mental health depends on individuals' coping resources. Adequate resources enable a person to withstand daily challenges, whereas inadequate psychosocial, economic, and practical resources increase vulnerability to emotional distress. Four types of resources protect against the harmful psychological effects of aging-related stress and may help to minimize late-life mental health disparities: psychological and cognitive resources, social support, socioeconomic resources, and genetic factors.

Psychological Resources: Coping Style and Cognitive Ability

"Coping" refers to our efforts to change or adapt to a stressful situation. Coping strategies generally fall into two categories: problem-focused and emotion-focused. Although people may use different strategies to cope with different problems, most also have a general repertoire of tactics they rely on. Problem-focused coping (PFC) involves trying to eliminate or change the situation causing us distress. People tend to use PFC when they see the situation as something they can change or improve. An older adult struggling with hearing loss can use a hearing aid, and someone with balance problems can use a cane. One study of older adults with vision loss found that using optical devices like magnifiers or closed-circuit TV helped to reduce depressive symptoms.[79] Of course, the capacity to obtain and effectively use devices in this way is contingent on tangible resources.

Emotion-focused coping (EFC), by contrast, focuses on allaying the psychological symptoms that may result from the stressor. People tend to use EFC strategies when they believe that nothing can be done to alter an unfortunate situation. EFC encompasses a broad range of strategies. Productive ones include confiding in a friend, finding humor in the situation, turning to prayer, or seeking professional help or medications to treat a negative mood. Unproductive strategies include ignoring or denying the problem or releasing negative feelings by drinking or lashing out at others.

PFC strategies are generally considered more effective than EFC strategies. People who use PFC go on to experience lower levels of psychological distress, whereas those who rely on EFC tend to report more sadness, worry, and hopelessness. However, in rare instances EFC may be more productive than PFC. PFC is ineffective when we have suffered an irreversible and irreplaceable loss, such as the death of a spouse or a diminished capacity to walk and breathe easily. We cannot bring a deceased loved one back to life, but we can soothe our grief by turning to friends for social support or distracting ourselves with happy memories of our late spouse. Older adults tend to use more EFC and less PFC than younger people, but this difference is almost wholly accounted for by the kinds of stressors that older adults face; many involve irreversible changes.[80] More highly educated persons and those with greater economic resources are more likely to use PFC because they possess both the means and the self-efficacious beliefs that help to effect change.[81] Coping style, then, becomes an engine of cumulative (dis)advantage: those with the richest economic and interpersonal resources are best equipped to alter or exit a stressful situation, whereas those with fewer resources are both more vulnerable to stressful contexts and less equipped to change them.

Cognitive functioning also is an essential resource for managing stress in later life. Older adults with superior memory, reasoning ability, problem-solving skills, and comprehension of complex concepts are less susceptible to stressful encounters, more effective at managing stress, and less vulnerable to depression and anxiety. High levels of cognitive functioning enable us to carry out meaningful activities, live independently, sustain supportive relationships, and participate fully in social life; these positive experiences, in turn, are linked with greater happiness and reduced loneliness.

Yet cognitive functioning in later life is powerfully shaped by cumulative advantages and disadvantages. Older adults with limited education tend to have lower levels of cognitive ability and earlier onset of cognitive decline, which make it difficult to creatively problem-solve in the face of stress. People with less intellectually complex jobs and less education have lower levels of perceived efficacy, which is an essential resource for engaging in problem-focused coping. Cognitive ability also is enhanced indirectly by positive health behaviors; people who exercise regularly and nonsmokers have better cardiovascular health, which in turn improves cognitive health.[82] It is not just the absolute level of one's cognitive capacities that are affected by social resources but also the pace of decline. Drops in cognitive functioning start earlier and are steeper for older adults who experienced deprivation and economic disadvantage earlier in life.[83] These disparities then contribute to socioeconomic inequities in later-life mental health.

That is not to say that those whose lives are marked by socioeconomic disadvantage cannot cope. They do, and many do so extraordinarily well, relying on creative problem-solving skills honed through years of overcoming challenge and structural obstacles. One recent study tracked more than 2,500 Americans over three years and found a curvilinear (upside-down U-shaped) association between the number of stressors experienced and both depression and anxiety symptoms. People who experienced very high levels of stress and those experiencing *no stress* fared the worst emotionally. Those who had suffered a modest pile-up of stressors developed coping skills that helped them to deal with new challenges that came their way. Those at the very low end of the stress-exposure curve had not developed such skills, while those at the very high end of the scale were simply overwhelmed by the onslaught of stressors.[84]

Other perspectives similarly propose that, with each passing year, older adults (regardless of socioeconomic background) acquire skills and capacities that allow them to roll with the punches in ways they would not have done years earlier. The attainment of wisdom and generativity (a concern for and desire to mentor younger generations) may help older adults respond to major challenges and daily nuisances with acceptance, perspective, and equanimity.[85] Older adults also develop an ability to find happiness in the "little things," such as a visit with a cherished friend; a tendency to align expectations with reality, thus minimizing the chances of disappointment and dashed hopes; and self-acceptance.[86]

Social Support

If mental health researchers were asked to name the single most important factor that distinguishes those who break from those who bounce back in the face of adversity, most would immediately say social support. Hundreds of studies affirm the importance of social ties as a resource that helps older adults to survive stressful times. A core component is emotional support, such as having a confidant who listens to their problems and feeling assured that family and friends will support them in times of need. Warm and supportive relationships with adult children, a spouse, siblings, and friends are a key to emotional well-being.

For older adults, however, the protective effects of social support are not a case of "the more the merrier." Having just one person with whom they can genuinely confide is considered the key to fighting loneliness and depression: each additional confidant adds only an incremental mental health benefit.[87]

Also crucial are instrumental and informational support—the practical assistance that older adults actually receive as well as the support they can anticipate during difficult times. Instrumental support encompasses tangible help such as rides to doctor's appointments or assistance with household chores while recovering from hip replacement surgery. Informational support, by contrast, involves the sharing of helpful information, such as getting a recommendation for a good cardiologist after suffering a first heart attack, receiving information on the pros and cons of long-term care insurance, or learning how to access free ride services available to local seniors. Such practical support helps to reduce anxiety symptoms as older adults manage their daily activities amid their own physical and cognitive health changes.[88] However, the capacity to access support from social networks is more limited for those who have sparser economic resources. As chapter 6 will show, older adults who have less education and who held lower-status jobs during their working lives tend to have smaller social networks, and thus the base of potential companions to whom they may turn for emotional or practical support is smaller.[89] And those network members often have challenges of their own that prevent them from providing support to elderly friends and family members.

Another source of social support, especially for older blacks, is religion, which encompasses direct support and encouragement from one's congregation as well as beliefs that provide solace and comfort. Blacks are more likely than whites to attend religious services regularly, to say that religion is very important in their lives, to pray regularly, to seek support from both fellow congregants and clergy, and to find solace in religious music and texts; each of these forms of coping may buffer the harmful effects of stress.[90] Older African Americans often report that they feel protected by a higher power and that God has a "divine plan" to watch over them. These beliefs may be especially protective for those facing stressors over which they have little control, like financial insecurity, disability, and poor neighborhood conditions or stressful life events like widowhood and other losses.[91]

Socioeconomic Resources

There is a kernel of truth to the old saying "money can't buy happiness." Most studies show that income, in and of itself, is a relatively weak predictor of happiness.[92] However, money can buy some reprieve in the face of stress. It is easier to adapt or bounce back when we have more financial and human capital resources at our disposal. Human capital resources such as education and connections to people in power, concrete financial resources like income and housing wealth, and subjective factors like feelings of financial security can help to mute the effects of stress on older adults' mental health. At the same time, the mental health–depleting consequences of stress may be intensified for those struggling with poverty and financial worries.

The Nobel Prize–winning economists Daniel Kahneman and Angus Deaton examined whether the psychological toll of stressors common in later life, including diabetes, marital dissolution, caregiving, and living alone, was more acute for those living in poverty (less than $1,000 in monthly income) compared to those living with adequate means (more than $3,000 in monthly income).[93] They found clear evidence that poverty exacerbates the emotional consequences of both chronic and acute stressors. Among those who suffered from serious headaches, 70 percent in the lowest income category yet just 38 percent in the higher income category reported high levels of worry and sadness. Of those who lived alone, nearly 60 percent of those living in poverty reported high levels of sadness and worry, yet the proportion was just half that (31.5 percent) among solo dwellers with adequate income.

Similarly, another team of researchers tracked how older adults' mental health changed with the onset of new disabilities, and whether these patterns varied based on their financial resources.[94] Using data from the HRS, the researchers found that older adults who had wealth above the median level showed smaller decrements in mental health when they experienced a new disability. By contrast, their counterparts with low levels of wealth had steeper declines in emotional well-being, consistent with cumulative disadvantage perspectives. In other words, disability is more distressing for those with fewer financial means to adapt, and money enhances mental health only when an older adult can put those resources to use in the face of stress. To tweak the old adage, money can buy happiness and conquer sadness, but only if it can be used to make a distressing situation less so for older adults.

Genetic Factors

When centenarians like Goldie Michelson talk about their long life spans (and supermodels boast about their slender physiques), they often thank their "good genes." Two genes have garnered the most attention as risk factors for mental health problems. The serotonin transporter gene (also known as SERT or 5-HTTLPR) has a "short" variant that is implicated in depression and anxiety disorders. Similarly, DRD4-7R, the "impulse control" gene, is a variant of a dopamine-processing gene called DRD4 and is linked to externalizing aspects of mental health, including drinking and aggression. Genes explain much more variation in early-onset versus later-onset mental health symptoms, underscoring the power of social contexts in shaping the mental health of older adults.[95]

Researchers have firmly established that genes matter for overall risk of mental health problems and are now investigating the extent to which these associations vary across social contexts. For instance, scientists are now asking whether a genetic predisposition amplifies the effect of adversity on depression risk, consistent with cumulative risk perspectives.[96] Intense spousal caregiving duties may drive anyone to have a glass of wine to unwind, but the risk of heavy drinking may be greater for those with the DRD4-7R gene. Likewise, an unsteady recovery from hip replacement surgery may demoralize anyone, but the risk of major depression may be even higher for those with the short SERT allele.

Scientists also are exploring resilience, evaluating whether social and economic advantages can overpower a genetic predisposition to depression and other mental health conditions. Research on gene-environment interactions and older adults' mental health is still in its nascent stages, although emerging evidence suggests that having social and economic resources sufficient to manage stress over the life course may be powerful enough to diminish the impact of genetic risk factors on late-life depression. A study based on twin data from a sample of World War II veterans in their seventies and eighties showed that even if an older adult had a genetic predisposition toward depression, that risk was diminished considerably for those who possessed the social and economic resources to manage adversity or seek effective mental health treatment.[97] These results suggest that, while social stressors and disadvantage can intensify the linkage between genetic risk and mental health symptoms, protective social contexts can minimize this link.

Minimizing Mental Health Disparities: Promising Policies and Practices

Psychological distress may be inevitable for older adults when adversities pile up, yet depression and suicidal ideation are not. Access to timely mental health care, including visits with a practitioner or receiving antidepressants or other medications, can be broadened through public policies that treat mental health care as essential to older adults' well-being. One of the most important advances in helping Americans of all ages seek help for mental health conditions is the Mental Health Parity Act, which was signed into law in 1996 and then replaced by the

Paul Wellstone and Pete Domenici Mental Health Parity and Addiction Equity Act (MHPAEA) in January 2010. These laws broadly state that health insurers must cover treatments for mental health conditions, just as they would physical illness. These changes extend to older adults in particular, with the Medicare Improvements for Patients and Providers Act (MIPPA), which required Medicare to increase its coverage of outpatient mental health services as well as coverage of medications, including antidepressants. Since the implementation of MIPPA in 2010, Medicare started paying 80 percent of the costs of older adults' psychological therapy, a substantial boost above the 50 percent coverage just two years earlier.[98]

The Affordable Care Act (ACA), established by President Barack Obama in 2010, ushered in additional programs to extend the detection and treatment of mental health problems among older adults. Expanded Medicare coverage for annual wellness visits includes screening for depression and other mood disorders, problematic substance use, and cognitive impairment. During the Medicare-reimbursed wellness visit, the practitioner also reviews the patient's risk factors for depression and will make referrals for counseling as needed.[99] The future of the ACA is under threat, yet continuation of screening and assessment, at a minimum, is essential to protecting the mental health of older adults in the United States.

While the MHPAEA and ACA are important steps toward improving the mental health of the nation's most vulnerable elders, they are not a guarantee that disparities in untreated depression or other mood disorders will disappear. Screening and more generous reimbursement schemes are important first steps, yet these benefits are effective only if older adults have access to trained professionals willing to see them. One recent study in the *Journal of the American Medical Association* found that just 55 percent of psychiatrists (versus 89 percent of other physicians) said that they were willing to take on new Medicare patients; their reluctance was due to the low reimbursement rates combined with the often lengthy and repeated visits required for effective treatment.[100]

Expanding the pool of potential mental health workers and reaching out to older adults, rather than waiting for older adults to seek medical or psychiatric treatment, may be especially effective in treating older African Americans and men, many of whom are reluctant to pursue treatment on their own. Community agencies like senior centers, residential facilities, and religious organizations could play a pivotal role in outreach and education—dispelling myths, destigmatizing depression and substance use, and educating family members on how to detect mental health symptoms among their aged relatives. Enlisting professional mental health workers to reach out to older adults in their homes may also be fruitful, although this would require creative changes and expansions to current Medicaid and Medicare policies. Visiting nurse and home care agencies could play a crucial role in diagnosing and providing services to homebound older adults, although under current reimbursement schemes, home care agencies are restricted by private and public insurance regarding the number of visits they can provide. Mental health conditions require regular and ongoing treatment, so increasing private and public reimbursement of home-based mental health services may help to better address the unmet care needs of the most vulnerable older adults. Practices that help to detect and treat older adults' mental health symptoms are essential to their daily quality of life, social relationships, and ultimately their survival.

As with physical health, however, disparities in older adults' mental health will not be fully eradicated merely by enhancing access to care. The sources of older adults' stress also must be targeted. Economic precarity over the life course is at the root of persistent strains ranging from chronic health problems to vulnerability to ageism, as well as to the use of maladaptive coping strategies like smoking, drinking, or stress eating. Policies that improve the economic well-being of poor and near-poor adults during their working years, like EITC, or in later life, like SSI benefits, may help to reduce stress and enhance their access to effective coping resources. But mental health is more than the absence of distress—it also encompasses "a state of well-being in which an individual realizes his or her own abilities . . . and is able to make a contribution to his or her community."[101] Programs that provide opportunities for older adults to share their skills and wisdom, pursue new challenges, and contribute to their families and communities (to the extent that their health and resources allow) are essential paths to enhancing older adults' sense of mattering, purpose, and happiness.

Chapter 6

The Loved and the Lonely: Social Relationships and Isolation in Later Life

If everything we knew about older adults' social relationships were gleaned from prime-time television, we might believe that widows and divorcées are surrounded by quick-witted friends and a steady stream of dashing suitors, as portrayed on the 1980s sitcom *The Golden Girls*. Or that older married couples live a stone's throw away from their adult children, enjoying regular family dinners while doling out sage advice to their adoring grandchildren, like the Johnson family in the sitcom *Black-ish*. A bleaker portrait looms on the long-running satirical cartoon *The Simpsons:* Abraham "Grampa" Simpson is callously dumped into the nursing home Springfield Retirement Castle, where he and his fellow residents are forgotten by their kin—even on family-centric holidays like Thanksgiving.

Cultural portrayals of older adults' social relationships sensationalize the extremes—the loved and cherished at one end, and the lonely and isolated at the other. But the reality is more nuanced and marked by intriguing paradoxes. Being alone does not necessarily mean that one is lonely. Family caregiving demands can be both a blessing and a burden. Some frail older adults are caring for (rather than being cared for by) their children and grandchildren, despite romanticized notions of the multigenerational home as a protective haven for older adults. And the people who hurt older adults the most are precisely the ones entrusted with their care. Televised images of older adults and their families also conceal another important reality: getting married (and staying married) has become a privilege enjoyed largely by white and middle-class adults in the late twentieth and early twenty-first centuries, so rising numbers of blacks and lower-income adults are growing old without the social and economic support of a spouse.[1]

Marriage and romantic partnerships, parenthood, grandparenthood, and friendships are among the most intimate aspects of older adults' lives, yet the extent to which they are sources of joy, distress, or something in between is a product of complex social factors. Gender, race, and socioeconomic status shape fundamental aspects of family structure, including whether, when, whom, and how often one marries; how one's marriage ends; whether, when, and how often one becomes a parent, stepparent, or grandparent; and how often and at what ages one experiences the deaths of family members. Family structure, in turn, can bring (or deny) older adults important benefits, like an added source of income and pension benefits, economies of scale (the money saved by splitting food, housing, and utility costs), an additional set of hands to do household chores, and a caregiver when one's health starts to fade.

One key aspect of family structure, marital status, is especially important for older adults' economic security, because it is tightly tied to the Social Security benefits they receive. Social Security provides a bigger financial boost to married persons and widow(er)s relative to divorced and never-married people (especially women) and penalizes those who had short-term marriages or who were married to partners with sporadic work histories, experiences that are especially common among black women.[2] Race, class, and gender also shape subjective and emotional aspects of personal relationships, such as marital happiness, whether older adults feel supported or drained by their children and grandchildren, and whether their social ties are plentiful or scarce, emotionally uplifting or depleting. As such, social relationships are a mechanism contributing to race and socioeconomic disparities in late-life well-being.

In this chapter, I describe how older adults experience key social relationships (or the lack thereof), including marriage, intergenerational relations, and social networks encompassing friends and acquaintances. I underscore race, gender, and socioeconomic disparities in social ties and discuss the implications of these patterns for older adults' emotional, physical, and financial well-being. I then discuss the dark side of social relationships, shedding light on three common problems experienced by older adults: social isolation and loneliness, elder mistreatment, and intensive caregiving. Nearly all older adults are susceptible to these stressful experiences, yet their risk and impact are heightened for those who are already the most socially and economically vulnerable.

Social Relationships and Late-Life Well-being

Social relationships are essential to health, happiness, and longevity. Both common sense and the classic Eagles song tell us that "love will keep us alive." Volumes of research dating back to the *Suicide* study of the pioneering sociologist Émile Durkheim provide incontrovertible evidence that social ties—whether with a romantic partner, children, friends, members of one's religious community, or even virtual social ties—sustain us.[3] Conducting the first population-based study of social ties and health, Durkheim examined death certificates obtained from parishes in Europe and found that spouses and parents were less likely to commit suicide compared to unmarried and childless adults. The key protective factor, he concluded, was the sense of belonging and meaning that comes from being integrated into a community. People who lack strong social ties, by contrast, were seen as socially and morally adrift, without the protective supports provided by family and community. This "excessive individuation," according to Durkheim, brought about feelings of melancholy and meaninglessness—both of which are precursors to suicide.

Contemporary research confirms that social relationships are critical to survival, especially for older adults. As paid work obligations diminish and the need for assistance with daily activities increases, social relationships become an increasingly important aspect of everyday life. But it is not merely the presence of social ties that enhances older adults' well-being: the quality and nature of these relationships and the broad constellation of overlapping relationships in which they are embedded also shape everything from daily mood to life expectancy. Social relationships are critical to older adults' well-being in their own right, yet they are also a key pathway contributing to (or mitigating against) race, gender, and socioeconomic disparities. Three key relationships—marriage, relationships with children and grandchildren, and social ties beyond the family—are especially central to older adults' well-being.

Marriage and Marital Dissolution

A satisfying and nurturing marriage is essential to good health, happiness, and longevity. Older adults who are married or who have a long-term romantic partner enjoy better physical and mental health and longer lives than their peers who have never married, are widowed, or are divorced. This pattern holds for men and women, straight and LGBTQ persons, black and white, those in first marriages and remarriages, legally married and cohabiting partners, and rich and poor.[4] Hundreds of social science, epidemiologic, and biomedical studies show that, relative to their unpartnered peers, older adults in stable and supportive romantic partnerships have lower rates of nearly all chronic illnesses, disability, mental health problems, and substance use, as well as more rapid recovery from injury, quicker wound healing, stronger immune systems, and lower mortality from all causes.[5]

Yet these advantages, referred to as the "marriage benefit," are not available equally to all older adults. Blacks and those with fewer economic resources are less likely than whites and more economically advantaged adults to get married and stay married. These gaps have widened steadily since the 1960s, reflecting structural factors like declining employment prospects and rising incarceration rates for black men, as well as cultural beliefs regarding the importance of stable employment and homeownership as prerequisites for marrying.[6] The eminent sociologist Andrew Cherlin has argued that marriage has become a "marker of prestige," such that "the purchase of a home, and the acquisition of other accoutrements of married life" allow us to show off the "attainment of a prestigious, comfortable, and stable style of life" befitting responsible married adults.[7]

It is not simply getting married that is a marker of privilege, but staying married. Blacks and lower-SES older adults are especially likely to become widowed, reflecting well-documented race and socioeconomic disparities in mortality risk. Divorce rates also diverge on the basis of race and class. The main reasons divorced couples give for ending their marriages are stressors that are especially common among economically disadvantaged families, including financial strain, substance use, and relationship conflict.[8] The chances of remarrying also differ by race and SES: in 2013, 60 percent of whites but just 48 percent of blacks had remarried following widowhood or divorce, while 60 percent of college graduates but just half of high school dropouts had wed a new partner.[9]

Disparities in marital status are especially pronounced among the baby boom and Generation X cohorts, yet stark gaps also are evident among older adults today. As figure 6.1 shows, 72 percent of white men age sixty-five and older are currently married compared to just 54 percent of black men. An even more pronounced gap emerges for women: 44 percent of white women yet just 23 percent of black women age sixty-five and older are married (figure 6.2). Among both men and women, blacks are more likely than whites to be widowed, divorced, or never married. And though lifelong singlehood is quite rare for current generations of older adults, it is twice as common among black men and women (8.7 and 9.4 percent) relative to white men and women (4.4 and 4.1 percent). Given the centrality of marriage to older adults' health and economic well-being, race gaps in family structure are a powerful mechanism contributing to later-life inequalities.

Researchers point to three broad reasons why married older adults enjoy greater health, wealth, and happiness than their unmarried peers:

Figure 6.1 Marital Status of U.S. Men Age Sixty-Five and Older, by Race, 2010

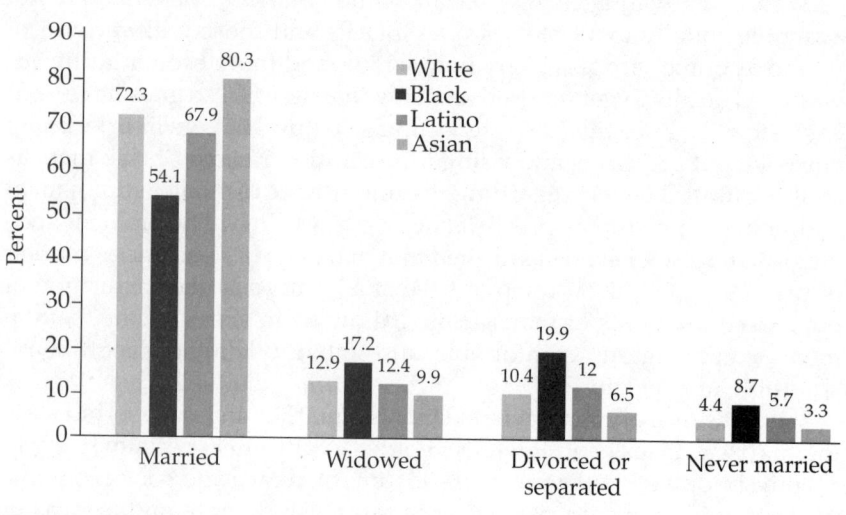

Source: U.S. Census Bureau 2014, table 5-2.

Figure 6.2 Marital Status of U.S. Women Age Sixty-Five and Older, by Race, 2010

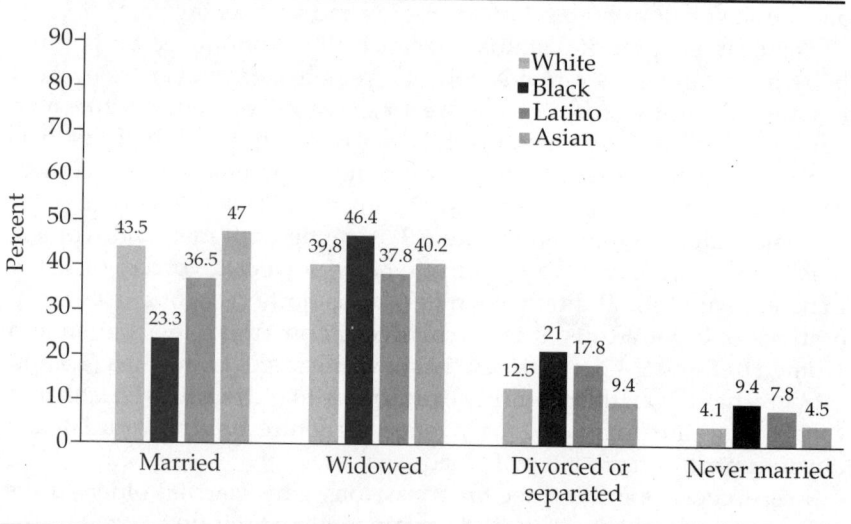

Source: U.S. Census Bureau 2014, table 5-2.

the direct benefits of marriage; the stress of marital dissolution; and social selection. First, marriage provides ongoing social, emotional, and economic benefits that enhance health and longevity, both directly and indirectly. Spouses (and cohabiting partners) enjoy economies of scale, so their pooled income and savings go further in covering expenses for shared resources like healthy food, secure housing, and heating bills. And when both partners are working for pay (or did so in their preretirement years), two incomes go further than one in covering daily expenses and providing a financial cushion in the event of a health crisis or other emergency.

Spouses also offer each other social and emotional support, a critical factor in sustaining health. This is especially important for older adults, who may need assistance as they recover from illness or injury or as they manage complex medication regimens. Studies consistently show that married older adults are more likely than single people to survive following major medical treatments such as chemotherapy and heart surgery, because they have a partner who can help them through the difficult recovery process.[10] Spouses also serve an important social control function by monitoring each other's health behaviors and encouraging healthy lifestyles. That friendly reminder to take the blood pressure medication each morning, to get a good night's sleep, or to forgo that second cookie or glass of scotch goes a long way toward keeping older adults healthy.

The psychosocial benefits of marriage and romantic partnerships are universal; partnered older adults uniformly fare better than the unpartnered. Yet a deeper exploration reveals that the magnitude of these benefits varies, with the largest gains accruing to those who already enjoy the greatest social and economic advantages. For instance, the social control function of marriage is more protective for men than women, because wives are more likely than husbands to take on the role of caregiver—a product of gender-typed socialization earlier in life. Women encourage their partners to eat nutritious meals, eschew smoking and drinking, wear their seat belts, and seek timely medical care and preventive tests like cholesterol screenings.[11] That is why recently widowed older men are more likely than married men to die of accidents, alcohol-related deaths, lung cancer, and chronic ischemic heart disease, but not from causes less closely linked to health behaviors.[12] Not surprisingly, parallel trends are not detected among women.

Likewise, the economic benefits of marriage are not equivalent for all. Among working-age adults, marriage provides greater economic security to whites and middle-class persons relative to blacks and lower-income adults, especially women. Given historically high rates of unemployment, underemployment, workplace discrimination, and low wages among black men, many older black women have worked for pay throughout their lives, often as a couple's primary breadwinner. As a result, the economic gains to marriage, as economists call it, are considerably less for black women relative to their white counterparts.[13] And because black, Latino, and working-class men are less likely than white and professional men to hold full-time jobs that provide health and pension benefits, marriage is less likely to bring these important benefits to their spouses.[14]

These differential economic returns to marriage persist into the retirement years, through the benefits that older adults receive from Social Security. The Social Security program, established in 1935 and revised in subsequent decades, was designed for an era in which most Americans married for life and maintained a traditional male breadwinner–female homemaker arrangement. Marriages typically ended through widowhood rather than divorce. Consistent with these early to mid-twentieth-century notions of families, Social Security provides more substantial benefits to married and widowed people relative to single and divorced people.[15] It also offers more generous benefits to those who maintained breadwinner-homemaker (rather than dual-earner) arrangements and to those who married for life rather than a brief spell.

Social Security also privileges families in which the breadwinner had a stable work history, with at least ten years of earnings. These rules ultimately translate into leaner Social Security benefits for black women relative to white women, given their lower rates of marriage, higher rates of divorce (and shorter marriages), and tendency to have maintained dual-earner arrangements. These rules also penalize those who have divorced, as they receive spousal benefits only if their marriages lasted ten years; even then, divorcées receive just half of what their ex-spouse's worker's benefits would be (although widows and widowers receive 100 percent). Never-married older adults receive benefits based solely on their own work and earnings histories; this is a particular problem for women, whose earnings consistently lag behind men's.[16] Although Social Security provides a critical source of income security for nearly all older adults, the program is most beneficial for married older adults, who already enjoy a position of privilege relative to their unmarried peers.

A second explanation for the superior health and well-being of married older adults relative to their divorced and widowed counterparts is that married people have been spared the health-depleting stress of divorce or widowhood. The stress of marital dissolution can take a significant toll on older adults' physical and mental health, and ultimately their survival. Many older widows had been providing round-the-clock care to their ailing spouse for the months leading up to the death. During that time, they may have neglected their own health problems or succumbed to the physical wear and tear of spousal caregiving, both of which may hasten their own deaths.[17] Although tabloid headlines often characterize bereaved spouses as "dying of a broken heart," the reality is far less romantic. Widow(er)s may die shortly after their spouses either because of shared risk factors, like poverty and poor health behaviors, or from the strain of caregiving and accompanying neglect of their own health. Widowhood, in turn, generates subsequent stressors that can further undermine well-being, like managing household chores alone, worrying about the late spouse's costly hospital and funeral bills, and trying to settle the estate.

Divorce also is fraught with stressors, from alimony battles and frayed ties with extended family members to the underlying problems that triggered the divorce in the first place, such as partner abuse or infidelity. Divorce also has substantial financial consequences, albeit different ones for men and women. The economic consequences of divorce have been widely debated, yet most recent estimates show that women experience a 25 to 40 percent drop in their standard of living, whereas men experience anywhere from a 10 percent gain to a 10 percent drop—the latter impact being limited to men whose wives were the family's primary breadwinner.[18]

Although divorce historically has been considered a young or midlife adult's transition, gray divorce or divorce among those age fifty and older is the most rapidly growing type of divorce in the United States. In 2010, more than one out of every four divorces occurred to a couple in which one or both spouses was age fifty or older.[19] Many divorced and widowed people eventually remarry and receive the marriage benefits discussed earlier—an effective cure for the stress of dissolution. Some researchers have even speculated that those who remarry in later life enjoy an added psychological boost, reflecting a mood-uplifting "honeymoon" effect, a more equitable division of household chores than they maintained in their youthful marriages, and a better sense of how to be a good spouse, drawing on hard-earned lessons from their first marriages.[20] Others opt for a "living apart together" (LAT) relationship, which is essentially a marriage-like relationship yet each partner retains their own independent home. Some will cohabit, living together without legalizing their union—often as a way to protect their investments and the pensions benefits received from their late spouse.[21] Yet these advantages of repartnership are most likely to be enjoyed by the most advantaged widow(er)s and divorcées, reflecting the selective nature of marriage and remarriage.

The final explanation offered for (re)married older adults' superior health and longer lives relative to their unmarried peers is social selection. Physically and emotionally healthy, financially stable people are considered more desirable partners and as such are more likely to get married, stay married, or remarry. Conversely, those with physical or mental health problems, bleak employment prospects, or a history of substance use are less likely to marry in the first place and are more likely to divorce or become widowed if they do marry.[22] The liabilities that inhibit someone from marrying, staying married, or remarrying are precisely the same factors that can take a long-term toll on well-being. In these complex ways, marriage and repartnering are not only a product of social inequality but a factor subsequently contributing to disparities.

Lifelong Singlehood

Lifelong singlehood is rare. According to U.S. Census Bureau estimates, shown in figures 6.1 and 6.2, just 5.9 percent of adults age sixty-five and older in 2010 had never married. This proportion is expected to increase to as many as 25 percent among future cohorts of older adults, however, starting with the Generation X cohort born in the late 1960s and 1970s and the millennials born in the 1980s and 1990s. Although single-for-life is an increasingly common status, the stigma associated with it persists. Ask a twenty-something single person why they want to marry or find a life partner someday and many will offer a variant on the theme "I don't want to die alone." Even if these words are uttered somewhat tongue in cheek, fears of aging alone are fueled by cautionary tales of lonely spinsters like *Great Expectations'* Miss Havisham and socially awkward bachelors like Chauncey Gardner in the 1979 film *Being There*.[23] In a recent Gallup Poll, 88 percent of unmarried Americans age eighteen to thirty-four said that they wanted to someday marry. Yet that proportion fell to less than one-third among single adults age fifty-five and older.[24] This precipitous drop reflects the fact that older adults (especially older women) grow to accept and even embrace their single status, rounding out their lives with other meaningful relationships and experiences and often forming "families by choice."[25]

Whether lifelong singlehood is a mechanism contributing to disparities in late-life health and well-being is a tricky question, because the pathways into and consequences of singlehood differ dramatically by gender among current cohorts of older adults. Certainly, lifelong singlehood is accompanied by significant economic disadvantages for both men and women, including lower household incomes, fewer assets, and more modest pension and Social Security benefits, relative to their married peers.[26] In 2014, never-married men and women age sixty-five and older were roughly five times as likely as their married counterparts to live beneath the poverty line (23 and 21 percent, respectively, versus 4.5 percent). This stark disparity is largely a product of single adults' lower household income over the life course, without the advantage of the economies of scale enjoyed by couples. It also reflects the structure of Social Security benefits, which rest solely on single workers' own income—despite the fact that they consistently earn less than their married counterparts. One recent analysis of HRS data showed that the average Social Security benefit of never-married men and women in 2010 was just shy of $12,000, while the mean benefit for their married peers—whether in a first marriage or a remarriage—topped $22,000.[27]

Financial disparities notwithstanding, lifelong singlehood is a largely positive experience for older women, although the situation is bleaker for men. Most studies conclude that single older women report physical, emotional, and social well-being that is just as good as that of their married counterparts and even better than that of their divorced or widowed peers.[28] Conversely, lifelong single men report poorer physical and mental health, fewer friendships, less social support, more loneliness, and an elevated mortality risk relative to their married, divorced, and widowed peers.[29]

This gender gap partly reflects the fact that never-married men and women differ in important ways, and these differences bear upon their physical and mental health. For current cohorts of older adults, women are positively selected, whereas men are negatively selected into lifelong singlehood. Stated more simply, among birth cohorts that reached young adulthood in the mid-twentieth century, men with stronger socioeconomic prospects were more likely to marry, whereas women with promising educational and career prospects were less likely to. Never-married older men tend to have less education and poorer-quality jobs, liabilities that make them "less marriageable," in the words of the sociologist William Julius Wilson.[30] Low socioeconomic status, in tandem with the lack of support from a spouse, intensifies single men's risk of health problems in later life. In sharp contrast, current cohorts of older unmarried women have higher-than-average levels of education and other resources that may protect their health in the longer term. For women who came of age in the mid-twentieth century, staying single afforded them the opportunity to pursue a college education, or even an advanced degree, and to enter rewarding professions (even if their earnings lagged behind those of their male counterparts). The expectations surrounding marriage at that time would have made it difficult for women to simultaneously hold the role of wife and mother while also pursuing their own personal and professional goals.[31]

Older single women also are comfortable and pro-active in seeking social support from friends and family as well as formal services like meal preparation and ride services.[32] Less is known about the ways in which unmarried men adapt to the challenges of aging, due in part to their small numbers. Because single men disproportionately experience physical and financial disadvantages throughout the life course, they are less likely than their female counterparts or married men to survive until old age. Those who do survive until later life are particularly vulnerable, isolated, and lonely because they have few ties to family or friends, a concern we revisit later in this chapter.

We also know surprisingly little about the ways in which socioeconomic status and race shape the social and emotional experiences of never-married older adults. Some evidence suggests that single black older women fare quite well emotionally. One study of 530 older unmarried adults in the greater Washington, D.C., area found that never-married black women reported lower levels of "single strain" than their white peers; single strain reflects one's agreement with statements like "There's no one to share day-to-day experiences."[33] Because older black women are more than twice as likely as their white peers to be lifelong singles, they may more easily find support among other single women in their communities. Black women also are more likely to have children outside of marriage, and they may rely on their children as well as other friends, relatives, neighbors, and members of their religious congregations for support.

Intergenerational Relationships

Intergenerational relationships refer to a person's ties to the generations above and below—parents, children, and grandchildren. I focus here on older adults' relationships with their adult children and grandchildren because these ties are particularly consequential for well-being and are a mechanism through which race, class, and gender inequalities are perpetuated. Although relationships with parents shape nearly every aspect of life through childhood and adolescence, they play a relatively modest role in the daily lives of older adults, simply because most do not have surviving parents. Few studies document precisely when adult children lose their parents, yet the evidence generally shows that most adults have lost both of their parents by the time they reach their midsixties, with this transition happening earlier for blacks and high school dropouts.[34] As a result, parents tend not to have a direct effect on the daily lives of most older adults, with one major exception. Older adults who have a surviving parent often must manage difficult and health-depleting caregiving demands, as described later in this chapter.

Parent-Child Relationships

Roughly 85 percent of older adults today are parents. Parents' emotional well-being takes a notorious and precipitous dip when their children are young and needy, but by the time these children are grown, parents and child-free older adults have similar levels of physical and emotional health.[35] Yet when researchers delve more deeply into the nuances of parent-child ties, they find that older adults derive health benefits from parenthood when their interactions with children are close, warm, and supportive and they can rely on their children for modest levels of assistance without being stifled or suffocated by excessive support.[36]

In general, older blacks and women report more close-knit and supportive relationships with their children than do whites and men.[37] Black older adults are more likely than whites to live in two- and three-generation households and to be involved in their grandchildren's day-to-day activities. Women's closer-knit relationships with their children reflect gender differences in parents' engagement with their children over the life course, a divide that is particularly pronounced for current cohorts of older adults. Not only do women have more frequent contact and more supportive ties with their children at every stage of the life course, but these ties persist or even strengthen when family changes occur.[38] Older women tend to grow more dependent on and close with their adult children upon widowhood, although comparable patterns are not evident among men.[39] Older fathers' ties with their adult children grow even more tenuous upon divorce, partly because they are more likely than women to remarry and may turn to their new wife for most of their emotional and social needs.[40]

Few studies explore social class differences in parent-child relationships, yet emerging research suggests that lower-income older adults have more strained ties, owing in part to an adult child's problems, exemplifying the life-course theme of linked lives. Intergenerational ties may become strained or even estranged when the adult child faces a significant problem like a divorce, a serious legal problem, or substance abuse.[41] For the most part, these problems are more likely to strike families with fewer economic resources. Children from better-off families are more likely to graduate from college; both education and the rewarding career prospects it brings are an important hedge against difficulties like unemployment and substance use.[42] Adult children's problems tend to be more distressing to mothers than fathers because they feel a greater sense of responsibility for how their children turn out.[43] Lower-income older adults also are less likely to receive financial support from their children (but more likely to receive practical assistance from them), yet much of this gap reflects the financial struggles of the children themselves, who simply do not have the disposable income to help their parents—even if they would like to do so.[44]

Grandparent-Grandchild Relationships

For most older adults, grandchildren are a source of joy and pride. Bumper stickers implore motorists to Ask Me about My Grandchildren. Roughly 70 percent of older adults have at least one grandchild, and for most, the experience is largely if not wholly positive.[45] Especially for older adults who have warm and close ties with their children, grandparenthood provides an opportunity to share love, advice, and a sense of family history with the younger generation without the hassles of serving as the primary disciplinarian.[46] For older men who prioritized work responsibilities over family earlier in life, the role of grandfather offers a fresh opportunity to nurture, mentor, and guide a child. (To wit: another popular bumper sticker tells us that Grandchildren Are God's Way of Giving Us a Second Chance). Because older adults are living longer than ever before, many will enjoy active years with their grandchildren that prior generations never could have dreamed of.[47] Grandchildren bolster the emotional well-being of older adults, especially when they experience other age-related losses, like the deaths of spouses, siblings, and friends, and as they exit the paid workforce. Researchers agree with older adults that playing with and caring for grandchildren "helps keep them young."[48] Some studies even suggest that reading to and playing with grandchildren may be a hedge against cognitive declines.[49]

Despite stereotypes of grandchildren who never call or write their grandparents, statistics show high levels of engagement. According to one national survey conducted by the American Association of Retired Persons (AARP), two-thirds of grandparents see a grandchild at least every two weeks, and more than 80 percent are in touch with a grandchild regularly whether through email, telephone, Skype, or mail.[50] Most grandparents view their role as playmate or mentor rather than disciplinarian. The activities that grandparents see as their main responsibility are spoiling the children, teaching them family history, and giving them treats or special gifts.[51]

Visiting with grandchildren may indeed be a source of joy, but the more time-intensive task of caring for those children can be a burdensome responsibility that falls disproportionately on older women. Grandmothers often provide child care so that their sons and daughters can work or attend school full-time without worrying about (or having to pay for) child care. Yet the hours that older women dedicate to feeding, tutoring, chauffeuring, and disciplining their grandchildren is time taken away from leisure activities in retirement, or from work hours among those who are still employed. According to data from the HRS, 30 percent of retirement-age women and 22 percent of men are providing grandchild care, with women investing more hours, for longer time periods, and in activities that are more direct care than fun play.[52] That is one reason why near-retirement-age women providing grandchild care are especially likely to cut back on their work hours or exit the labor force before they reach retirement age.[53] These work cutbacks (and accompanying sacrifice of earnings and pension contributions) are yet another factor linked to older women's economic precarity relative to men, whose work lives are less affected by family demands. Exiting the labor force early to care for grandchildren and the accompanying early receipt of Social Security benefits prior to full retirement age permanently reduces the benefit that one is eligible to receive by as much as one-third. The experiences of forty-eight working grandmothers, as detailed by the sociologist Madonna Harrington-Meyer, vividly illustrate the life-course principle that choices are made within highly constrained circumstances.[54] Although grandmothers may indeed find "joy" in child care, others admitted that they were "drowning in exhaustion and debt" in an effort to help their adult children juggle their own work, school, and family demands. Putting their children's needs before their own, the working grandmothers felt "obliged, needed, even forced, to provide care."[55]

Grandparenting experiences are powerfully shaped by socioeconomic status and race. Relative to wealthier persons and whites, the transition to grandparenthood comes earlier—often as young as one's thirties or forties—among people from disadvantaged economic backgrounds, blacks, and Latinos.[56] Young adults with fewer years of schooling typically become parents earlier than their more-educated peers. Their children, in turn, may face compromised prospects for higher education or professional careers and are likelier to follow in their parents' footsteps by bearing children early. Consequently, those from disadvantaged backgrounds become grandparents at younger ages and are more likely to serve as surrogate parents to their grandchildren when their own children face struggles that limit their capacity to parent.[57]

Custodial grandparenting, or caring for grandchildren on a full-time basis, is one of the most rapidly growing concerns facing older adults today—especially older African American women and those from economically disadvantaged backgrounds.[58] The share of U.S. children living in a grandparent's household has more than doubled over the past four decades, from 3 percent in 1970 to 7 percent in 2010.[59] An estimated 2.9 million older adults are currently raising their grandchildren. The challenges of custodial grandparenting exemplify the life-course theme of linked lives. The main reason why older adults are raising their grandchildren is that the middle generation is either unable or unavailable to provide adequate care. The rise in skip-generation families, comprising just a grandchild and grandparent, is largely due to several sweeping social problems that have disproportionately struck economically disadvantaged and black families over the last four decades: the War on Drugs, rising rates of incarceration, the HIV/AIDS epidemic, and the lingering effects of the Great Recession. Since the 1970s crackdown on illegal drugs, incarceration rates in the United States have risen dramatically and are now among the highest in the world. Law enforcement policies like the "three strikes rule" implemented in the 1990s effectively removed large numbers of African American men and, to a lesser degree, women from their communities and imprisoned them.[60]

Since the 1990s, the crack and HIV/AIDS epidemics, as well as prolonged military deployments, have also disproportionately affected young men and women of color. These conditions have contributed to the premature death, incapacitation, and imprisonment of young people who might otherwise be caring for their children. In the early 2000s, many young parents were unable to get back on their feet financially after losing jobs in the Great Recession. Some victims of layoffs could not afford their own homes or were evicted from their apartments, forcing them to place their children in the safe environment of a grandparent's home.[61] And in the 2010s, the heroin and opioid crises have left growing numbers of children (especially poorer and rural white children) either orphaned or abandoned, forcing their grandparents to step in as primary caretaker.[62] The stress that an older adult feels when taking on the daunting responsibility of custodial grandparenting is amplified by the distress of witnessing their child's drug, financial, or legal problems.[63]

Researchers paint a consistently bleak portrait of custodial grandparenting. Custodial grandparents often feel overwhelmed by their responsibilities, and they report more physical and mental health problems, poorer-quality sleep, lower levels of satisfaction with the grandparenting role, poorer health behaviors, and isolation from other friends and family.[64] These harmful effects persist even when the grandparents' other risk factors, such as low income or education, are controlled.[65] Some custodial grandparents feel stigmatized, isolated, or ashamed because of their child's struggles with addiction, crime, or illness. Grandparents living with school-age children are also exposed to childhood colds, which are especially dangerous for older adults who already have compromised immune systems. And keeping up with an energetic child or disciplining a headstrong teen can be particularly difficult for older adults whose energy, stamina, and physical strength are waning. For

Figure 6.3 Children Under Age Eighteen Living with a Grandparent, by Race-Ethnicity and the Presence of Parent(s), 2012

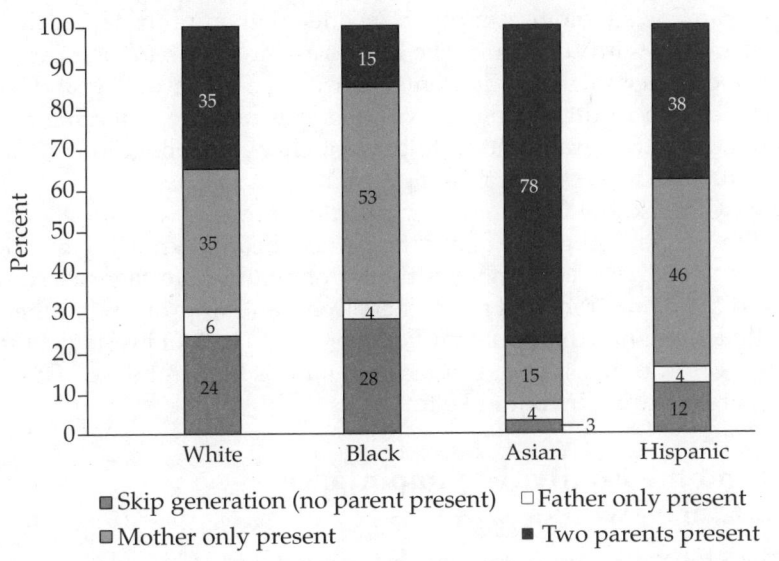

Source: Ellis and Simmons 2014.

many grandparents, grandchildren bring new and unanticipated expenses, such as clothing, furniture, extra food, school supplies, and medical bills, straining their already stretched incomes.[66]

Most custodial grandparents are still working for pay and may struggle with work-family balance at precisely the time when they would prefer to be contemplating retirement. Some suffer a further financial hit when they cut back on their work hours, take a more flexible job, or quit work altogether in order to manage their new role as caretaker. Reentering the labor force when their grandchild no longer requires round-the-clock care can be difficult if not impossible, given pervasive ageism in the workplace.[67] These work-family strains may compound the financial and physical challenges that these vulnerable older adults faced even prior to becoming custodial caregivers. According to one national study, 21 percent of custodial grandparents live beneath the poverty line, 25 percent have a disability, and 40 percent have cared for their grandchildren for more than five years—rendering it a chronic strain (figure 6.3).[68]

Yet custodial grandparents can and do find purpose, growth, and satisfaction in their role. Perhaps the most famous custodial grandparents are the couple lovingly referred to by the gold medal–winning Olympic gymnast Simone Biles as "Mom and Dad." Simone's grandfather, Ron Biles, and his wife Nellie adopted the gymnast and her sister when Simone's biological mother was deemed an unfit parent due to her struggles with addiction. The Bileses are not alone in their capacity to thrive as custodial grandparents. Many develop new skills and competencies as a result of their unexpected return to the parenting role.[69] As one custodial grandparent told researchers at Generations United, "I'm making it. Well, not making it, but I got my head above water. Thank God I know how to doggy paddle, because if I didn't, I would have drowned a long time ago."[70] Some take heart in knowing that they are doing all they can to enhance their grandchild's life chances. As one custodial grandparent told researchers Deborah Sampson and Katherine Hertlein: "I'm just thankful that I am able to do it. . . . I just look at it as an opportunity to make a difference in a kid's life, and if I could do it for more children, I would like to."[71]

Beyond the Family: The Importance of Social Networks

Older adults' lives are embedded in social networks that extend beyond the family. Casual acquaintances—like a former coworker, the daughter of one's best friend, a member of one's religious congregation, or a high school classmate with whom one reconnected on social media—might be an occasional dinner companion or a sounding board during times of stress, even though they seldom sign on for heavy-duty caregiving tasks. For older adults, daily life also is enriched by what the developmental psychologist Karen Fingerman calls "consequential strangers."[72] The postal carrier who checks in to see if an older adult is taking in her mail each day. The cashier at the local diner who worries if a retired gentleman doesn't come in for his daily coffee. The bank teller who notices if an older adult is suddenly withdrawing large sums of money from his or her savings account. All of these people contribute, directly and indirectly, to older adults' quality of life.

Both traditional wisdom and classic theories of aging, like disengagement theory, suggest that older adults' social networks grow smaller with each passing year. Social networks inevitably shrink as friends and neighbors move out of their longtime neighborhoods into assisted living facilities, loved ones die, and happy hours with coworkers come to a halt upon retirement. Yet a diminishing social circle also may be a desired and normal part of healthy aging, according to the Stanford University psychologist Laura Carstensen. She argues that older adults' days are numbered, so they may choose to conserve their emotional energy and maintain close ties only with those nearest and dearest to them. This perspective, called socioemotional selectivity theory (SST), suggests that a large circle of acquaintances may be less personally meaningful and less protective for an older adult's well-being than a small inner circle made up of spouse or partner, children, and his or her closest friends and siblings.[73] According to SST, our social networks shrink over time because we intentionally invest only in our closest ties as we age, and we let our less meaningful ties slip away.

Yet recent analyses of National Social Life, Health, and Aging Project (NSHAP) data challenge the core assumptions of SST and show that many older adults retain or even add new members to their social networks. The sociologist Benjamin Cornwell and his colleagues traced changes in older adults' social networks over a five-year period and found that a remarkable 80 percent added at least one person to their social circle and more than half (59 percent) met a new confidant with whom they could share their private thoughts and feelings.[74] Surprisingly, a higher proportion of NSHAP participants reported a net gain (38 percent) versus a net loss (27 percent) in the size of their social networks. Those who had added new confidants to their social circles went on to show improvements in physical health, mobility, cognitive functioning, and psychological well-being, while those whose social networks had shrunk experienced a slight decline in physical (although not emotional) health. The NSHAP data challenge SST in another way. It is not just new confidants who enhance older adults' well-being: adding more distant ties or consequential strangers to one's circle also is beneficial. New relationships with neighbors and distant acquaintances can be particularly protective for recent widows and widowers, who may relish having new social ties and a new social circle apart from their families. Other studies show that online social ties also enhance older adults' emotional well-being and reduce loneliness, in part because virtual contact facilitates telephone and face-to-face interactions.[75]

So how do we reconcile these two contradictory sets of patterns? SST holds that older adults' social circles shrink, that distant social ties are cast aside as they age, and that a small, close-knit social circle is most essential to their health and well-being. Yet recent data show that older adults are more likely to expand rather than reduce their social circles, that social networks may grow through the addition of distant and virtual ties, and that these ties to new acquaintances are beneficial to health and well-being. Digging more deeply into the data, it is clear that these changes in social networks vary by race, gender, and socioeconomic status. In general, blacks, men, and those with limited socioeconomic resources have fewer social ties than whites, women, and those with richer socioeconomic resources.[76] Older adults whose lives are marked by disadvantage also experience more turnover, meaning that they both lose *and* gain more network members over time. This rapid turnover can create problems, especially for older adults who are losing close and enduring ties and replacing them with tenuous or ephemeral ties that they cannot necessarily count on in times of need.

In the NSHAP, blacks and older adults with lower levels of education lost more confidants than their white and college-educated peers during the five-year observation period.[77] These losses largely reflect a greater number of deaths to family, friends, and acquaintances in more-disadvantaged communities. Yet blacks and those with lower levels of education also added new acquaintances, contributing to instability and churning in their networks. Such churning reflects the long-standing disadvantages experienced by blacks and lower-income adults, including unstable employment and a continually shifting pool of temporary or seasonal coworkers, as well as lower rates of homeownership and less stable housing, leading to an ever-changing set of neighbors.[78] As the sociologist Matthew Desmond observed in his study of a poor urban community in Milwaukee, because the network ties of socially disadvantaged adults are often temporary and "disposable," these older adults are less likely to turn to these fleeting acquaintances in times of serious need.[79]

The extent to which more versus fewer, stable versus unstable, and new versus long-standing ties are protective for older adults' well-being also depends on precisely who is in their network. In short, it depends on the mix or relative balance of close versus distant ties, as each brings distinctive benefits to older adults. Women have not only larger networks than men but more connections to family, friends, and neighbors, whereas men maintain more ties to former coworkers. That is one reason why women benefit more from their social ties: friends and family are more likely than former coworkers to offer practical support and a supportive ear.[80]

Older women's social networks have another benefit: women are more likely than men to befriend people who do not know each other already. According to network analysts, these more distant acquaintances, or "weak ties," serve the important bridging function of exposing older adults to information, events, and experiences that they might not find in a more tight-knit network.[81] If an older woman spends most of her time with lifelong friends who all know each other, eat at the same restaurants, have the same doctors, shop at the same grocery store, and rehash the same tidbits of gossip, they may not branch out, learn, or expand their horizons. Although a more distant or "outsider" acquaintance may not be a source of regular emotional or practical support, she may well provide a connection to new opportunities and ideas.[82]

Women's more varied social ties also help explain why they tend to adjust better emotionally to stressors like widowhood and feel less urgency to remarry after their spouse dies.[83] Many older women's social needs are met through their extended social networks, but men, by contrast, rely almost exclusively on their wives. If their marriage ends, widowers and divorced men tend to invest their time and emotional energy in seeking out a new romantic partner rather than establishing a larger social circle of golf buddies or acquaintances with whom to share an occasional beer. The sociologist Deborah van den Hoonaard conducted in-depth interviews with twenty-six older widowers in the United States and Canada and found that men often saw their close friendships and casual acquaintanceships wither away after their wives died because their wives had done the work of sustaining those bonds.[84] Many of the men shared sentiments similar to those of widower Stan, who recalled that the couple's friends were really his "wife's friends. . . . I hardly hear from them now. You don't even get a Christmas card."[85] Other widowers acknowledged that they could have done more to sustain their friendships; as Keith admitted, the demise of the friendships "was kind of a gradual thing. I don't blame them. I just probably haven't followed up on it. . . . You just sort of drift away."[86]

Network analysts have also found race differences in who makes up older adults' enduring social ties; blacks' networks, for instance, include a particularly high proportion of family members.[87] Some researchers have noted that blacks' reliance on family members is rooted in lifelong experiences with discrimination and racism: family members, close friends, and fellow church members are more likely to be trusted and welcomed into one's network, whereas more distant ties are viewed with skepticism or distrust.[88] These close-knit ties are one explanation for why older blacks adjust more easily to some late-life stressors like widowhood.[89] Yet these tight-knit ties have a potential downside: if a member of an older adult's inner circle becomes ill or faces a crisis, that may limit his or her capacity to provide the support that the older adult needs.

The Dark Side of Older Adults' Social Relationships

For most older adults, social relationships are a source of comfort, companionship, and support. When four thousand older adults in the United States of Aging Survey were asked to name the one thing that they consider most important for maintaining a high quality of life, the top response was "staying connected with family and friends." Nearly half named social relationships as the key to happiness, surpassing the second most popular answer, "having financial means," which clocked in at just 30 percent.[90] These statistics are not surprising considering that 78 percent also said that they were satisfied with their relationships with family and friends, while just 40 percent were satisfied with their finances or health.

Yet a more pessimistic interpretation of these statistics is that more than one in five older adults may be either suffering from a lack of meaningful relationships or entrenched in relationships that are a source of strain, stress, or even outright mistreatment. Three aspects of older adults' social relationships are potential sources of harm: the loneliness and isolation they may experience, the abuse and mistreatment they may suffer, and caregiving strains. All three are chronic stressors that are especially likely to strike the older adults who are already most vulnerable and subsequently intensify their vulnerability.

Social Isolation and Loneliness

Loneliness and social isolation can be emotionally and physically damaging to older adults. One of the most gripping and heartbreaking portrayals of social isolation was described by the sociologist Eric Klinenberg in his book *Heat Wave*.[91] He examined the painful question of why poor black older men accounted for a disproportionate share of the more than five hundred Chicago residents who perished in the city's 1995 heat wave. Klinenberg points to social isolation as a pivotal factor. Many victims had few family members or friends to check on them, and some did not have even acquaintances who took a passing interest in their well-being.

While *Heat Wave* reveals the most dramatic consequences of social isolation, quieter forms of isolation and loneliness pervade the lives of millions of older adults—even those who may have a spouse, children, and friends. A recent AARP survey of three thousand midlife and older Americans found that one-third admitted to feeling lonely.[92] Studies taking a wider view of the life course show that rates of loneliness decline steadily between adolescence and later life, but then spike up among the oldest-old in their eighties and beyond.[93]

The ebbs and flows of loneliness over the life course are tightly tied to the ways in which social roles and activities change with age. Recent retirees often are young and healthy enough to spend their newfound free time with friends and family or pursuing hobbies and activities that enrich their social circles. With advanced age, the deaths of friends and family and the diminished capacity to travel, volunteer, or participate in social activities may render older adults isolated and vulnerable. Yet loneliness reflects more than the number of people in one's life or the time spent with others. The widely used UCLA Loneliness Scale asks respondents to agree or disagree with statements such as "I feel starved for company," or "My social relationships are superficial."[94] Their answers show that loneliness can also be the feeling or belief that one's social and emotional needs are going unmet.

Conceptual writings on loneliness also distinguish between emotional and social loneliness, or the difference between feeling alone and being alone. Emotional loneliness refers to a lack of intimacy and closeness in one's relationships. An older adult who has a stale marriage or chilly relationships with his or her children might feel a sense of "utter aloneness" even when surrounded by others at a lively family dinner.[95] By contrast, social loneliness refers to dissatisfaction with the size of one's social network and frequency of interactions.[96] The two types of loneliness may go hand in hand: widow(er)s, those living alone, or those living far away from their friends and families consistently report higher levels of both types of loneliness than persons who are more socially integrated.[97] Yet even those who are socially integrated may feel emotionally isolated. One in four married older adults report emotional loneliness, and these rates are even higher for those whose spouses are chronically ill, who have a dissatisfying (or nonexistent) sexual relationship, or who have infrequent or conflicted conversations.[98]

Researchers have documented race, age, and socioeconomic disparities in feelings of loneliness, yet these gaps are partly accounted for by other social disadvantages, consistent with cumulative inequality perspectives. Older adults in their eighties and beyond experience spikes in loneliness, yet these patterns largely reflect their high rates of widow(er)hood and living alone, as well as the physical and sensory declines that limit their meaningful social engagement. Likewise, blacks, Latinos, and those with fewer years of education report more loneliness than whites and highly educated persons, but these patterns reflect other risk factors for loneliness, such as having a small social network, being in poor health, living alone, experiencing high levels of stress, and receiving low levels of emotional support from one's spouse. The gender gap in loneliness is largely accounted for by qualitative aspects of their relationships: women are not as lonely as men because they give and receive more emotional support and tend to have close and supportive relationships beyond the marital dyad.[99]

Loneliness and social isolation are serious public health concerns because they are linked to sleep problems, poor cardiovascular health, elevated blood pressure, depressive symptoms, compromised immune function, and cognitive decline, each of which carries long-term consequences for mortality risk.[100] Experts predict that both emotional and social loneliness will become even more pressing social concerns as the large baby boom cohort enters old age. Some have suggested that baby boomers and members of Generation X hold unrealistically high expectations for what their social relationships should provide, such as the belief that their romantic partner should be a soulmate who meets all their emotional needs. If these lofty expectations go unfulfilled, then future cohorts of older adults may be particularly vulnerable to emotional loneliness.[101]

At the same time, baby boomers are more likely than their parents' generation to divorce, to stay single for life, to have fewer children, and to live miles away from their children who have traveled to distant locations to pursue their own career goals.[102] As a result, they may be particularly susceptible to social loneliness. Gerontologists have coined the term "elder orphans" to describe those older adults who are essentially aging alone. They have no spouse or romantic partner, have outlived both parents, and are either childless or have children who live far away and do not visit. They also lack friends or neighbors who regularly visit. According to one recent analysis of HRS data, an estimated one in five older adults are elder orphans or at risk of becoming one in the coming decades.[103] The loneliest and most isolated older adults are most vulnerable to two particularly harmful aspects of social relationships: abuse and neglect, and the strains of intensive caregiving.

Elder Mistreatment

We would like to believe that we live in a society that respects older adults and treats them with kindness and dignity. Yet contemporary news reports (and mounting statistical data) show that elder mistreatment is all too common and that those who are already the most isolated and vulnerable are most likely to be victimized. The forms and varieties of mistreatment continue to expand as technology creates new opportunities for the unscrupulous to prey on their victims. Telemarketers may scam lonely older adults like Richard Guthrie of their life savings. Guthrie, a ninety-two-year-old World War II veteran, had entered a few lotteries, so his name and contact information appeared in a consumer information firm's database. The company promptly sold Guthrie's contact information to fraudulent telemarketers, who tricked the lonely widower into disclosing his banking and personal information and ultimately raided his account of all his savings. A devastated Guthrie recounted, "I loved getting those calls. . . . Since my wife passed away, I don't have many people to talk with. I didn't even know they were stealing from me, until everything was gone." Guthrie is not alone; the Federal Trade Commission (FTC) estimates that 10 to 15 percent of older adults each year are the victims of consumer fraud.[104]

Older adults' bodies and dignity also are preyed upon, often by the people they and their families have entrusted with their care. In the past decade, home health aides and nursing home assistants have made a game out of taking humiliating photos of older adults and posting these images on the internet "for laughs." In 2016, the Centers for Medicare and Medicaid Services (CMS) started to discipline nursing homes whose workers did so.[105] This federal crackdown occurred only after one nursing assistant in New Jersey posted a photo of a nursing home resident's genitals on Facebook. And two aides at an assisted-living facility in Green Bay, Wisconsin, uploaded to Snapchat a collection of photos showing older residents undressing, sitting on the toilet, defecating, or vomiting. These cruel acts of betrayal were just two of the dozens of infractions detected.[106] This viral abuse is not the only form of mistreatment that happens at nursing homes. An estimated one in five nursing home residents have been mistreated by a fellow resident (dubbed R-REM, or resident-to-resident elder mistreatment), while one in four are physically or emotionally mistreated by nursing home staff.[107]

While these shameful acts have captured national media attention, it is the less sensationalist, more private forms of abuse that are most common yet the most difficult to combat. Elder abuse occurs most frequently at the hands of those closest to older adults, especially their spouses, adult children, grandchildren, and other relatives. Because older adults often are close with or dependent upon the people mistreating them, they are reluctant to report these incidents to the authorities for fear that their abusers will retaliate.[108] This fear and paralysis was dramatically recounted by the late Oscar-winning actor Mickey Rooney, who shared his own experiences of abuse when he testified to the Senate's Special Committee on Aging in 2011. In his emotional testimony, ninety-year-old Rooney stated that his stepson confiscated his mail, medication, and food and made him a "prisoner in [my] own home. . . . My money was stolen from me, by someone close. When I asked for information, I was told that I couldn't have any of my own information. I was literally left powerless."[109] Although any older adult is hypothetically at risk of abuse, those with the fewest social ties and poorest physical and cognitive health are particularly vulnerable to abuse and are most reticent about reporting it.

Definitions and Trends Elder abuse typically takes one of five forms: physical abuse, sexual abuse, emotional or psychological abuse, financial exploitation, or neglect. Physical abuse encompasses any violent act that causes pain or impairment, such as hitting, force-feeding, or improper use of physical restraints or medication. Sexual abuse refers to nonconsensual intimate contact, or sexual contact when the older adult is incapable of giving consent. Emotional abuse is a broad category covering any act causing psychological anguish, such as threats, insults, or humiliation. Legislators recognize that an otherwise loving yet occasionally frustrated caregiver may blurt out a curse word at the care recipient from time to time, so some states stipulate that at least ten such acts within a year are the minimum criteria for establishing emotional abuse.[110] Neglect is a pervasive yet difficult-to-detect behavior that refers to a caretaker's failure to meet the older adult's basic needs, such as depriving the older adult of adequate food and water, willfully preventing the older adult from getting necessary medical care, not keeping him or her clean, allowing the apartment or home to fall into a state of squalor, or keeping the older adult socially isolated. Financial exploitation involves the mismanagement or misuse of an older adult's money or assets for personal gain. While Richard Guthrie was exploited by strangers at a telemarketing firm, Mickey Rooney was victimized by his own stepson, who allegedly siphoned money from Rooney's assets and monthly income to purchase luxury cars and vacations for himself.

Elder abuse is distinct from other forms of violence against older adults, such as street crimes or assaults; abuse refers to instances of mistreatment within a trusting relationship between a victim and perpetrator who know one another. More than half of all emotional abuse and sexual abuse incidents, and three-quarters of physical mistreatment cases, are perpetrated by family members.[111] That is why statistics on abuse and mistreatment are so difficult to obtain and confirm: older victims may be too frightened to report their mistreatment to authorities or they may not know whom to report to. Some are afraid to tell their physicians or social workers because they fear a breach of confidentiality. Others feel ashamed and embarrassed or may convince themselves that the mistreatment was justified because they were making demands on their abuser. It is not uncommon for victims of elder abuse to say things like, "I know it's hard, taking care of an old sick person like me. I can't blame him for getting angry." And for members of historically marginalized groups, these obstacles are even more daunting. LGBTQ older adults are particularly reluctant to report abuse for fear that their abuser will divulge their sexual identity, or because they anticipate being dismissed or mistreated at the hands of formal service providers.[112] Undocumented immigrants may not disclose their abuse to the legal authorities who could help them, out of fear that they or their abuser could be deported.

Despite the many challenges of measuring and documenting elder abuse, most experts agree that 10 percent of older adults experience some form of abuse each year.[113] Data on elder mistreatment typically come from two sources: reports from social service and health care providers, and population-based studies. Formal reports to adult protective services (APS) offer dramatically lower counts of abuse than self-reported survey data, despite the fact that nearly every state has mandatory reporting laws.[114] Levels of underreporting to or by authorities also vary based on the type of abuse. Physical abuse is well defined and may leave a visible imprint, such as bruises or scrapes. As such, it is more likely to be reported to authorities than more ambiguous types of mistreatment, like neglect or emotional abuse. About one in three cases of physical abuse are reported to authorities, compared to just 16 percent of cases of sexual abuse and 8 percent of emotional abuse cases.[115] One study comparing self-report and documented case data in New York found self-reported cases of financial abuse to be a stunning forty-four times higher than the number of documented cases reported to authorities.[116]

Self-reported survey data are especially valuable because they also include other personal information that helps researchers not only identify which older adults are at elevated risk of abuse but also shed light on the identity of the abuser. One of the most widely cited surveys is the National Elder Mistreatment Study (NEMS), which collected data from more than six thousand community-dwelling adults age sixty and older.[117] The NEMS asked older adults about their experiences of mistreatment by persons both known and unknown to them. Another important data resource is the National Social Life, Health, and Aging Project, a survey of roughly three thousand older adults age fifty-seven to eighty-five that includes detailed questions on mistreatment.

Rates of abuse in these surveys are fairly low, yet the data consistently show that emotional abuse is most common, followed by financial exploitation and neglect. The NEMS finds that in the past year roughly 5 percent of older adults reported emotional abuse, financial abuse, or neglect, while 1.6 percent reported physical abuse and fewer than 1 percent reported sexual abuse.[118] Yet surveys have their limitations. Older adults who have the greatest vulnerabilities (such as not being fluent in English), who have severe cognitive or physical limitations, or who have mental health problems may be less likely to participate in a survey or complete the questions on a potentially disturbing topic like abuse.

Differentials and Risk Factors Experts claim that "elder abuse knows no boundaries—older adults of all ages, genders, races, incomes and cultures experience abuse."[119] The data bear this out, albeit in an indirect manner. Basic descriptive studies show that self-reported elder mistreatment is more common among women than men, among the oldest-old than the young-old, and among blacks and Latinos than whites.

However, multivariate analyses show that these differences are no longer statistically significant after health status and social support are controlled.[120] That means that traditional dimensions of social stratification do not play a direct role in an older adult's risk of abuse. Rather, members of historically disadvantaged groups are at greater risk of the two factors most strongly linked to experiences of abuse: poor physical and cognitive health, and social isolation.[121] As detailed in earlier chapters, ethnic minorities, those with lower levels of education, and oldest-old adults are more likely to suffer cognitive impairment and physical limitations, which render them vulnerable to abuse. Because of women's longevity, they are more likely than men to become widowed and live alone for many years, and also to experience age-related health declines that put them at risk of mistreatment.

Cognitive impairment is one of the most powerful risk factors for abuse, especially financial abuse. As their mental acuity fades, older adults have reduced capacity to manage their financial affairs independently and may show poor judgment or increased reliance on so-called helpers who take advantage of them.[122] Severe cognitive impairment also places older adults at risk of physical and emotional abuse: nearly half of all older adults with dementia have experienced emotional abuse, physical abuse, or neglect.[123] One of the main reasons for this high rate of abuse is that some older adults with dementia become physically and verbally aggressive toward their caregivers, who may react by shouting, insulting, withholding food, or physically restraining them. Some overwhelmed caregivers may threaten to put the dementia patient in a nursing home or vow to stop providing care—threats that can be demoralizing and frightening to the older adult.[124] This behavior on the part of the caregiver is hardly defensible, but it does signal a powerful wake-up call that policies and practices are needed to help dementia caregivers who may lack the skill, physical stamina, or emotional strength to provide quality care to their loved one. Moreover, it is also important to recognize that most beleaguered caregivers do not hurt their family members; to the contrary, caregivers themselves are often victimized by their loved one's loss of impulse control when he or she develops dementia.[125]

Social isolation is another major risk factor for abuse. Older adults with low levels of social support are three times as likely to experience abuse, relative to those with sufficient levels of support.[126] One reason why social support buffers against abuse is that it gives older adults someone they can turn to for help and assurance. Those with more extensive social networks also have more eyes and ears focused on them, alert for early signs of abuse, and ready to intervene when such signs are detected. Older adults who have denser social networks—a greater number of friends and relatives who know one another—also are less likely to be victimized.[127] Yet some studies find that the causal direction is the reverse: it is not just that isolation puts older adults at risk of abuse, but also that older adults in abusive situations have fewer friends and confidants because their abuser prevents them from maintaining those ties. Just as with physical and sexual abuse of children, abusers may try to isolate the victim in order to conceal the abuse, limiting the victim's capacity to reach out for support or to escape the situation.[128]

Social isolation is highly patterned, as described earlier. Isolated older adults in rural areas are particularly susceptible to abuse and neglect and less likely to receive the supports they need. Rural women have especially high rates of physical and emotional victimization and neglect, compared to their urban counterparts.[129] Compounding this disparity, rural women also may be less likely to seek and receive care. In a fascinating study of rural Appalachian communities, Pamela Teaster and her colleagues found that poor older women were especially reluctant to report abuse in tight-knit communities because their abusers, local service providers, and emergency responders were all likely to know one another, heightening the feelings of embarrassment and fear of retaliation.[130] Geographically isolated older adults also face obstacles to seeking virtual support or information, whether through email, social networking sites, or websites like AARP or the National Center on Elder Abuse (NCEA). More than half of rural residents lack high-speed broadband, which residents of urban areas take for granted.[131]

Elder abuse and mistreatment present a powerful example of cumulative adversity, in that those in poor health and with the least social support are most vulnerable to abuse. This abuse, in turn, elevates victims' risks of physical symptoms, such as pain or injury; symptoms of psychological distress, including fear, depression, hopelessness, anxiety, and suicidal thoughts; and further social isolation, dependence, and withdrawal due to embarrassment, demoralization, and shame. The psychological distress experienced by older abuse victims may exacerbate their underlying health problems, ultimately increasing their risk of death.[132]

The mistreatment of older adults is pervasive and potentially deadly, yet difficult to track and treat. A major turning point in fighting elder abuse occurred in 2010 when President Barack Obama signed into law, as part of the ACA, the Elder Justice Act, which provides federal funding to "prevent, detect, treat, understand, intervene in and, where appropriate, prosecute elder abuse, neglect and exploitation." The act is fairly comprehensive, and it targets detection, prosecution of abusers, and investments in education, research, and surveillance. It makes grants available to train law enforcement, legal professionals, and others on the front lines of care in detecting abuse; creates a national database for tracking abuse in long-term care facilities and carrying out background checks on the employees of care facilities; and requires that abuse perpetrated in long-term care facilities be reported immediately to law enforcement.[133] However, much of this work happens under state adult protective services, which is largely funded by social services block grants (SSBGs) made to states. As of June 2018, the current administration's proposed fiscal year 2019 budget would eliminate SSBGs.[134] Although it would continue to provide $5 million in federal funds for training and education aimed at elder abuse prevention, few funds will remain for further training and education once the SSBG program is zeroed out.[135] As the large cohort of baby boomers enters later life, the need for programs targeting elder mistreatment will become all the more essential.

Caregiving Strains

Nearly everyone will be a caregiver at some point. Whether preparing dinner for a bedridden friend, picking up prescription medications for an ill parent, or helping a frail spouse to shower and get dressed each morning, an estimated 40 million Americans today are providing care to a family member or friend.[136] Caregiving is different from merely lending a helping hand; it is help given expressly because a loved one has a significant physical, psychological, or developmental need. Many older adults are caregivers themselves because their friends, siblings, and spouse are their age-peers, and with age comes an increased risk of physical and cognitive impairments that may stop them from functioning as independently or energetically as in the past. For married older adults, spousal caregiving is an essential part of the marital bargain. More than 80 percent of older spouses are the primary caregiver to their partner, and three-quarters of them do so without additional help.[137]

At every stage of the life course, women are more likely than men to be caregivers. Women, even those with full-time jobs, are more likely than men to tuck their children into bed, wash their clothes, wipe their noses, and drive them to doctors' appointments.[138] Men and women follow these gendered patterns throughout their lives, and they converge only among the oldest-old. Although men provide care to their ailing wives and parents, women disproportionately bear the brunt of caregiving work. Women dedicate more hours per week to the care recipient and provide care for longer time periods. According to recent estimates, women spend an average of 6.1 years—nearly 10 percent of their adult lives—in caregiving activities, whereas men spend just 4.1 years, or 7 percent of their adult lives, providing care to others.[139]

The specific caregiving tasks performed also vary by gender, with women taking on the most time-intensive and physically and emotionally draining tasks. Researchers classify caregiving tasks into assistance with activities of daily living (ADLs) and instrumental activities of daily living (IADLs). The former includes help with the most basic activities that need to be accomplished each day, like walking, bathing, dressing, toileting, brushing teeth, and eating. The latter includes more complex activities that enable the patient to lead a full and independent life, such as cooking, driving, using the telephone or computer, shopping, keeping track of bills and finances, and managing daily medication regimes.[140] Women are more likely than men to provide help with both sets of tasks, although the gender gap is a bit narrower for IADLs. That is another reason why midlife and retirement-age women are more likely than men to drop out of the paid workforce when they are providing care: tasks like feeding and bathing must be done every day and cannot be neglected, whereas tasks like paying bills are less frequent and urgent. Caregiving in later life, like providing child care in young adulthood, is a key reason why women earn less during their working lives, leading to a reduction in their Social Security benefits and pension wealth, as well as an increased risk of late-life poverty, especially after being widowed.[141]

Less is known about race, ethnic, and SES differences in caregiving, yet data generally show that older blacks and Latinos invest more time in caregiving than whites. One analysis of 116 studies of racial differences in caregiving found that blacks were more likely than whites to help with ADLs, although no differences were detected for IADLs.[142] Part of the reason is that blacks, on average, suffer more numerous, more frequent, and earlier onset health problems than their white counterparts. As a result, their family members and friends often are pulled into caregiving at younger ages and thus help their ailing loved ones with basic daily tasks for long stretches of time.

Yet broad explorations of racial differences conceal more complex patterns of intersectionality, with race, gender, and marital status together shaping caregiving experiences. One study found that older black and white men are equally likely to provide care for an aging parent, yet black women are much more likely than white women to provide this care. This gap is largely due to marital status differentials. Older black women are less likely than white women to be married, so they spend less time in spousal caregiving and more time in parent caregiving, which is particularly demanding given a parent's advanced age.[143]

Race and ethnicity affect more than just for whom or for how long one provides care; they also shape the lived experience of caregiving, reflecting cultural differences in how older adults think about providing care. Social gerontologists have observed a "cultural justification for caregiving," or the belief that providing care to loved ones is an essential part of a person's role as a family member.[144] That is one explanation offered for why older blacks are less likely than whites to say that they feel burdened by providing care; they adhere more strongly to the cultural justification belief.[145] In this worldview, caregiving is not viewed as punishment but rather as a way for younger family members to show love and gratitude to those in the family upon whom they relied when growing up.

Yet the cultural expectation to provide care also poses challenges for older adults, especially Latinos. Older Latinos are more likely to provide care to aging family members than whites are, and they are reluctant to rely on institutional care. To put one's elderly parent or spouse "in a home" would be seen as shirking one's duty as a devoted son, daughter, or spouse—a concern that is especially deeply felt in immigrant families.[146] Older Mexican American women in particular are socialized into the gender role of *marianismo*, which emphasizes traits like femininity, duty, and a sense of responsibility to one's family. One recent qualitative study of forty-four older Mexican American women caregivers in Southern California found that, even though they dedicated themselves to time-intensive family caregiving, upholding the value of *marianismo*, at the same time many found this sense of duty to be draining and overwhelming. A caregiver named Luz Maria explained why she provided care to her mother, despite its intrusion on her other activities and goals: "It's an obligation that I feel that I alone have to do for my mother. . . . Like the Ten Commandments indicate, you must obey your father and mother so that you live a good life. So I am doing this." Another caregiver admitted, "I don't have a life. My parents have consumed my life. I can't go [out] at the drop of a hat. I had my freedom [but] I have no freedom [now]."[147] These competing feelings of dutiful obligation and entrapment partly account for the disproportionately high number of depressive symptoms reported by older Latina caregivers.[148]

Only a handful of studies explore socioeconomic-status differences in caregiving, yet the emerging consensus is that older adults with less education, less income, and poorer-quality jobs are more likely to provide all types of care, to do so for longer hours, and to carry out these tasks for longer periods of time. Older adults with limited financial resources often cannot pay for home health aides or the high costs of nursing home and assisted living facility supports.[149] For older adults who are still in the workforce, juggling low-wage work and caregiving is difficult if not impossible. Workers earning an hourly wage lose their pay when they take time off to provide family care. They also are unlikely to have flexible schedules, sick leave, family leave, paid vacation days, or other benefits that might help lessen the load of caregiving. For many of these older workers, there is only one way to resolve the juggling act between paid work and caregiving—quitting work and dedicating their hours to unpaid family care, which further threatens their financial stability.[150]

The Impact of Caregiving on Health and Well-being Caregiving affects nearly every aspect of older adults' lives. Older workers are more likely to stop working or to reduce their work hours so that they can fulfill their caregiving responsibilities. The time spent on caregiving also reduces (or eliminates) the time spent on other meaningful activities that older adults look forward to in their retirement years, such as visiting with friends and family, volunteering, attending religious services, traveling, and social activities like going to the movies.[151] The chronic stress of caregiving takes short- and long-term tolls on physical, emotional, and economic well-being and also can amplify the health declines that are a part of normal aging. Older caregivers are more likely than noncaregivers to report depression and anxiety, poorer self-rated health, more sleep problems and fatigue, appetite loss, weight loss, and greater risk of cardiovascular disease and death.[152] Caregiving takes an especially profound toll on those who perceive their experience as stressful; older caregivers who report high levels of psychological strain have mortality rates 50 percent higher than rates for their counterparts who do not describe their caregiving as distressing.[153]

Most studies show that caregiving is more harmful to older adults' physical health than their emotional health, for three main reasons. First, caregiving may impede positive health behaviors and increase negative ones. Caregivers have scarce time to exercise, sit down to a healthy meal, sleep eight hours a night, take needed medications, or seek care for their own health concerns.[154] Many aged caregivers neglect or minimize their own health concerns, which they may view as less important than the health concerns of the care recipient. One study of dementia caregivers found that nearly one-third neglected to take their own medications, and half did not keep their own doctors' appointments.[155] Some stressed-out older caregivers may cope by turning to cigarettes, alcohol, or unhealthy comfort foods. Each of these behaviors, in turn, renders one susceptible to other symptoms and illnesses.

Second, caregiving tasks can be physically strenuous at any age, increasing one's risk of musculoskeletal injuries, backaches, muscle strain, scrapes, and bruises. Yet these strains are especially damaging among older adults who are already experiencing health declines (especially among oldest-old caregivers, as discussed later). A slender woman lifting her husband out of bed puts her own health at risk, as does an arthritic caregiver constantly bending and reaching in order to clean house or prepare meals. These hazards are intensified for those of limited means, whose run-down homes may present added risks. Homes or apartments with very small rooms, clutter, uneven floors and stairs, cracked sidewalks, and tubs and toilets without grab bars put caregivers at risk of falls or other dangerous mishaps.[156]

Third, many caregivers derive a genuine sense of purpose, competence, and emotional closeness that helps to counterbalance or even overshadow the emotional distress that can accompany chronic stressors like caregiving. The caregiving expert Richard Schulz has written widely on the positive aspects of caregiving, noting that many older adults derive a sense of purpose from caregiving, and others even develop a sense of mastery as they learn and apply new skills.[157] One recent analysis of the National Survey of Caregivers (NSOC) found that more than half reported an increase in their ability to deal with difficult situations with an accompanying boost to their self-confidence.[158] Caregivers also report a sense of personal gratification and appreciate the opportunity to "give back to" their loved one for all the support they received in the past. Some studies show that men report greater benefits than women, as well as a more profound sense of growth. Because of their larger size and lower risk of arthritis, men tend to suffer fewer injuries or aches from the physical aspects of caregiving, like lifting up or carrying the care recipient. Additionally, current cohorts of older men often were socialized to be very "results-oriented," and they derive a sense of accomplishment from their daily caregiving tasks. Men who are caregivers also may attract more praise and support from others, because men typically are not expected to be caregivers.[159]

High-Risk Caregiving The personal impacts of caregiving, like any other chronic stressor, vary based on specific aspects of the experience. Three subgroups of older caregivers may be particularly depleted (and least rewarded) by their experience: oldest-old caregivers, "reluctant" caregivers who have strained or tenuous relationships with the care recipient, and dementia caregivers. For each of these rapidly growing subgroups, caregiving rewards may be few and far between, and the harmful effects on their bodies and psyches may be overwhelming.

Older adults age seventy-five and older are one of the most rapidly growing groups of caregivers in the United States. According to the National Caregiving Alliance, more than three million adults age seventy-five and older are now helping their loved ones with daily ADL and IADL tasks and providing increasingly difficult medical and nursing care at home.[160] About half are caring for a spouse, while most others are caring for their siblings, friends, or neighbors. Just 8 percent are caring for their superannuated parents. These numbers are expected to rise even higher in future cohorts as more adults survive into their eighties, nineties, and beyond.

Caregiving is particularly hard for very old adults for several reasons. First, caregiving is not a short-term or fleeting task for them. Because the people they are caring for are also, on average, very old, the care recipient's needs are particularly high. The typical caregiver age seventy-five or older has been in his or her role for nearly six years, spending an average of thirty-four hours per week on care—ten hours more per week than younger caregivers. That is just one hour short of a full-time job. Those caring for a spouse are essentially a live-in care provider who is on call 24/7. Those providing round-the-clock care have more sleep problems and less regular mealtimes. They may skimp on the nutritious meals that they once shared with their spouse, and they are less likely to tend to their own health concerns. Older caregivers also have fewer financial and social resources than their younger or working-age counterparts. Most older adults are living on limited incomes and their assets dwindle with time, so these senior caregivers are less likely than their younger (or employed) counterparts to have the means to pay for assistance. Very old caregivers also have fewer unpaid helpers; the friends and siblings to whom they might otherwise turn also are very old and may be too ill to pitch in.[161]

Second, the most senior caregivers are grappling with severe health problems of their own. Because most caregivers, especially very senior caregivers, are women, they may struggle with the physical demands of providing care. Walking up and down the stairs carrying meals to their loved one's bedroom, lifting him or her, and helping with toileting, bathing, and showering can be particularly difficult for a small or physically frail septuagenarian or octogenarian. For the oldest-old caregivers, the physical strains of caregiving are exacerbated by their impaired sense of balance, limited motion due to arthritis, and weakness due to age-related changes in muscle mass.[162]

An older adult's relationship with the care recipient also shapes whether he or she experiences distress or emotional uplift. Despite compelling data on the positive aspects of caregiving, emerging research suggests that those emotional rewards are hard to come by for older adults caring for family members who were unkind, abusive, or distant earlier in their lives. A fascinating analysis of Wisconsin Longitudinal Study data by the sociologists Jooyoung Kong and Sara Moorman delved into the caregiving experiences of older adults whose now-dependent parent had been abusive earlier in life.[163] Overall, caregivers had more physical and mental health symptoms like insomnia, trouble concentrating, sadness, and lethargy relative to their peers who were not caregivers. Yet these harmful effects were much stronger among those caring for a parent (typically a mother) who had been abusive or neglectful roughly fifty years earlier, when the caregiver was an adolescent.

Caregiving hurts most when one resents the care recipient. Practitioners refer to these older adults as "reluctant caregivers"—they experience stress, resentment, and anger at caregiving rather than feelings of closeness and warmth. Others experience guilt over these feelings of resentment yet cannot divulge their ambivalent feelings for fear of being a "bad" son, daughter, or spouse; the silence can then compound the distress triggered by the caregiving burden.[164] A *New York Times* article on these reluctant caregivers elicited more than a hundred emotionally charged comments, mostly from older adults describing how they tried for decades, often unsuccessfully, to reconcile their lingering hurt with their sense of obligation to their abusive family member. As one poster poignantly shared, "I had a mother no one would want. I took care of her by providing others to care for her, and limiting my exposure to her to what I could bear. And cutting short visits when she was unpleasant. . . . When she died, I watched and was sorry for her miserable life."[165]

Caregiving is also particularly difficult when the care recipient is suffering from dementia. An estimated 15 million Americans, mostly older adults themselves, are caring for a loved one with dementia. The challenges are immense and persistent. The average length of time a patient lives with Alzheimer's disease or severe dementia is about seven years, yet some patients live as many as twenty years with the condition, making it the quintessential chronic stressor for their caregivers. Dementia patients may become agitated and verbally or physically aggressive toward their caregivers. As their mental capacities diminish, they may leave the burners on the gas stove turned up and then walk away, or they may wander outside of the family home without warning, triggering panic in their caregivers. Others may yell, bite, throw things, curse, or behave in a sexually inappropriate way. Some may sit still as if in a coma, registering barely any eye movement, causing their caregivers to harbor guilty thoughts like, *Maybe he'd be better off dead.*

The strains of caring for a dementia patient may push an older caregiver to act in an overly aggressive manner toward their loved one. While this does occur, the much more common phenomenon is that the dementia patient's symptoms and reactions do harm to the caregiver. The most common reason why dementia caregivers decide to place their loved one in a nursing home is that they can no longer handle the role of caregiver and are fearful for their own safety. For instance, one Montana resident told the *New York Times* that since her husband was diagnosed with Alzheimer's disease three years earlier, he had started to become more angry and irritable, often sleeping with a loaded gun. Similarly, octogenarian Long Island resident Phyllis Edelstein became worried when her retired dentist husband Richard began to lash out at and strike people. When he jumped up and lunged toward the television one afternoon, in an effort to fight with the "bad guy" on the screen, Phyllis knew she had no choice but to place her once mild-mannered husband into a nursing care facility.[166]

Given the intense emotional and physical strains of dementia caregiving, it is not surprising that these caregivers have more physical, cognitive, and mental health problems and an elevated mortality risk relative to their counterparts who are providing care to loved ones suffering from other types of illness. An estimated 60 percent of dementia caregivers rate their emotional stress as high or very high, and 40 percent suffer from depressive symptoms. One reason for the poor health of dementia caregivers is that the experience can be all-consuming: they spend significantly more hours per week providing care than nondementia caregivers do, they have elevated out-of-pocket costs for health care, and they report greater impacts on their everyday life in terms of employment complications, less time for leisure and self-care, and more conflicts with family members.[167] Perhaps most importantly, dementia caregivers often neglect their own symptoms and health care concerns because they feel that their aches and pains are inconsequential in comparison to what their loved one is experiencing. Fully three-quarters of dementia caregivers say that they are concerned about their own health, and as many as 20 percent have cut back on or missed their own doctor's appointments because they could not get away from their caregiving duties.[168]

The psychological strains associated with dementia caregiving are profound, regardless of the caregiver's race, gender, and socioeconomic status. Yet this toll is buffered somewhat for those with greater economic resources, who can afford to place their loved one in a special memory care facility. African Americans find some solace in their religious beliefs and are buoyed somewhat by their feelings of obligation and devotion to their families. Yet dementia caregiving, and caregiving more generally, is and will continue to be a stressor that afflicts millions of older adults and requires public resources to help protect beleaguered caregivers. Federally funded programs like the National Family Caregiver Support Program and the Lifespan Respite Care Act provide resources to states to help family caregivers by increasing the availability of respite care, supporting caregiver education and training, and offering additional services like local support groups and home modifications. These programs are significantly underfunded, however, and their future is uncertain.[169] The reauthorization of the Lifespan Respite Care Act was introduced in May 2017, yet further action has not yet been taken.[170] Additionally, states vary widely in the resources that they offer Medicaid beneficiaries to help pay for family caregivers to assist their aging relatives.

New policies are continually evolving to address caregiver needs.[171] In May 2017, the bipartisan bill called Credit for Caring Act was introduced, with the goal of helping caregivers stay in the workforce and have greater financial stability. The legislation would provide a nonrefundable federal tax credit of up to $3,000 for eligible family caregivers who work and use their own money to help care for a loved one. Although the future of this bill is uncertain, policymakers from both sides of the aisle agree that some forms of public support for caregivers will become increasingly important as the large cohort of baby boomers reach old age, a serious public health concern revisited in chapter 9.[172]

Good social relationships—including loving marriages, supportive children, devoted grandchildren, rich friendships, and even casual ties to neighbors and service providers—are essential sources of happiness, connectedness, and concrete support in older adults' lives. At the same time, social relationships also can be a source of strain, demands, and even physical harm, especially among the most vulnerable older adults. Social ties, from the most intimate to the most casual, are a critical mechanism contributing to disparities in older adults' well-being. Lower-income persons and blacks are less likely to marry and stay married, and as a result they may be deprived of an important source of economic, practical, and emotional support. At the same time, they also are more likely to find themselves in demanding family situations like custodial grandparenting or doing intensive caregiving. Other stressful aspects of social relationships like abuse and mistreatment are especially likely to befall those who already are the most physically frail and socially isolated. In these ways, social ties are both a product of and perpetuator of social disparities.

Chapter 7

The Home Front: Residential and Community Experiences of Older Adults

At the Mather, a senior community of luxury condominiums in the tony Chicago suburb of Evanston, Illinois, residents savor meals of free-range chicken, house-made gelato, and other gourmet dishes prepared by the facility's three-star chef. At the nearby Montgomery Place Continuing Care Retirement Community in Chicago's Hyde Park neighborhood, residents enjoy amenities like an herb garden, a weekly farmers' market, a heated indoor pool, and an arts and crafts studio—an atmosphere that makes Montgomery Place feel more like an Ivy League college campus than an urban retirement community.[1] Married couples take evening strolls on the pristine grounds, while widows and widowers enjoy the company of their neighbors at activities like movie nights, lectures, and group outings to local museums.

Just a few miles away from the bucolic settings of the Mather and Montgomery Place sit run-down apartment buildings and public housing projects in some of Chicago's poorest neighborhoods, like North Lawndale. Many older adults—most of them African American, and many of them living alone—call these dilapidated high-rise buildings "home."[2] With unpredictable heating, ventilation, and air conditioning (HVAC) systems, and malfunctioning elevators, these apartments were the site of a horrific public health crisis that struck during the swelteringly hot month of July 1995: an estimated 520 older adults died of heat-related conditions.

Where, with whom, and how comfortably older adults live vary dramatically as a consequence of both earlier experiences—including wealth accumulation, residential discrimination, and social ties—and macroeconomic factors that make some regions more or less desirable and resource-rich. In this chapter, I describe the living arrangements of older adults, the roots and personal consequences of such arrangements, and the impact of older adults' homes and neighborhoods on their health, well-being, and social integration. I begin with an overview of older adults' living arrangements, such as whether they live in their own home or apartment, an assisted living facility, or a nursing home, and I highlight the ways in which their personal resources and public policies guide these arrangements. I then describe four aspects of place that are powerful mechanisms through which disparities in older adults' health, mobility, independence, and social participation are sustained and exacerbated: compositional factors, meaning who lives in their neighborhood; physical aspects of the built environment; crime and neighborhood disorder; and vulnerability to disasters. Finally, I provide a glimpse into the lives of those who have fallen through the cracks—older adults who are living on the streets, in a shelter, or in prison. Their lives provide a chilling example of how cumulative disadvantages over the life course can rob older adults of their health, well-being, safety, and dignity.

This chapter shows that community is essential to older adults' well-being. Some regions provide top-notch resources, amenities, and social services, whereas others fail to provide the basic services that older adults need to age comfortably in the space they have long called home. In these complex and varied ways, where older adults live is both a consequence of and a powerful engine driving social inequalities.

Defining Home: Where Older Adults Live

A common stereotype in the United States is that selfish and ungrateful adult children callously dump their aging parents into nursing homes when they are too old or frail to care for themselves. That stereotype flies in the face of data showing that nearly all older adults live in their own homes or apartments up until very advanced ages, when they require services and supports that outstrip what their family members and caregivers are capable of providing. Nearly all (98 percent) adults age sixty-five to seventy-four live in the community—meaning in an independent home or apartment. That proportion declines with age, yet even among the oldest-old, those age eighty-five and up, independent living is the most common housing arrangement. As figure 7.1 shows, 93 percent of those age seventy-five to eighty-four and 77 percent of those age eighty-five and older live on their own. Living "on one's own" does not necessarily mean living alone, nor does it always mean being wholly self-sufficient. It simply means that these older adults live in a home in the community, some residing with their spouse or an adult child, and

Figure 7.1 Older Adults Living in Long-Term Care, Community Housing with Services, or Traditional Community, by Age Group, 2013

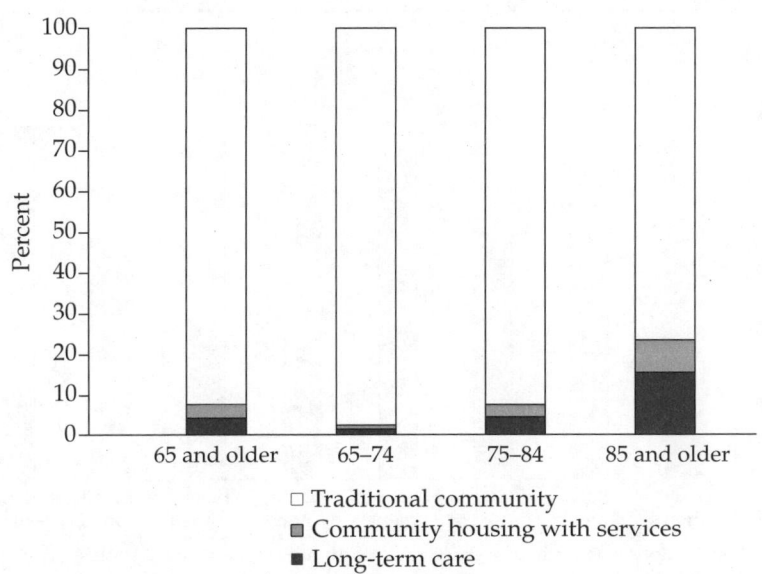

□ Traditional community
▨ Community housing with services
■ Long-term care

Source: Federal Interagency Forum on Aging-Related Statistics 2016.
Note: Older adults who live in "community housing with services" live in a retirement community or apartment, senior housing, a continuing care retirement community (CCRC), an assisted living facility, a board and care facility, or a similar setting, and they also report that they had access to one or more services such as meal preparation, housekeeping services, or medication assistance. "Long-term care facilities" refers to residences that are certified by Medicare or Medicaid; to facilities that have three or more beds, are licensed as nursing homes, and provide at least one personal service; or to the provision of round-the-clock supervision by a nonfamily paid caregiver.

some receiving at least some help from family, paid caregivers, or community services like Meals on Wheels.[3] However, women, and especially women of color, are roughly twice as likely as men to live alone (36 versus 20 percent), reflecting the race and gender patterns of family structure described in chapter 6 (see figure 7.2).

Older adults who dread the thought of living long-term in an institution will seldom have that fear realized. Although half of older adults will spend at least some time in a skilled nursing facility, most will do so either in a short-term stint for rehabilitation or during the final days or weeks of their lives; roughly 20 percent of older adults die in a nursing facility.[4] Even among the oldest-old, however, only 23 percent live in an institution for extended periods. Physical health matters more than age for residential arrangements; two-third of adults age sixty-five

Figure 7.2 Adults Age Sixty-Five and Older Living Alone, with Nonrelatives, with Other Relatives, or with a Spouse, by Age and Sex, 2014

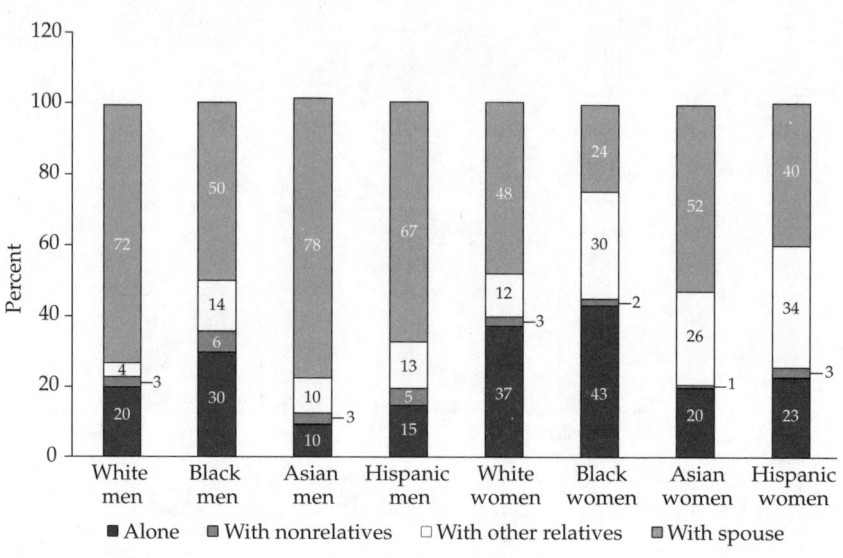

Source: Gibbs et al. 2012.
Note: "Living with other relatives" indicates that no spouse is present. "Living with nonrelatives" indicates that no spouse or other relatives are present.

and older with three or more ADL limitations live in a long-term care setting.[5]

The term "nursing home" is used colloquially to describe institutional living, although institutional living is actually a broad category encompassing several different settings. An estimated 3 percent of all older adults (and 8 percent of those age eighty-five and older) live in a residential community that feels like a private home yet also offers amenities like meals, laundry service, and assistance with medications. These communities include assisted living facilities (ALFs) and continuing care retirement communities (CCRCs). Many are designed to look like private homes, with elegant living rooms, pianos for weekly recitals, artwork decorating the hallways, beauty parlors, and manicure services.

Another 4 percent of those age sixty-five and older (and 15 percent of the oldest-old) live in long-term care facilities, which include nursing homes. Nursing homes fall along a continuum, from those that feel like an antiseptic hospital to others designed to look and feel as much like home as possible. What makes long-term care different from community housing with services, such as ALFs, is simply the level of services provided. Long-term care facilities typically provide twenty-four-hour, seven-day-a-week supervision because their residents are older or have more intensive medical needs. These facilities may include a special wing for dementia patients, often described euphemistically as "memory care" homes.

No single residential arrangement is ideal for older adults. Rather, the quality of their experiences living in their own homes, long-term care facilities, or community housing varies based on their economic resources, physical capacities, and social ties. Although most older adults desperately want to remain in their own home, this experience can be isolating and even hazardous for those who lack the social ties and physical accommodations that help them to thrive on their own. And even the most sterile nursing home can provide high-quality, attentive, patient-centered care and a sense of community for residents.

On One's Own: Living Independently in the Community

Living independently in their own home or apartment has long been considered older adults' most desirable housing option, as it enables them to age in place. "Aging in place" refers to the capacity to live in one's own home and community safely, independently, and comfortably. An estimated 90 percent of older adults say that they want to remain in their own home or apartment, where they have memories of raising their children and sharing family dinners.[6] They also want to remain in their community, where they have long-established routines like grocery store visits and morning walks with friends. Home and hearth are important sources of stability in later life, when unsettling events like retirement, the deaths of friends and family, and new health problems may create a sense of personal turmoil and uncertainty. Among adults age sixty-five to seventy-nine, roughly half have lived in their home for more than twenty years, and another 25 percent have lived there for ten to twenty years. Among those age eighty-five and older, 60 percent have lived in the same house for more than twenty years, and another 20 percent have lived in their home for ten to twenty years.[7] Such deep roots can be difficult to pull up for an older adult faced with the prospect of moving.

The phrase "living on one's own" is a bit deceptive because fewer than half of older adults residing in the community actually live alone, although this proportion creeps up with age. By age eighty, 60 percent of older adults live alone, and three-quarters of these solo-dwellers are women, reflecting their tendency to outlive their husbands.[8] Living in one's own home, whether alone or with a spouse, is desirable for many reasons. It can provide a sense of autonomy and independence for physically and cognitively healthy older adults. Decisions about what to eat for dinner, what time to wake up, what to watch on television, and how to arrange the living room furniture are truly one's own. And the personal possessions that fill an older adult's home are more than just "things"—they embody his or her identity and personal history. As Jane E. Brody wrote in a *New York Times* column, the most difficult part of leaving her home for an assisted living facility would be "relinquishing my independence and the incredible number of treasures I've amassed over the last half century. The junk would be easy, but parting with the works of art and mementos would be like cutting out my heart."[9]

Despite these many benefits, gerontologists caution that aging in place is not a guaranteed path to a happy, healthy, and autonomous old age. Rather, aging in place is desirable only when an older adult's home and community provide the accommodations and resources that enable him or her to live safely. A stately center hall colonial with slippery hardwood floors, loose area rugs, a grand curved staircase, and an elegant clawfoot bathtub is not ideal for an older adult with mobility problems. A run-down apartment with cracked bathroom tiles, dim lighting, or a broken hand railing on the front steps can be hazardous for a resident with an unsteady gait. Falls are a major public health concern for older adults. One in four older adults fall each year, and roughly 20 percent of those who fall sustain a major injury such as a broken bone or head trauma.[10] Experts say that 95 percent of older adults' hip fractures are the result of falls.[11] Falls are not due solely to environmental factors. Health conditions, including lower body weakness, dizziness, poor vision, and sharp or sudden drops in blood pressure, make people vulnerable to falls and balance issues. In addition, unsafe housing conditions can exacerbate the risks imposed by preexisting health conditions.

To age safely and well, private apartments and homes (especially multistory homes) need innovative design features or renovations to preserve older adults' security and independence. The wish list generated by gerontologists includes wide doorways to accommodate a walker or wheelchair, slip-resistant floors, lever-style door knobs and faucets because round knobs are difficult for arthritic hands to grasp and turn, remotely controlled lighting, walk-in showers, secure railings, smooth ramps, and (for the relatively few who can afford it) wheelchair lifts. Besides these accommodations to enhance mobility-related safety, other adaptations are needed for personal safety and peace of mind. Desirable amenities might include a twenty-four-hour help system, a mobile phone, surveillance cameras, and even GPS locators that help family members remotely track the whereabouts of their loved one.[12]

These adaptations are critical to older adults' physical health and security, but emerging evidence suggests that physical accommodations also are essential to older adults' social engagement and integration. A fascinating study based on National Health and Aging Trends (NHATS) data found that 6 percent of older adults living in their own homes are homebound, meaning that they rarely or never leave their homes. In raw numbers, that's 2 million older adults who do not leave their homes, compared to just 1.4 million who live in nursing homes. When the definition of "homebound" is expanded to include the semi-homebound— those who can leave their home only with great difficulty or with the assistance of another person—the ranks swell to 8 million.[13] Homebound older adults are particularly likely to suffer from physical or mental health conditions, including memory loss, dementia, and depression, to be poor, and to struggle with the English language, compounding their feelings of isolation.[14]

Design and environmental factors also compound an older adult's chances of being homebound. Stairs are one of the biggest impediments. An estimated 40 percent of homes in the Northeast, where housing stock is older, have no bathroom or bedroom on the first floor. Older adults living in run-down apartments with unreliable elevators cannot risk walking down several flights of stairs to leave their building. As a result, these older adults limit the amount of time they spend going downstairs, never mind going outside.[15] It is not surprising, then, that another analysis of the NHATS data found that assisted living facility residents left their homes more often than those living in the community.[16] Assisted living facilities provide supports like ramps, nursing aides, ride services, and single-level floor plans that help older adults leave their homes and participate in the larger social world.

Older adults from all rungs on the socioeconomic ladder struggle with aging in place, although the nature of those struggles varies. Wealthier older adults have the means to hire personal assistants and ride services, and they can afford to retrofit and make at least some structural changes to their homes. Yet they also tend to own larger houses that are physically difficult to navigate, and their larger lots and yards keep them at greater distances from neighbors than is the case for those living in smaller homes or apartments. Especially for those living alone, a cry for help may go unheard. Low-income older adults, by contrast, tend to live in poorer-quality housing situated in more run-down neighborhoods with not only a greater risk of crime, pollution, and other environmental hazards but also a greater vulnerability to threats of disaster, ranging from fires to hurricanes. At least some of the daily challenges faced by low-income older adults, however, are now mitigated by public programs offering home- and community-based services (HCBS) to those who are Medicaid-eligible.

HCBS encompasses services like homemaking and home health aides, personal care assistance, and day and residential habilitation services. Many state Medicaid programs have been investing more heavily in HCBS services over the past two decades, as these home-based services are seen as a desirable alternative to institutional care. Mounting evidence shows that increased spending on HCBS is linked with lower rates of nursing home use among older adults receiving Medicaid.[17] Although this is largely good news for those who can remain in their homes with some assistance, the shift of Medicaid funding away from nursing homes may create challenges for the frailest older adults or for those who live in subpar housing and would struggle to remain alone in their home. As I discuss later in this chapter, older adults, especially those of limited means, may not receive the skilled nursing care they need, especially if the medical requirements to receive Medicaid-covered long-term care grow more stringent as a way to curb program spending. A further concern is that nearly all HCBS beneficiaries receive services via a waiver, so there is no guarantee that an older adult will receive those services in the event of major policy or funding shifts. In sharp contrast, Medicaid coverage of long-term care is considered an entitlement, meaning that the government is required to provide these services to eligible older adults.[18]

Middle-income older adults, many experts argue, are caught in the most difficult position. Because they are not eligible for Medicaid benefits, they do not have access to HCBS programs. At the same time, most cannot afford the expense of paid help. To fill this gap, new community-based innovations have developed over the past decade. Gerontologists believe that one of the most promising is the "Villages" programs, designed to help older adults age in place. This initiative started in Boston in 2002 with the philosophy of "neighbors helping neighbors." Nearly 250 programs now exist throughout the United States, with another 125 sites under development. Although most are in urban or suburban regions, just over 20 percent of the sites are in rural areas, an important advance given particularly high rates of isolation among rural older adults.[19]

Villages programs are structured as community-based membership organizations through which volunteers and paid staff assist older residents with services such as transportation, technology training, home repairs, and grocery shopping. One Villages program in Washington, D.C., offers its members a volunteer note-taker who joins them on visits to the doctor, providing a second set of eyes and ears to absorb new information about diagnoses and medications.[20] In some communities, members receive other perks like discounted health and wellness services or referrals to health care providers. Rather than segregating older adults into age-based communities, Villages programs allow older adults to remain in their own home and have services brought to their door. Members pay modest annual dues of $500 to $1,000 on average, but those eligible for a needs-based discount may pay as little as $25 to $100 per year.[21] Evaluation studies find that participation in the Villages program improves quality of life, sustains social engagement, assists older adults (especially those living alone) as they transition from hospitals or rehab facilities back to their own homes, and supports daily living needs, especially transportation.[22] To some degree, however, the success of this program reflects social selection: older adults in better physical and financial health are especially likely to participate in a Villages program.

Despite their promise and escalating popularity, Villages programs are not a cure-all for the aging in place problem. The main criticism raised by policy analysts is that most participants thus far are middle-class, both because of the dues structure and because the program sites tend to be located in high- or middle-income neighborhoods. That is starting to change, however. For instance, the Office on Aging in the District of Columbia, after recognizing that most of the programs were clustered in the better-off neighborhoods, like Foggy Bottom, has awarded grants to help launch Villages programs in the city's lower-income wards.[23] Chicago's deputy commissioner for senior services also spearheaded the development of six Villages programs in lower-income neighborhoods, creatively enlisting volunteers from the community and using resources and supplies already in place in the city's nearly two dozen senior centers. Each of the six sites sets its own goals to meet local community needs, such as providing mental health services to older adults who have experienced emotional trauma caused by shootings.

Program administrators believe that the Villages and similar programs hold great promise and can meet the needs of residents from diverse economic backgrounds. At the same time, they acknowledge concerns about the financial sustainability of their programs, which are supported largely by dues, private donations, foundations, and local businesses' contribution of in-kind services like free or discounted office space.[24] However, several innovative community programs based loosely on the Villages models are developing strategies to provide services to lower-income older adults for a nominal fee, or none at all. For instance, in rural Plumas County, California, the Community Connections program charges members dues of just $10 a year and relies on volunteers sharing their skills through a time-bank model. Volunteers accrue credits in their time-bank accounts when they help members of their community, and they can use those banked credits to "pay" for assistance when they need it themselves. The model is based on the premise that everyone has skills and expertise to offer, whether preparing meals, gardening, picking up mail, or teaching computer lessons.[25] These programs enable older adults of lower income and fewer resources to participate, at the same time affirming their sense of competence, self-worth, and generativity.

Institutional Living: Aging in Assisted-Living and Long-Term Care Facilities

Institutional living gets a bad rap. Older adults plead with their children not to put them "in a home." The Gray Panther founder and aging activist Maggie Kuhn scathingly referred to senior housing facilities as "glorified playpens" that segregate older adults from the activities and social life of mainstream society. These sweeping generalizations ignore the fact that one's experience of living in an ALF or long-term care facility depends on the quality of the facility, one's relationships with staff, and whether the facility meets one's personal preferences and tastes. The term "senior living" may conjure up images of primly dressed older women playing mah-jongg, while *Lawrence Welk* reruns hum on the television. But older adults (at least those who can afford it) now have options to age in institutions that allow them to maintain their personal identities and live alongside like-minded peers. For instance, the Lillian Booth Actors Home in Englewood, New Jersey, is an assisted living and skilled nursing care facility that houses 124 former musicians, actors, writers, set designers, and even a few surviving vaudevillians. A very different crowd lives at The Escapees CARE Center in Livingston, Texas. Here older adults who are avid recreational vehicle (RV) travelers live in their own RVs, which are parked on the premises, and nursing care is brought to them there. Those who are ambulatory can take advantage of activities, classes, and social events in the main clubhouse, just as they would at a more traditional facility.

For all their appeal, these boutique assisted living facilities may simply be out of financial reach for lower- and middle-income older adults. Those of more limited means tend not to live in the newer, high-tech, beautifully decorated facilities that regularly host university lecturers and classical music recitals. Rather, they tend to live in small, older facilities that are colloquially referred to as "board and care" homes. These are no-frills homes that may serve older adults' physical needs with care and affection, but lack the luxuries that round out daily life in the higher-end homes.[26]

Continuing care retirement communities are a particularly desirable type of institutional living. To allow older adults to age in place as their symptoms intensify, CCRCs typically provide a continuum of services, starting with independent living apartments and moving up through assisted living units, skilled nursing units, and units providing intensive dementia care, all on the same campus. CCRCs are especially desirable for married couples who have very different care needs; a healthy spouse may reside in an apartment, while the other spouse is just a stone's throw away living in the dementia care wing.[27]

While arrangements like these sound ideal, the price of living in a residential long-term care community can be exorbitant. According to recent estimates, the median costs for living in a skilled nursing care facility top $90,000 per year, and costs go even higher if dementia care is involved. That figure is roughly three times the average annual income of most older adults. For spouses living in different parts of the CCRC, two different sets of fees are required. Although people have the option to purchase long-term care insurance when they are still young and healthy, only 10 percent of all older adults have done so.[28] Most middle- and working-class adults cannot afford the premiums, which average $2,000 to $3,000 per year. Those who can afford the insurance may not need it, because they typically have sufficient savings or housing wealth to pay for what long-term care they may need. Others think that they do not need long-term care insurance because they assume, often erroneously, that their children will take care of them. Finally, many believe, again erroneously, that their long-term care costs will be covered by Medicare.[29]

The fact is that Medicare does not cover long-term stays, but only very particular and time-delimited components of long-term care. For instance, Medicare will cover up to one hundred days of care in a skilled nursing facility, but only after a hospital stay of at least three days and only if the patient needs daily medical care, such as physical therapy after a knee replacement. While some medical aspects of care are covered, long-term residents without acute needs typically pay out of pocket. Low-income older adults who do not have the means to pay rely on Medicaid to cover their expenses. Yet many well-off adults ultimately rely on Medicaid as well, because most will exhaust all their savings on pricey long-term care and eventually become eligible for Medicaid. Medicaid is now the primary payer for older adults' long-term care, covering the expenses of more than 60 percent of nursing home residents at a total cost of $55 billion per year.[30] Policy analysts worry that these expenditures are not sustainable in the long term given the large cohort of aging baby boomers who will eventually need care, raising public concerns about how exactly older adults (and especially low-income older adults) will get the housing and care they need.

The intricacies of paying for long-term care and the role of public insurance are too complex to discuss at length here.[31] The most critical point is that, by federal law, Medicaid is required to cover nursing home care. Medicaid works closely with each of the fifty states to pay for their residents' long-term care costs by providing federal matching funds, with no preset limit. However, proposed cutbacks to Medicaid under the Trump administration include capping those matching funds, which would place a new and costly burden on states as they bear a larger brunt of their residents' costs. Older residents of historically poorer states like Mississippi and West Virginia may be especially vulnerable, as more than three-quarters of nursing home residents in these states (yet just 60 percent of residents nationwide) rely on Medicaid as their primary payer.[32]

State officials would ultimately decide how to cut costs, but federal slashes to Medicaid budgets would force states to make tough choices, such as lowering reimbursement rates paid to nursing homes, which could lead to cutbacks in staffing and poorer-quality care for residents.[33] Other cost-saving strategies might involve making it more difficult for people to qualify for Medicaid-covered nursing home care; in that event, more older adults struggling with health problems would have to rely on their own caregivers (or their own funds to cover their long-term care) until their condition was deemed debilitating enough to qualify for care. Still other solutions might include nursing homes requiring that residents or their family members pay for a portion of their care or placing limits on the types and duration of services that residents receive, similar to what Medicare already does. Faced with these constraints, nursing home administrators may opt to fill their beds with residents who can either pay their own way or rely on their long-term care insurance, leaving poorer adults with fewer options for residential care.[34] The well-being of frail elders may be further undermined if they opt instead to remain in their community, potentially putting themselves at particular risk of social isolation and even physical peril, especially those who live in run-down homes and neighborhoods.

Why Space and Place Matter for Older Adults

Where and with whom older adults live are highly consequential for their well-being, and what goes on beyond the confines of their own four walls—the spaces, places, and communities they inhabit—are particularly important for older adults. Comfortable, amenity-rich surroundings can lift older adults' daily mood and help them lead engaged, active, and healthy lives. Conversely, neighborhood poverty, crime, and environmental threats can be physically dangerous and emotionally demoralizing. Beyond the physical environment, what also matters are older adults' neighbors, who can either enrich or dampen their well-being. Emerging research shows that whether one lives in an age-segregated or age-integrated neighborhood can affect health and well-being in complex ways.

That neighborhoods and place affect our lives is one of the oldest discoveries of modern sociological research. The earliest studies done by the Chicago School sociologists in the early twentieth century emphasized the importance of "ecology," or those aspects of neighborhoods that affect everyday life.[35] Yet neighborhoods are especially consequential for older adults. Compared to younger people, older adults navigate a much narrower life-space—that spatial area in which a person moves about and interacts with the world. Our life-space constricts with age. Once older adults retire from the paid workforce, they spend more time in their immediate neighborhoods compared to younger people, who may commute long distances to work and for recreation. Physical mobility also declines with age, as older adults are less capable of walking or biking long distances. Older adults tend to cut back on their driving, forsaking nighttime or long-distance driving. The use of public transit also becomes difficult with advancing age; going up the steps to board a bus or down the stairs to hop a subway can be difficult for those with lower-body limitations. One recent study found that 20 percent of older adults had not left their city, town, or county in the past two months, owing in part to these mobility challenges.[36] Because their time is spent almost exclusively in the areas immediately surrounding their homes, neighborhood characteristics are an omnipresent influence on older adults' well-being.

It is not just that older adults have more intensive daily exposure to their neighborhoods; they also have longer lifetime exposure. Older adults typically have been living in their neighborhood for many years and thus have more long-lasting exposure to its sources of support or strain. For instance, longtime neighbors know each other's routines and habits and may check in if they notice that the eighty-year-old next door has not been taking her daily walks or has newspapers piling up on her front walk. Yet at the other end of the continuum, cumulative exposure to neighborhood stressors—whether noise or pollution or fear of crime—can take a significant toll on an older adult's emotional and physical health.

Because older adults spend such a large proportion of their time in the life-space surrounding their home, even a seemingly minor annoyance like honking car horns or unpleasant odors from a local factory may be a highly salient round-the-clock source of distress. And because of their more fragile physical state, older adults are more sensitive to even seemingly minor environmental nuisances. Uneven sidewalks can spell disaster for an older adult with an unsteady gait, while a traffic intersection with a blind spot can be hazardous to older drivers with waning visual acuity and slower reflexes.[37] Social scientists who study the impact of neighborhoods on older adults typically focus on four main features: population composition; physical and environmental characteristics; crime and disorder; and vulnerability to disaster and crisis.

Who Are the People in Your Neighborhood? Neighborhood Composition

One of the most frequently studied topics in neighborhoods research is whether the socioeconomic or age composition of a neighborhood affects the health, well-being, and social integration of its residents. For instance, if an older adult lives in a neighborhood where 80 percent of residents live beneath the poverty line, would her health, mobility, and feelings of safety differ from the health, mobility, and feelings of safety of a comparable older adult living in a neighborhood where just 10 percent live in poverty? Finding definitive answers to these questions is challenging because researchers need data on both an individual's personal characteristics, like socioeconomic resources, health, and feelings of safety, and area-level measures of characteristics, like neighborhood poverty.

Measures of neighborhood characteristics are calculated for a particular geographic unit that corresponds with official regions identified by the U.S. Census Bureau. One of the most commonly studied units is the census tract, which is roughly the size of a typical neighborhood and home to 2,500 to 8,000 people. Because census tracts are administratively defined regions for which the census obtains information such as the age, race, and income composition of each region's residents, they may not align with what older adults think of as their neighborhood. Studies also might use county-level indicators, which have limitations because counties can be very large and diverse. For instance, Essex County in New Jersey is home to both Newark, one of the poorest cities in the state, and Glen Ridge, one of the wealthiest.

Researchers exploring the impact of area-level compositional factors also must parse out the distinctive effects of the neighborhood versus the effects of an individual's own characteristics. Because low-income older adults tend to live in poor neighborhoods, researchers must use sophisticated statistical modeling approaches to identify whether neighborhood poverty, an older resident's own low income, or a combination of the two contributes to that resident's mobility limitations or memory problems.

Most studies focus on two main aspects of neighborhood composition: income or poverty levels, and age composition. Researchers have found that both factors are linked to older adults' health and mobility, with these patterns reflecting both social selection and causation processes. For example, the stress of living in a poor and run-down neighborhood may undermine older adults' health (causation). Conversely, unhealthy adults may not have the wherewithal to move out of a poor neighborhood (selection).

Neighborhood Characteristics

Poverty and Income Levels Older adults living in poorer neighborhoods, typically measured as the proportion living beneath the federal poverty line or below the median national household income, report more chronic health conditions, more functional limitations, poorer self-rated health, higher levels of allostatic load, and poorer cognitive functioning than their counterparts who live in wealthier neighborhoods. Studies based on HRS data find that older adults in wealthier neighborhoods are less likely to be obese, while those in poorer neighborhoods (especially women) are more likely to suffer from chronic conditions such as asthma, diabetes, cancer, arthritis, and high blood pressure.[38] These patterns persist even when residents' own socioeconomic resources are taken into account.

Neighborhood poverty undermines health in several ways. First, poorer neighborhoods tend to have a greater proportion of renters than owners and thus have higher levels of transience (frequent in-and-out movement of residents). High transience can weaken a neighborhood's cohesion and lessen the chance that longtime neighbors will look out for one another. Homeowners feel a sense of pride and community and may be more engaged than renters in trying to ensure that their neighborhood is safe and secure. Second, wealthier and more-educated residents are adept at using their social networks and power and may be particularly effective in demanding neighborhood services or fighting against changes they do not want. High concentrations of empowered and politically engaged residents may successfully demand prompt snow removal, additional stoplights at busy intersections, or speed bumps on streets where older adults walk. Third, wealthier communities have the financial means to attract and support businesses linked to health promotion, like gyms, top-notch medical centers, grocery stores, and restaurants.[39] Living in a neighborhood that provides a healthier food environment—like greater access to fruits and vegetables and fewer fast-food restaurants—is linked to residents' lower risk of high blood pressure, ischemic stroke, and other cardiovascular outcomes.[40] Wealthier neighborhoods also fare better on nearly all aspects of the built environment, from walkability to clean air to noise levels, features that can exacerbate the already powerful effects of economic factors on health.

Age Segregation: Do Birds of a Feather Flock Together? Do older adults fare better when they live in a neighborhood with other older adults? Or are they better off when their neighborhood includes more twenty-five-year-olds than seventy-five-year-olds? Over the past decade, researchers have started exploring the impacts of neighborhood age segregation, which refers to how diverse or similar a neighborhood is based on the ages of its residents. A neighborhood made up largely of dorms, frat houses, and student apartment complexes in Ann Arbor, Michigan, or Berkeley, California, would be highly age-segregated, as nearly all residents would be eighteen- to twenty-one-year-old college students. By the same token, neighborhoods like the high-rise apartments in the Bronx's Co-Op City or the one-level ranch homes in The Villages in Sumter County, Florida, are highly age-segregated because most residents are age sixty-five and older.

"Older" neighborhoods, or those regions that disproportionately house adults age sixty-five and older, have two very distinct flavors. One type of older neighborhood, like Co-Op City, is referred to as a naturally occurring retirement community, or NORC. These neighborhoods are "old" because their current residents moved in many decades earlier and never left. For instance, an apartment building that was inhabited largely by young parents in the 1950s has matured and now, sixty years later, has morphed into a NORC. NORCs, which are technically defined as neighborhoods where more than 40 percent of residents are age sixty-five and older, were not originally designed for older adults but instead have evolved naturally. For this reason, they vary in how well they can meet older residents' needs. Some NORCs are assisted by active local governments and social service providers who assemble supportive services programs (SSPs) that provide social services, health care management, education, recreation, and volunteer opportunities. More elaborate and well-funded programs might also provide adult day care, meals, transportation, home care, legal and financial advice, home safety improvements, mental health counseling, and disease management.[41]

By contrast, other NORCs, especially those in rural areas, provide little in the way of services and are desolate and lonely places to grow old. Rural areas are particularly hard hit because young people move out, seeking more lucrative or exciting opportunities elsewhere. As young adults leave, older adults account for a disproportionately larger share of the overall population. That is why rural and small-town census tracts are home to 21 percent of the overall U.S. population but 25 percent of all older adults. And twenty-one of the twenty-five "oldest" counties in the United States are classified as rural.[42] The exit of young people explains why rural states like Iowa and North Dakota and states with fading coal and steel industries like West Virginia and Pennsylvania are among the oldest states in the nation: more than 15 percent of all residents are age sixty-five and older. With dying industries, a sparse tax base, and few enticements for new businesses, financial resources to help support programs for older adults are scarce.

While NORCs are "old" because older people stay and younger people leave, other areas become "old" because older adults are moving in. A case in point is The Villages in Florida. This census-designated place began as an age-restricted community whose developer sold apartments and small ranch houses to older adults seeking warm weather and amenities like golf courses and pickleball courts. Today more than fifty thousand residents call The Villages home. In-migration to places like The Villages and the pink-and-white high-rise apartments along Palm Beach is the reason why Florida is the oldest state in the United States. Seventeen percent of Florida's residents are age sixty-five and older, and a whopping 43 percent of Sumter County, Florida, residents are of retirement age.[43]

The benefits to older adults of living in an age-segregated neighborhood are subject to debate and depend in part on the personal and public resources available in those communities. The traditional wisdom was that communities with large numbers of older adults, like The Villages, are best. A concentration of older adults provides a ready-made network of friends. Social services that assist older adults, like adult day health centers, ride services, and visiting nurse programs, are plentiful. Stores, restaurants, health care facilities, and services that cater to the needs of older adults are just a short ride away. Some argue, however, that a high concentration of older adults in a neighborhood, sequestered away from the rest of the world, is problematic. The eminent critical gerontologist Carroll Estes denounced living arrangements and social programs that "single out, stigmatize, and isolate the aged from the rest of society."[44]

Over the past decade, several dozen studies have explored the effects of neighborhood age composition on older adults' health and well-being. This work consistently shows that, after controlling for neighborhood socioeconomic status, living in communities with a large proportion of age-peers is good for older adults' physical and mental health, cognitive functioning, and social engagement.[45] The main explanation is that these neighborhoods are socially cohesive and provide access to peers who are a potential source of support. One intriguing study found that older widows and widowers living in neighborhoods with high concentrations of widow(er)s had lower mortality rates than their peers who lived in neighborhoods with lower concentrations.[46] Researchers suggest that older widow(er)s can seek support, companionship, and practical assistance from others who share and understand their situation.

Older neighborhoods also may have more ample formal support services and social programs to meet local older adults' needs.[47] One of the selling points of neighborhoods and housing developments designed explicitly to attract older residents, like The Villages, is the availability of services and amenities. NORCs also have the capacity to attract these services. Although NORCs were not originally designed as senior communities, they have matured into communities with a sufficient density of older residents to achieve the economies of scale that distinguish more traditional retirement communities. One older adult may not have the means to pay for services like home-delivered meals, personal care services, housekeeping, information and referral, and transportation services. Yet NORCs, especially those with a strong formal network of social workers and other professionals in place, can harness their bulk buying power to create and purchase services that would be otherwise unaffordable.[48]

There's No Place to Walk After Dinner: The Built Environment Chicago is home to roughly 280,000 older adults, yet it would be impossible to speak about a typical block that the Windy City's older residents call home. Even within this single city, where and how older adults live diverges dramatically across neighborhoods, which differ based on key aspects of the built environment. The social gerontologists Philippa Clarke and Linda George have observed that the built environment is distinguished by the "three Ds": housing density, diversity of land use, and design.[49] Housing density refers to the number of units in a particular geographic area. Diversity of land use refers to the mix of private homes, businesses, factories, and nonprofit organizations like churches or senior centers. These two conditions affect older adults' lives in subtle ways. Crowded neighborhoods are more susceptible to high levels of noise, traffic, and air pollution, all of which may harm older adults' physical, emotional, and cognitive health.

Design refers to aspects of a neighborhood's layout and land use, encompassing elements like walk lights at busy intersections that are long enough for older adults to safely cross the street, smooth sidewalks

Figure 7.3 Neighborhoods with Street and Sidewalk Lighting and Sidewalks, by Neighborhood Income Level, 2012

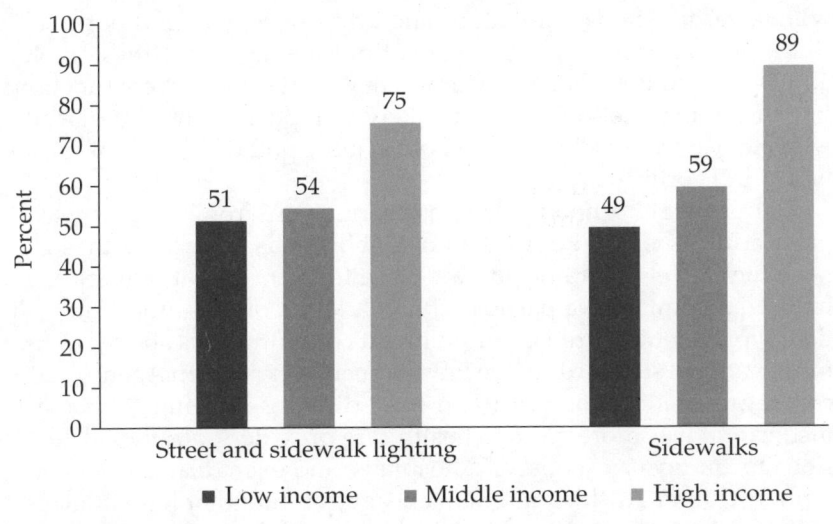

Source: Gibbs et al. 2012.

that are amenable to walkers, well-lit streets, and public ride services to local grocery stores and pharmacies. Poor neighborhoods, in particular, are plagued by threats that the human eye cannot detect: particulate matter, or the pollution generated by car exhaust and factories, can harm older adults' cardiovascular, pulmonary, and cognitive functioning.

At a minimum, the built environment can either limit or facilitate older adults' mobility and capacity to socialize. At the most extreme, however, dangerous aspects of the built environment can do harm and even hasten mortality among older adults. The threats imposed by the built environment are most extreme in poor neighborhoods, further contributing to disparities in the health and mobility of advantaged versus disadvantaged older adults. A recent study supported by the Robert Wood Johnson Foundation assessed the walkability of more than 10,000 streets in 154 communities across the United States. They found that people living in low-income communities are less likely to encounter sidewalks, clearly marked crosswalks, and traffic calming measures such as pedestrian-friendly medians, curb extensions, and traffic islands. As figure 7.3 shows, nearly 90 percent of high-income neighborhoods have safe sidewalks, compared to just half of low-income neighborhoods.[50]

A neighborhood's walkability is associated with better physical health outcomes for its older residents, even those with preexisting conditions. Walkability, typically defined as street connectivity, or having a higher number of intersections and fewer dead-end streets, is linked with fewer functional limitations and lower obesity rates. Poor-quality sidewalks can intensify the impact of preexisting disabilities on older adults' functioning. One study found that adults with severe functional impairments were four times as likely to report a mobility disability when they lived in neighborhoods with more potholes and broken sidewalks and curbs.[51]

Poorer neighborhoods also pose serious environmental threats to older adults' health. Poor urban neighborhoods, especially those that have high levels of traffic and are close to factories, oil refineries, and industrial plants, have particularly high levels of pollution. Air pollution, typically measured as air pollutant concentrations above the level of the national standards of the Environmental Protection Agency (EPA), can aggravate chronic heart and lung diseases, leading to increased medication use, more visits to health care providers, additional admissions to emergency rooms and hospitals, and even death. The demographer Jennifer Ailshire and her colleagues found that higher levels of pollution in the census tract in which older adults lived also increased their risk of poorer cognitive function.[52] These patterns were documented in two data sets, the HRS and the Americans' Changing Lives study, and were not explained away by the fact that more polluted neighborhoods tend to be poor. Pollution hurts older adults' cognitive function by taxing the cardiovascular system, which is connected to the brain through blood vessels. Cardiovascular and cerebrovascular disease, in turn, increase an older adult's risk of cognitive deficits, cognitive decline, dementia, or Alzheimer's disease pathology.[53]

It is not just physical hazards that can do harm—noise levels also matter. Noise levels, which are particularly high in lower-income urban neighborhoods and neighborhoods close to major highways, are linked with poor health outcomes, including elevated risk of heart disease, high blood pressure, and hospitalizations—even after controlling for individual characteristics like income and education. One recent study found that living in a neighborhood with average noise levels above sixty decibels (compared to average noise levels of less than fifty-five decibels) increased the risk of hospitalization by 5 percent for adults under age seventy-five, and by 9 percent among those age seventy-five and older. Living in a louder neighborhood also increased mortality risk by 4 percent.

A noise level of sixty decibels is not particularly loud—no louder than one would hear at a crowded restaurant or movie theater—yet cumulative exposure to this sound level day after day is especially consequential for older adults.⁵⁴ Exposure to noise affects the autonomic nervous system by increasing the heart rate and blood pressure. Noise can also affect the HPA (hypothalamic-pituitary-adrenal) axis, increasing cortisol, the stress hormone. All of these physiological responses, if persistent, can lead to inflammation and compromised heart health. Noise also impairs sleep, and poor sleep is linked with poor cardiovascular health.

Preying on the Vulnerable: Older Adults' Crime Victimization

Violent crimes against older adults regularly grab news headlines, in part because these crimes betray our moral beliefs that older adults should be treated with respect and dignity and that the vulnerable should not be victimized. A 2017 string of violent robberies and a sexual assault at a senior housing facility in Long Beach, California, was particularly disturbing, as the assailant preyed on older adults in their own apartments.⁵⁵ As disturbing as these reports are, they represent the exception rather than the rule. Federal crime statistics show that older adults are far less likely than younger people to be the victims of violent street crimes, including rape or sexual assault, robbery, aggravated assault, and simple assault. Between 2000 and 2013, the nonfatal violent crime victimization rate among adults age sixty-five and older was 3.6 per 1,000, just a fraction of the rate for youths age twelve to twenty-four (50 per 1,000) and young adults age twenty-five to forty-nine (28 per 1,000). Yet perceptions of crime and safety may be nearly as consequential to older adults' daily lives as actual crime rates. Perceived safety and fear of victimization are two of the main reasons why older adults, especially those living in poor neighborhoods, confine themselves to their homes.⁵⁶

Perceptions of danger also are linked to physical health and functioning, albeit indirectly. Analyses of HRS data show that older adults living in neighborhoods that they perceive to be safe are more likely to recover from a mobility limitation because they socialize with neighbors and engage in outdoor physical activity, such as taking walks and gardening, which bolsters their strength and recovery.⁵⁷ The worries and persistent feeling of peril that older adults experience in unsafe neighborhoods also take a physiological toll, which carries short- and long-term consequences for their immune function, cardiovascular health, and general well-being. Cumulative exposure to stress—including the stress of living in an unsafe neighborhood—hastens biological processes of aging such as telomere shortening.⁵⁸ Given that poorer and African American older adults are disproportionately located in neighborhoods that are either dangerous or perceived to be dangerous, neighborhood safety is yet another mechanism contributing to disparities in health and well-being over the life course.

Disaster and Its Impact on Older Adults Weathering the Storm

Hurricane Katrina devastated New Orleans and the surrounding Gulf Coast region when it struck in 2005, taking an estimated 1,800 lives. In the decade that followed, a string of natural disasters touched all corners of the United States: the Joplin, Missouri, tornados in 2011; Hurricane Sandy, which ravaged the East Coast in 2012; and a torrent of wild fires, mudslides, floods, droughts, and blizzards. The frequency and intensity of natural disasters striking the United States and worldwide escalated dramatically in the late twentieth and early twenty-first century, exemplified by the deadly hurricanes that struck Florida, Puerto Rico, and the Gulf Coast in just a three-week span in 2017. Experts predict a continuation and even heightening of these trends—an unequivocal consequence of climate change. A recent report by the United Nations' Intergovernmental Panel on Climate Change (IPCC) reported that an increase in greenhouse gases in the atmosphere is likely to boost temperatures over most land surfaces. Although climate scientists cannot predict the future with 100 percent certainty, the consensus is that rising temperatures will increase the risk of droughts, more intense storms—including rainier monsoon seasons and more aggressive tropical cyclones with faster and more dangerous wind speeds—and more frequent heat waves such as the Chicago heat wave chronicled by Eric Klinenberg.[59] Temperature increases also may give rise to melting glaciers and ice caps, which could lead to rising sea levels, making coastal flooding more severe when storms hit shore.[60]

While natural disasters and extreme temperatures have far-reaching impacts for all people, their homes, and their communities, these impacts are all the more devastating for older adults, especially those already suffering from compromised health and financial insecurity. Older adults make up 12 percent of the overall U.S. population, yet they consistently represent anywhere from one-half to three-quarters of all deaths following natural disasters like hurricanes.[61] Consider a few facts about the death tolls from the most lethal recent disasters in the United States. Roughly two-thirds of the estimated 1,800 people who died in Hurricane Katrina were age sixty-five and older. More than half of the 117 who succumbed to Hurricane Sandy were older adults. The average age of people dying of heat-related deaths during Chicago's 1999 heat wave was seventy-five.[62]

It was not simply the frailty of old age that killed these victims; most of their deaths were a direct consequence of environmental and social factors that the victims could not overcome. In Hurricane Katrina, two-thirds of older victims either drowned or died from illness or injuries brought about from being trapped in their homes, surrounded by water. The remaining one-third fell to injuries, infections, and other health conditions brought on or exacerbated by the difficult evacuation process. The physical wear-and-tear of evacuation hastened the fatal effects of preexisting health conditions like heart disease or weakened immune systems. Some frail older adults sought medical care in local hospitals that had lost power and could not provide life-sustaining treatments like oxygen.[63] A similarly bleak portrait emerged from Superstorm Sandy, most of whose victims drowned in their own homes.[64] People like eighty-five-year-old Rose Faggiano, seventy-two-year-old David Gothelf, and ninety-year-old George Stathi—all of Queens, New York—succumbed to rising water levels in their homes and could not escape in time.[65] And in 2017's Hurricane Irma, fourteen residents of a Florida nursing home between the age of seventy-one and ninety-nine died of heat-related causes after the facility's air conditioning failed.[66]

Disaster experts say that deaths occur following hurricanes and floods because local residents fail to evacuate promptly. Yet for older adults, this is less a matter of willful defiance and more a matter of an inability to comply with evacuation orders. Poor and socially isolated older adults are least capable of evacuating. Some stay put because they have nowhere to go and no one to help them move. Older adults with cognitive impairments may not fully understand the severity of the risk and may require help in making timely decisions. The notion of relocating to an area where one has no social ties and must start over again is just too much for some older adults to bear. Some cannot afford the cost of moving, and many lack the help required to relocate. In a Harris Poll, 25 percent of adults age seventy-five and older said that they would require help evacuating if required to do so, with 60 percent saying that they would need help from someone outside the household, as they lacked such a helper.[67]

Others do not want to abandon the few meager possessions they have, a legitimate concern for destitute older adults. For socially isolated elders whose main source of emotional support is a pet, evacuation to a shelter may mean a separation (often permanent) from a faithful friend, as shelters are not dog- and cat-friendly. American Red Cross emergency facilities will not accept pets because they create challenges in meeting health and safety regulations; the Red Cross makes exceptions only for the service animals of those with disabilities.[68] That is why pet owners are half as likely as those without pets to evacuate during a storm.[69]

For older adults who stay in their homes and communities, services and supports may not be readily available. During a major disaster, local medical resources like hospitals and EMT services may be overwhelmed and out-of-state assistance like disaster relief teams may face obstacles reaching remote, isolated, or frightened older adults. Pharmacies often are closed or without power, and older adults may lack the transportation, money, or assistance needed to obtain additional medications. Some older adults, especially those with cognitive impairment, immigrants, and others who have experienced mistreatment at the hands of local authorities, may distrust social service organizations and thus rebuff their offers of support.[70] For others, support services provide only a short-term fix. In Hurricane Katrina, the city of New Orleans received federal and state money that paid for buses, trucks, and trains to relocate local residents to government-funded shelters. Yet the stress of the move and uncertainty about what the future would hold after leaving the shelter kept many frail and socially isolated adults in their unsafe homes and communities.[71]

Natural disasters like Katrina may be episodic, but climate experts agree that extreme temperatures are increasingly normal conditions that are here to stay. Extreme temperatures like heat waves and long-lasting cold spells are especially harmful to older adults, who are vulnerable to hypothermia and hyperthermia. A loss of electrical power during a storm may mean the loss of air conditioning or adequate heat and also may prevent the use of necessary medical equipment, like nebulizers or home oxygen treatments.[72] Some older adults who suffer from circulatory, nervous system, or rheumatic conditions like arthritis or hardening of the arteries also are at a heightened risk of a condition called Raynaud's syndrome. When exposed to extreme cold, the small blood vessels in their hands and feet may narrow, stopping healthy blood flow. If older adults do not warm up quickly enough (or seek timely treatment), they may face amputation of a hand or foot.[73] Some older adults who lose their heat or cannot afford to pay their heating bills during a cold snap may resort to using gas stoves to warm up their homes—a dangerous decision that may lead to death from carbon monoxide poisoning. That was the tragic end for septuagenarian husband and wife James and Edna Saylor, who died in their apartment in a McKeesport, Pennsylvania, senior housing project.[74] During a long and unseasonably cold spell in early October, the couple had turned up the heat on their gas stove and opened the door to warm up their apartment when the building's heating system stopped operating properly.

Public assistance has been available to help some low-income older adults pay for their heating oil and air conditioning. In 2017, more than 7 million low-income households, 40 percent of which included an older adult, received roughly $4 billion in assistance from the Low-Income Energy Assistance Program (LIHEAP). The federally funded program, established in 1986, distributes money to the states to assist poor residents who spend a disproportionately high share of their income on heating or cooling their homes. The funds have helped older adults weatherize their homes and pay for regular heating or cooling bills. The program is not perfect: it operates on a first-come, first-served basis, leaving some out in the cold, literally. Still, it has been particularly helpful to poor older adults in the Northeast, where 80 percent of homes require costly heating oil. In 2018, the passage of the omnibus appropriations bill included continued funding for the program. Although policy analysts estimate that LIHEAP benefits average just $350 per household, this assistance is critical to older adults on fixed incomes, whose annual heating costs average $650 for gas heat and as much as $2,000 for oil heat in the winter.[75]

Through the Cracks: Aging on the Streets or in Prison

For a small yet escalating number of older adults, the later years will not be spent in a longtime family home, a retirement community in Florida, or an assisted living facility. For nearly a half-million adults age fifty-five and older, most of whom are black, come from disadvantaged economic backgrounds, or have struggled with mental illness, "home" is either the streets, a homeless shelter, or prison. Surviving on the streets or in a cell block is difficult even for the young and healthy; for older adults, these settings are particularly cruel, as they undermine one's safety, security, sense of dignity, and ultimately survival.

Aging on the Streets: Homeless Older Adults

Fans of R&B music were stunned to learn of the death of chart-topping singer Colonel Abrams, who died of diabetes-related complications at age sixty-seven on Thanksgiving Day 2016. More shocking than his death was the fact that this artist, who had once performed with Prince, died penniless and homeless on the streets of New York. According to a fund-raising webpage set up by his friends, the Colonel had fallen on hard times financially. His diabetes symptoms kept him from regular work, and the costs of medical care ate up his savings because as a freelance musician he had lacked health insurance.[76]

While the particulars of this tragedy may be unique to Colonel Abrams, in many ways his experience is fairly typical of homeless adults. It is difficult to document precisely how many older adults live on the streets or in homeless shelters in the United States, although a recent report from the U.S. Department of Housing and Urban Development (HUD) estimates that 306,000 persons over age fifty were homeless in 2014, a 20 percent increase since 2007. People age fifty and older make up one-third of all homeless adults. Depending on the particular city, as many as 80 percent of homeless older adults are African American, nearly all of whom are men.[77] Older adults who are new to the streets have often suffered a major health crisis or job loss that turned their once-stable lives upside down, while many of the long-term homeless have struggled with physical or mental health troubles for decades.

It is easy for armchair observers to ask incredulously, "How did these people end up on the streets?," but data clearly show how tenuous secure housing can be, especially for older adults living on a limited income. A study from Harvard University's Joint Center for Housing Studies found that one-third of adults over fifty, and slightly more than one-third of those over eighty, are "rent-burdened": they pay more than 30 percent of their income for housing.[78] In pricey cities like San Francisco or New York, more than half of older residents' income regularly goes to keeping a roof over their heads.[79] That leaves little money for essentials like food and medications. And if medication costs are very high, like Colonel Abrams's diabetes treatments, then monthly rent and utility bills may go unpaid.

Most homeless older adults have been living on the street for decades, victims of layoffs during the 1970s recession, the deinstitutionalization of mentally ill patients and funding cuts for mental health services during the Reagan era, cutbacks for funds for federal housing, and the crack cocaine epidemic of the 1980s. Veterans, especially from the Vietnam War, are particularly likely to be homeless, accounting for roughly 15 percent of those on the streets; many of these veterans suffered physical and mental health impairments while serving their country.[80] It is less likely for someone to become homeless in their fifties or older, but rising numbers of older adults have fallen into difficult financial straits in the years since the Great Recession of the early 2000s. Rising housing costs and declining vacancy rates in major U.S. cities like New York, Los Angeles, and San Francisco keep private housing, even dilapidated single-room occupancies (SROs), out of older adults' price range.[81] For older adults living paycheck to paycheck, a single event can be the trigger for homelessness. Job loss, a major health condition, the death of a loved one who helped foot the household bills, a house fire, a funeral, medical expenses, or a run-in with the law may be all it takes until one's meager savings disappear and the rent goes unpaid.[82]

Some supports are available for homeless older adults, although these programs may provide too little too late. Federally subsidized low-income housing projects give preference to older adults, and Social Security benefits like Supplemental Security Income for older adults and disabled persons start at age sixty-two. But housing subsidies and SSI benefits may arrive too late to improve the fates of homeless elders. Experts say the average life span for a homeless person living on the street is sixty-four years, roughly fifteen years younger than the U.S. average expectancy.[83] One fascinating study in Oakland, California, found that homeless older adults in their late fifties and early sixties had more trouble with ADLs like bathing, dressing, and eating than eighty-year-olds who had housing. They also had higher rates of cognitive and visual impairment, urinary incontinence, depression, and falls. These geriatric conditions were fairly similar across different subgroups of homeless adults, including those who camped out on the streets, moved between shelters and SROs, or occasionally crashed with family and friends. Shelters may be frightening for older adults who feel threatened by younger and more aggressive bunkmates. Family may be a source of abuse and humiliation rather than love and support. The strains of living on the streets or sleeping on a family member's floor, combined with the health problems that got them there, hasten the aging process so that homeless midlife adults and frail elders more than three decades their senior suffer in similar ways.

Graying Behind Bars: Older Adults in Prison

An unprecedented number of Americans are aging and ultimately dying behind bars. An estimated 165,000 adults age fifty-five and older are currently living in state and federal prisons, a number that has increased fivefold over the past two decades.[84] Older adults now make up roughly 10 percent of the U.S. prison population, a steep increase since 1993, when they accounted for just 3 percent. By 2030, an estimated one in three inmates will be age fifty-five or older.[85] The one-third of older prisoners serving a life sentence will almost certainly die behind bars. From a population health perspective, older prisoners may not seem a significant concern. After all, prisoners make up a tiny fraction of the overall aged population. Yet these older adults exemplify the indignities of cumulative disadvantage. Most prisoners come from economically and socially disadvantaged backgrounds, belong to ethnic minority groups, and suffer from mental illness and addictions at disproportionately high rates. Prison, like the streets, is a difficult if not impossible place to age well.

Doing time is hard for anyone, but it is especially so for older prisoners who are frail, have mobility, hearing, cognitive, and vision impairments, and suffer from chronic illnesses. Walking a long distance to the dining hall, sleeping on a thin mattress with a threadbare blanket, climbing to a top bunk, or standing for count can be a struggle for some older frail prisoners. The feelings of paranoia and confusion that are a normal part of dementia may be particularly dangerous in prison, as an ailing inmate may wander to another person's cell or provoke fights and arguments while in a state of agitation.[86] Incontinence and the need for help with dressing and toileting may be a source of embarrassment and, at worst, an invitation for victimization at the hands of predatory cellmates.[87]

For older inmates, there are two paths to prison—committing a crime as a young adult and then growing old in prison, or committing a crime later in life and being admitted as an older adult. Roughly 40 percent of older inmates today were admitted after they turned fifty-five, and nearly all had done time in the past. The other 60 percent are aging in prison, having entered years earlier and remaining in prison for long spells due to strict sentencing practices introduced in the United States in the 1970s.[88] That was precisely the time when the large cohort of baby boomers reached their teens and twenties, the ages at which criminal behavior tends to peak. Offenders who would have received short sentences, or "skid bids," in earlier eras instead found themselves locked up for decades if not life. Among the best known of these tough sentencing laws was New York's Rockefeller Drug Laws, which were implemented in the early 1970s, promptly followed by Michigan's 650-Lifer Law. These unforgiving "tough on crime" practices were widely criticized for treating drug offenses as on par with murder, and they were ultimately rolled back. Still, the damage was done, with unprecedented numbers of young adults—overwhelmingly black men—already sentenced to spending their lives behind bars.[89]

The 1990s and 2000s ushered in new policies that further fueled the growth of the older prison population. In 1995, the federal government implemented a policy commonly referred to as the "three strikes rule": courts would impose harsher sentences on those convicted of an offense if they had been previously convicted of two serious criminal offenses. The intent of these laws was to keep repeat offenders in prison and away from potential victims, but what they did was put more aging ex-cons back in jail. Older convicts who had been released from prison and were living in the community had had more time than younger people to build up long criminal records and to have two strikes under their belts already—leading some judges to dole out longer sentences for a third offense.[90] That, along with the sheer size of the baby boom cohort, is why more than four times as many prisoners age fifty-five or older were admitted to state prisons in 2013 than in 1993 (26,000 versus 6,000).

Decades of mass incarceration have subjected unprecedented numbers of older adults to aging in institutions that are designed for young men and are particularly cruel to aging minds and bodies. Human Rights Watch warns that prisons are ill equipped to provide the health care, appropriate housing, and other services that aging prisoners need.[91] Because prisons are legally responsible for providing health care to inmates, the aging of the prison population could overtax their budgets and personnel. A report from the Vera Institute for Justice estimates that older inmates make five times as many trips to health care facilities as their younger counterparts and consequently cost three to nine times as much to incarcerate.[92]

Some prison systems have no choice but to build new facilities for frail or cognitively impaired inmates. The Fishkill Correctional Facility in Dutchess County, New York, is one of just a few facilities nationwide dedicated to inmates with dementia. More facilities like Fishkill will be needed in the future, an unintended consequence of extended sentences. With one-third of older inmates and 10 percent of inmates overall serving life sentences, the need for dementia and end-of-life care in prisons will escalate in the coming decades.

Given the challenges of providing suitable housing, medical care, and security for aging inmates, some prison advocacy groups believe that older frail prisoners should be granted compassionate early release. Compassionate release is a process through which inmates become eligible for immediate early release on the grounds of extenuating circumstances. Historically the criterion for early release was dementia or terminal illness, although the Bureau of Prisons recently expanded this to include advanced age (age sixty-five or older) and being the sole possible caregiver for a family member.[93] Compassionate release is different from parole in that release is not based on a prisoner's behavior but rather on medical or humanitarian grounds. Older adults, some advocates believe, should not wither away in prison and should instead return to the community to die. Supporters of early release programs point out that recidivism rates plummet as ex-convicts reach old age.[94] The recidivism rate—the proportion returning to prison within one year after release—is nearly 50 percent for young adults yet just 3.2 percent for older adults. Once released, older inmates tend not to commit more crimes.

Despite humanitarian, logistical, and financial reasons for compassionate release, these reprieves are seldom granted. Data from the Bureau of Prisons indicate that just 312 of the 5,400 petitions submitted between 2013 and 2017 were approved, with average waits of six months. During that same period, 266 applicants died in custody.[95] The main reason petitions are denied is that "truth in sentencing" laws prohibit people with certain convictions, like sexual offenses, capital murder, or some drug offenses, from ever receiving compassionate release.[96] Both Democratic and Republican legislators have been urging the Bureau of Prisons to speed up or loosen up the process, efforts that reflect both humanitarian concerns and fears about the current and projected costs of housing and providing health care to the swelling ranks of older and ill prisoners.

Yet even if these releases were easily granted, returning to the community may provide little comfort for older convicts. Research on older prisoners' release is scarce, although the evidence generally shows that upon release, whether through compassionate leave, parole, or at the end of their sentence, some older convicts have nowhere to go. The longer one stays in prison, the more tenuous are one's social ties in the community. Family relationships are often frayed or nonexistent. Going back to work is not a realistic option for those with few marketable skills or with physical and cognitive frailties. Adapting to new technologies, from smartphones to computers to cars and public transit, can pose challenges. Some who require ongoing care cannot secure a bed at a nursing home or long-term care facility, as administrators have concerns about admitting residents with a criminal past (especially in cases of sexual assault) or with a substance abuse problem. Although social service agencies provide important transitional services, such programs require adequate federal or private funding. For these reasons, older ex-convicts often end up on the streets.

The experience of older prisoners is an extreme case, yet it powerfully demonstrates that the physical and social environments in which older adults live are both a product of cumulative (dis)advantages over the life course and a force contributing to disparities in older adults' well-being.

= Chapter 8 =

Is Death the Great Equalizer? Disparities in Dying

Theologians, poets, and scholars have proclaimed that death is "the great equalizer."[1] All people, according to scripture, "share a common destiny . . . the good and the bad, the clean and the unclean . . . will die" (Ecclesiastes 9:2–3). In "Death the Leveller," the seventeenth-century poet James Shirley observed that death erases the inequities that existed during life:

> Death lays his icy hand on kings:
> Sceptre and Crown
> Must tumble down,
> And in the dust be equal made
> With the poor crooked scythe and spade.[2]

Despite such eloquent claims about the inevitability and universality of death, it is not an egalitarian transition. At what age and of what causes a person dies are tightly tied to social, economic, and geographic (dis)advantages over the life course.

Researchers have only recently started to investigate disparities in the quality of dying among older adults. According to bioethicists, death quality encompasses many dimensions, such as whether the dying person takes their last breath at home surrounded by family and friends or alone in a hospital room. Death quality also reflects whether those final days are marked by pain versus comfort, medical care that matches rather than betrays the wishes of the dying, autonomy versus acquiescence in end-of-life decision-making, and family cooperation versus conflict. This chapter provides a historical sketch of death and dying in the United States and suggests reasons why inequalities in older adults' dying experiences are a uniquely contemporary phenomenon. I describe the core components of good versus bad deaths and show the complex ways in which these experiences are linked to markers of social inequality and public policies, especially Medicare reimbursement practices.

I also argue that while death is inevitable, a bad death is not—even for older adults whose lives have been marked by persistent disadvantage. I describe strategies and policies that may help older adults die peacefully and on their own terms. These strategies include advance care planning (ACP) and other tools, like physician orders for life-sustaining treatment (POLSTS), that convey a patient's preferences to both loved ones and health care professionals. ACP is available to all adults, in theory, yet in practice these tools are used far less often by African Americans, the poor, and socially isolated older adults than by whites, the wealthy, and socially integrated older adults.[3] This lack of ACP, in turn, renders patients less likely to receive treatments they want and more likely to receive futile, costly, and uncomfortable treatments they had hoped to avoid.

A Brief History of Dying in the United States

Death today rarely comes suddenly, quickly, or painlessly. We may cling to the dream that we will die suddenly, doing what we love, like Jane Little, an eighty-seven-year-old bassist with the Atlanta Symphony who collapsed and died while performing onstage in 2016, or seventy-year-old actor-director Orson Welles, who died suddenly of a heart attack in 1985 the morning after discussing his life's work on *The Merv Griffin Show*. Most older adults' deaths are much less dramatic and far more difficult. Of the more than 2.6 million deaths in the United States in 2016, nearly 80 percent were to adults age sixty-five and older, and most of them died of long-term chronic illness, such as heart disease, cancer, respiratory disease, stroke, Alzheimer's disease, or other diseases that slowly destroy the mind and body.[4] Older patients suffering from chronic illness may survive for months, if not years, following their initial onset of symptoms. The "living-dying interval" that follows is marked by spells of pain, breathlessness, difficulty swallowing, emotional distress, fatigue, frailty, and the gradual fading of cognitive capacities.

This modern phenomenon, where dying unfolds slowly over a protracted time period, is sometimes referred to as "the failure of success."[5] More people than ever before are surviving into their eighties, nineties, and beyond, and a very long life span is now considered a clear indicator of "success" when evaluating the health of a society. Yet a prolonged life span often is accompanied by compromised quality of life, which is widely considered an indicator of "failure." Today more adults will die slowly from aging-related conditions and be kept alive via technological interventions that are deemed futile—that is, they do not improve a patient's health, well-being, comfort, or prognosis.

Difficult, drawn-out deaths from chronic illness are a uniquely modern phenomenon. This shift in how adults die has its historical roots in the epidemiologic transition. From the eighteenth century through the early twentieth century, most deaths were caused by infectious diseases, like diphtheria and pneumonia, and struck quickly after a person fell ill. Infectious diseases were generally egalitarian, striking rich and poor, men and women, young and old.[6] Take, for example, the deaths of the founding fathers and early presidents of the United States. As Atul Gawande writes in *Being Mortal*, George Washington developed a throat infection and died the next evening.[7] John Quincy Adams, Millard Fillmore, and Andrew Johnson all died within two days of suffering strokes, while Rutherford B. Hayes died three days after his heart attack. Even those with chronic illnesses died much more quickly than their counterparts do today. Ulysses Grant was diagnosed with throat cancer and, despite treatments, died a year later. James Monroe and Andrew Jackson suffered for several months before succumbing to a condition now believed to be tuberculosis. In stark contrast, Ronald Reagan announced publicly in 1994 that he had been diagnosed with Alzheimer's disease and then suffered for ten years before dying in 2004.

The Medicalization of Death and Dying

Technological and medical advances are largely responsible for the shift from a short and swift death to a protracted dying process. Throughout the twentieth century, improved sanitation and nutrition, immunizations for communicable diseases, effective treatments for infections, and other medical advances dramatically reduced mortality rates among young people, and life expectancy increased accordingly. These trends were accompanied by an important cultural transformation: the medicalization of aging and dying. Aging and dying were once accepted as natural parts of life. Today aging is seen as something to be cured, and death as something to be staved off. The National Academy of Medicine's "Grand Challenges" program, along with the proliferation of anti-aging lotions, diets, vitamins, fitness regimens, and magazine articles with catchy titles like "Extending Life: 7 Ways to Live Past 100" and "12 Tips for a Longer Life," reflect the expectation of the contemporary cultural zeitgeist that we should search for the elusive cure for aging and death.

Medicalization influences how older adults die today in two distinct ways. First, people now die in different locations than they did in the past. In the eighteenth and nineteenth centuries, death happened at home, where family members, clergy, and community members would provide care to the dying person. In the twentieth century, by contrast, death moved from the home to hospitals and long-term care institutions, where chronically ill older adults receive high-tech medical treatments intended to increase their life span, such as ventilators and feeding tubes, as well as round-the-clock monitoring by skilled nursing professionals.[8] This highly medicalized death stands in stark contrast with the "good death" to which patients and their loved ones aspire.[9]

Second, medicalization has created a context in which dying patients and their families cede health care decisions to physicians. With the rising prestige of the medical profession in the twentieth century, patients began to believe that their doctors were authorities who should not be challenged.[10] As the Institute of Medicine (IOM) recounts, for most of the twentieth century older adults with advanced chronic illnesses "relied almost unquestioningly on their physicians' judgments regarding treatment matters, trusting that physicians would act in their patients' best interests as a matter of professional and personal ethics."[11] This tendency to go along with doctor's orders rather than assert one's own preferences or share decision-making varied by race and socioeconomic status, and that remains true today: blacks, Latinos, and older adults with lower levels of literacy and education and less ease in interacting with medical professionals are less likely to assert their own values and preferences when meeting with clinicians.[12]

For older adults today, delegating decisions to health care providers often involves acquiescing to invasive life-extending interventions, even if they would prefer less aggressive treatment. Through much of the twentieth century, medical education emphasized saving and sustaining patients' lives. As the pioneering palliative care physician and MacArthur Foundation "genius grant" recipient Diane Meier observed in the *British Medical Journal*, "medical students are taught to do things, not how to know what not to do."[13] Consistent with this training, physicians often are reluctant to withhold life-extending treatments and may shield patients from dire prognoses.[14] Telling a patient, "I'm sorry, but there's nothing more we can do," may be seen as an admission of failure. Physicians' reluctance to withhold treatment also reflects that, as human beings with emotions, they may not be ready to admit that a patient's death is imminent. Physicians who have close and warm relationships with their patients may be highly motivated to keep them alive, especially if they believe that the dying patient is not yet ready to say good-bye to his or her family.[15] More cynical interpretations are that costly and aggressive treatments are financially lucrative for health care institutions, and that fears of malpractice lawsuits impel physicians to over- versus undertreat.

Although physicians' training and professional mission support the use of life-extending treatments, national survey data show that patients want the exact opposite. In 2013, Pew Research Center surveyed more than four thousand Americans about their end-of-life treatment preferences.[16] More than 70 percent of those age sixty-five to seventy-four and 62 percent of those age seventy-five and older said that they would want their doctor to "stop treatment so they could die" if they had "a disease with no hope of improvement and were suffering a great deal of pain." Such desires to avoid life-extending treatment are consistent with accumulating evidence about the problems with many life-extending technologies. Medical researchers and practitioners alike recognize that many aggressive treatments are futile and may take an emotional, physical, and financial toll on patients and families.[17]

According to a recent estimate, one in five critical care clinicians believe that their patients receive care that is futile.[18] And while reliance on feeding tubes has declined dramatically over the past two decades, their use persists even though they do not prolong patients' lives, sometimes cause infections, and have been strongly criticized by major professional organizations, including the Alzheimer's Association.[19] The economic costs of end-of-life care also pose a substantial burden to older adults, their families, and the federal government. In 2017, an estimated 13 percent of the $1.6 trillion spent on health care overall, and one-quarter of the $675 billion in Medicare spending, was for people in their last year of life.[20] Together, the epidemiologic transition, the "failure of success," and forces of medicalization have conspired against a good death—especially for older adults who may lack social and economic power.

Attaining a Good Death

The notion of a good death may seem subjective, reflecting highly personal preferences and values, yet survey data show that most Americans share a similar vision of what a good death looks like. A research team led by Karen Steinhauser surveyed two thousand people across four different categories: seriously ill patients, recently bereaved family members, physicians, and other care providers, such as nurses and chaplains.[21] More than 90 percent of people across the four groups rated twelve out of forty-four possible death attributes as very important at the end of life. These twelve attributes reflected four broad end-of-life goals: being comfortable and free of pain; maintaining one's dignity; being knowledgeable about and prepared financially and emotionally for death; and having positive relationships with care providers. These perceptions map closely onto the Institute of Medicine's definition, which describes a good death as "free from avoidable distress and suffering for patients, families, and caregivers; in general accord with patients' and families' wishes; and reasonably consistent with clinical, cultural, and ethical standards."[22]

Approaches to Studying Inequities in Death and Dying

Is the idealized good death, marked by dignity and comfort, truly attainable? New research on death quality reveals both stark disparities and some universalities. Yet studying dying experiences is difficult and distinct from many other aspects of older adults' well-being because self-report data are seldom if ever available. In short, dead people cannot report on the care, support, and medical treatments they received at the end of life. Instead of self-reports from decedents, two main types of information are used to study death quality.

The first is interviews with proxies, or people who are knowledgeable about the dying person's end-of-life experience, typically a widow(er) or adult child. This approach also is referred to as a mortality followback method. Surveys like the Changing Lives of Older Couples (CLOC), a study of widowhood, ask widows and widowers how painful or prolonged their late spouse's death was.[23] Likewise, the National Health and Aging Trends (NHATS) survey asks proxies whether the decedent and family members were treated with dignity and respect, and whether the dying patient's personal care needs were met during the last month of life.[24]

These assessments, like most retrospective survey data on emotionally charged topics, may be affected by recall bias. Bereaved family members who are particularly grief-stricken, depressed, anxious, or carrying unresolved anger may describe the death in more critical terms, whereas those who were closely involved in caregiving may offer more positive appraisals, perhaps as a way to affirm their belief that they did all they could to help ensure a peaceful death for their loved one.[25] Methodological studies that compare reports from multiple proxies, such as spouses and children, or that compare proxy reports with medical record data find that proxy reports of subjective aspects of the dying process, such as the patient's level of pain or psychological distress, may be biased. However, their reports are much more reliable in evaluating concrete or observable conditions, such as the services received or whether the patient struggled with breathlessness.[26]

A second method for assessing death quality is to use formal medical claims data or medical records. The widely used Dartmouth Atlas, a highly respected source of information on objective indicators of death quality such as hospice use, place of death, medical expenditures, length of hospitalization, specific services used, and intensity of medical care, is based on information on Medicare beneficiaries obtained from the Centers for Medicare and Medicaid Services. These data also include very basic information on the decedent's demographic characteristics, such as age, race, sex, and geographic region. Using these data, researchers can examine patterns like racial and ethnic differences in the number and duration of hospitalizations, intensive care unit (ICU) admissions, hospice use, and whether death occurred at home or in a hospital.[27] These two types of data resources can be used to explore disparities (or similarities) in four main dimensions of death quality: place of death, pain and pain management, use of hospice care services, and subjective and interpersonal aspects of end-of-life care, like being treated with dignity. To date, most of this research has focused on race differences rather than socioeconomic differences, owing in part to the unclear meaning of SES among very old and terminally ill patients.[28]

Most older adults at the end of life are retired rather than employed. Some might have transitioned from a lifetime job such as construction worker or waitress to a less physically demanding job, like store cashier, when their health started to decline. Most rely on Social Security as their primary income source, and many have depleted their savings to pay for medical or nursing home care. The handful of studies that do obtain information on SES may not necessarily capture the socioeconomic position that individuals occupied for most of their adult lives.[29] Thus, I focus primarily on race and regional differences in place of death, pain management, hospice use, and a broader range of social factors that might influence subjective death quality indicators, such as social isolation.

Place of Death

Whenever I give lectures on death and dying—whether to community groups, academic audiences, or even eighteen-year-old college students—I often ask, "How would you like to die?" Without fail, one clear answer emerges from the crowd: "When I'm very old . . . at home, in my own bed, surrounded by loved ones." The specific details may vary— some would like a Schubert string quartet playing in the background, others want a prime rib feast as their final meal, while others name favorite activities that would fill their final day, like a quiet moment at the beach with their spouse and dog. My informal poll results map closely onto national survey data: 75 to 80 percent of American adults say that they would like to die at home, and similar proportions of older adults with chronic diseases say that they would like to avoid hospitalization and intensive care at the end of life.[30] However, statistics on where older adults die show that the common desire for a home death is seldom realized. In 2009, just one in three died at home, and nearly 60 percent died in an institution, whether an acute care hospital (25 percent) or a nursing home (28 percent).[31] Even though most Americans say that they do not want to be hooked up to machines at the end of their life, one-third of all recent decedents spent time in an ICU in their final month.[32]

Most adults want to die at home for personal and spiritual comfort, to avoid the sterile and impersonal hospital or nursing home environment, and to spend their final moments with loved ones. Caregivers also say that they prefer that the dying person take his or her final breath at home.[33] Experts agree that a home death is better than an institutional death for the patient and family, especially if in-home hospice services are used. One study of cancer patients and their caregivers found that patients who died in an ICU or hospital experienced more physical and emotional distress and poorer quality of life compared with patients who died at home with hospice. For their caregivers, as well, ICU deaths were associated with heightened risk of post-traumatic stress disorder (PTSD) and prolonged grief disorder.[34]

Dying in an institution can be particularly distressing for older adults who need transfers in care at the end of life and are moved from home to a hospital or nursing home and then to an ICU in their final days. Within the last three months of life, dying patients average 3.1 transfers.[35] These abrupt shifts often lead to fragmented patient care when the old and new care teams have limited communication about the patient's health conditions, treatments, and personal history.[36] Such moves also can be disruptive and disorienting for dying patients and their families, as they must adjust to unfamiliar surroundings, new treatments, and new teams of care providers.[37]

The privilege of dying at home, like most other privileges, is linked to race and socioeconomic status. Yet these patterns are complex and closely tied to the severity of one's health condition, the treatments required, the availability of support systems to provide care at home, and public policies that dictate the kinds of treatments and services Medicare will cover. First and foremost, whether an older adult dies at home or in an institution depends on his or her health trajectory—that is, the timing and level of health symptoms. Medical researchers generally agree on three common dying trajectories for older patients with progressive chronic disease. As figure 8.1 shows, terminal illnesses, such as cancer, are distinguished by a steady progression of symptoms and a clear terminal phase. Deaths from organ failure (such as heart or respiratory failure) are marked by a gradual decline punctuated by roller-coaster-like up-and-down episodes of deterioration, recovery, and a seemingly sudden or unexpected death. Frailty refers to deaths from

Figure 8.1 Proposed Trajectories of Chronic Illness and Death

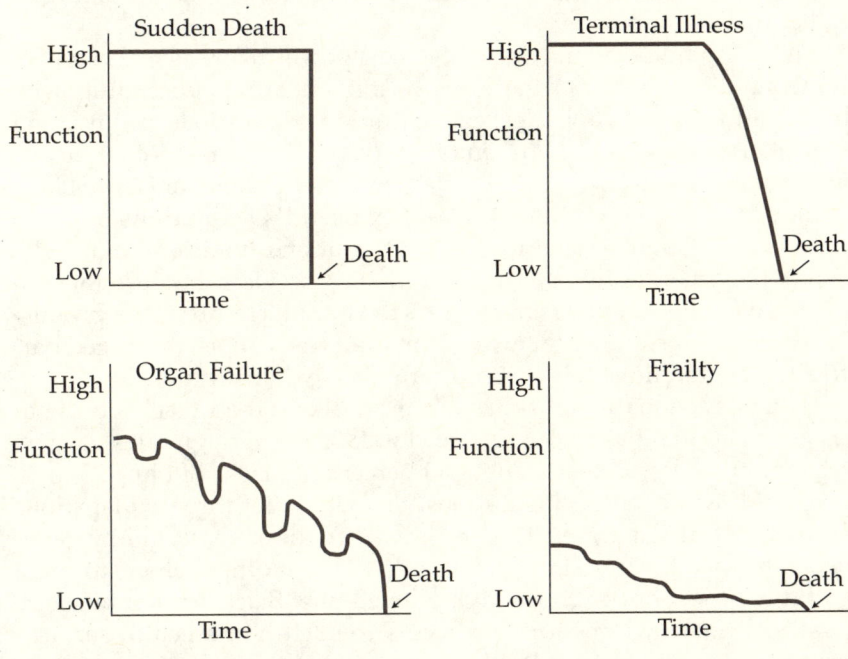

Source: Lunney, Lynn, and Hogan 2002.

dementia or extreme old age: in these cases, the patient experiences a prolonged and gradual decline or "dwindling."[38] A fourth, sudden death, is very rare in older adults and might be due to a sudden heart attack. In general, older adults whose disease progresses in a generally steady and predictable way, like cancer or dementia, are more likely to die at home, often using hospice services. By contrast, patients in the second category, who experience unpredictable up-and-down symptoms, are more likely to die in an institution.[39]

Second, a home death is more likely for those who have social support and whose caregivers have the schedule flexibility that allows them to carry out their tasks. One study of 350 terminally ill cancer patients found that those whose relatives took at least two weeks off work in the three months preceding their death were more likely to die at home, compared with patients whose relatives took off fewer than three days.[40] Another study based on 1.5 million patients from thirteen countries found that older adults with a greater number of family caregivers were five times as likely to die at home.[41] Socially isolated older adults without a spouse, children, friends, or other loved ones to provide informal care often have no choice but to spend their final weeks in an institution rather than at home.

Third, location matters. One of the most powerful predictors of where someone dies is whether there is a hospital nearby; older adults who live in an area with a greater concentration of hospitals and nursing homes are more likely to die in one.[42] In sharp contrast, older adults living in rural areas with few hospitals or nursing homes are more likely to die at home without the services they need.[43] Older adults living in rural areas also may need to move into nursing homes prematurely, before they require the full menu of nursing services, because they do not have family caregivers nearby. As their adult children seek promising career opportunities far away from their rustic roots, their aged parents left behind must rely on paid formal care or institutions.[44]

Fourth, race matters. Whites are more likely than blacks to die at home, a gap that has widened since the 1980s. Although rates vary by region and cause of death, about 40 percent of blacks but just 25 to 30 percent of whites die in institutions.[45] Experts offer three explanations for these racial disparities. The first is cost. To die at home, family members often need to invest in home health aides or other helpers to assist with the tasks of caring for a dying loved one. Blacks and Latinos are less likely than whites to have access to such home health services through private insurance.[46] Although some Medicare coverage is available, the conditions are strict. If a doctor orders in-home health care, Medicare may pay for only part-time or "intermittent" care from a home health aide. This equals roughly three ninety-minute visits a week during the period of illness. And many of the most common daily needs of frail older adults are not covered. For instance, Medicare does not cover personal care services, such as bathing and dressing, if that is the only care required. In sharp contrast, Medicare and Medicaid provide fairly generous coverage of nursing home care, which contributes to blacks' and Latinos' more frequent use of nursing homes at the very end of life.

The second reason for the race gap in home deaths is that terminally ill blacks are less likely than whites to have a family caregiver who is available to assist with transportation, homemaking services, and personal care. Having a family caregiver is closely tied with demographic factors, such as being married or having children living nearby, as well as economic factors, like having a family member who can afford to take time off work or cut back on work hours in order to provide care. Data from the Assets and Health Dynamics among the Oldest Old (AHEAD) show that white older adults are most likely to turn to a spouse (28 percent) or adult children (41 percent) for assistance with their daily activities and personal care, whereas black adults named adult children

(42 percent) and a nonfamily member (30 percent) as their main caregivers. Hispanics were most likely to rely on family members, with 52 percent relying on children and 20 percent relying on a spouse.[47] These gaps partly reflect family structure: blacks are less likely than whites and Hispanics to marry and stay married, and they may give rather than receive care from family members, even in later life.[48]

Whether an older adult relies on family members or nonrelatives for personal care matters because the type of tasks each performs differ. Older adults (especially women) generally prefer that close family members assist with dressing, bathing, bedpans, and other very personal tasks, while friends, neighbors, and members of one's religious congregation may be called on to help with less intimate tasks, like giving rides or delivering the occasional meal.[49] The personal care tasks are essential to helping a terminally ill older adult to remain in his or her own home.

The third reason for the race gap in home deaths is African Americans' and, to a lesser extent, Hispanics' preferences for aggressive care at the end of life—care that can only be delivered in an institutional setting. Ethnic minorities are more likely than whites to say that they want resuscitation and intubation (a breathing tube), and therefore they end up spending more time in the ICU than whites. Yet, as we shall see, blacks' stated preferences for more aggressive care may not capture their actual desires but may instead reflect fear of a health care system that historically has deprived them of treatments they wanted and needed.[50] Other studies suggest that ethnic minorities, especially those with lower levels of literacy, do not understand what end-of-life treatments entail—often because physicians fail to keep them informed.[51]

Pain and Pain Management

Pain is considered one of the core aspects of a bad death, yet most dying older adults experience some pain. One-half to two-thirds of older patients experience some pain during their last month of life, with considerably higher rates among those with arthritis, musculoskeletal conditions, depression, and cancer.[52] One review of fifty-two studies conducted over a forty-year period showed that one-third of older patients rated their pain as moderate or severe.[53] Recent surveys find that 75 percent of older adults have multiple sites of pain and that one in four experience pain that they describe as "dreadful" or "agonizing."[54] Shortness of breath, or dyspnea, is another common source of discomfort, with 50 to 60 percent experiencing breathlessness in the final two weeks of life.[55]

Pain and dyspnea are undesirable outcomes in their own right, yet they are also at the root of other psychological and interpersonal difficulties. Pain and breathlessness impair older adults' daily functioning, reduce their capacity to socialize or get exercise, increase their risk of depression, and reduce their psychological well-being.[56] Pain also takes a toll on caregivers; both witnessing loved ones in pain and trying (often unsuccessfully) to soothe that pain are among the most distressing burdens identified by the family caregivers of dying patients.[57] Family caregivers also may worry that they lack the knowledge or training to help administer pain medications to their loved one and fear making potentially fatal errors.[58]

Severe pain at the end of life is not inevitable, however, and can be treated effectively with medication. Studies of dying patients in their own homes and in nursing homes show that the use of opioids, including morphine, increases the patient's quality of life and does not hasten death unnecessarily.[59] A recent analysis of NHATS data showed that just 25 percent of proxies reported that their loved one had "unmet need for pain management" and just 21 percent reported "unmet need for dyspnea" in the last month of life.[60] However, the extent to which pain is appropriately treated varies markedly by race, with blacks experiencing considerably more unmet need (that is, inadequately treated pain) than whites.

One analysis of twenty years of data found persistent black-white gaps in the prescription of analgesic painkillers: blacks were only two-thirds as likely as whites to receive such prescriptions for chronic painful conditions like backaches and migraines, and they were also less likely to receive painkillers for traumatic injuries or surgery.[61] Studies based on Medicare data show that expenditures for older adults' pain medications were lower in geographic areas with high proportions of black residents, whereas studies analyzing workers' compensation claims show that less money was spent on painkillers for injured black versus white workers, and that the duration of the prescriptions (and payment) were considerably shorter.[62] Many factors account for this disparity, ranging from the implicit prejudices held by care providers to institutional racism such as pharmacies in historically black or poor neighborhoods failing to stock adequate supplies of pain medications.

Some researchers have suggested that health care providers may (unwittingly) hold implicit attitudes about race—such as the belief that blacks are more likely than whites to abuse drugs—that make them reluctant to prescribe analgesics to blacks. Others contend that physicians—the majority of whom are white or Asian—are less adept at empathizing with patients who look different from them and less able to accurately gauge their pain. Recent studies suggest that older black and, to a lesser extent, Hispanic patients are more likely to have their pain underestimated by health care providers and are less likely to have pain scores documented in their medical record compared to whites. As a result, dying African Americans and Hispanics are less likely to receive opioid analgesics and more likely to have their pain untreated compared to white patients.[63]

One particularly disheartening study suggests that doctors' underestimation of pain in African American patients reflects inaccurate if not outlandish beliefs about blacks' superior ability to tolerate pain. In a study of medical students and residents, Kelly Hoffman and her colleagues found that 14 percent of second-year medical students believed that "blacks' nerve endings are less sensitive than whites," while 42 percent believed that blacks have "thicker skin than whites."[64] Although the proportions endorsing these beliefs declined considerably by the students' final year in medical school, the researchers argue that these stereotypical beliefs and biases are a crucial mechanism behind the disproportionately high levels of untreated pain among African Americans at every stage of the life course.[65]

Racial disparities in the appropriate use of pain medication for dying older adults also may reflect institutional racism, a form of racism carried out in the practices of social and political institutions. Although the intent of such practices may not be explicitly racist, the outcome is unequal on the basis of race or ethnicity. In the case of pain medications, pharmacies, especially those in poor, urban, and historically African American neighborhoods, may not stock opioids if they believe they are at risk of theft. Yet these practices ultimately keep much-needed medications out of the hands of dying older adults who desperately need them.

One study of 188 retail pharmacies in Michigan characterized a pharmacy as having "sufficient" opioid analgesic supplies if it kept in stock at least one long-acting analgesic, one short-acting analgesic, and one combination opioid analgesic.[66] The researchers classified neighborhoods as predominantly white or predominantly black based on whether more than 70 percent of residents were white or black, respectively. Pharmacies in the minority zip code areas were fifty-two times less likely to carry sufficient opioid analgesics than pharmacies in white zip code areas, regardless of income. A similar study of New York City pharmacies yielded similar albeit less extreme results.[67] The researchers examined 176 pharmacies, randomly selected from all pharmacies in the city, and documented whether they stocked morphine and other opioids like fentanyl patches and oxycodone. Just 25 percent of pharmacies in predominantly black neighborhoods had opioid supplies that were sufficient to treat patients in severe pain, compared to 72 percent of pharmacies in predominantly white neighborhoods. The study investigators attributed these patterns to fear on the part of pharmaceutical companies and business owners that these medications would be stolen by local addicts. Yet even when local crime rates were taken into consideration, the disparities persisted, revealing that perceptions of the kinds of people who lived in the neighborhood were more powerful influences on business decisions than the actual crime rates.

In informal interviews with New York City pharmacists, some pharmacists told the *New York Times* that they did not stock the drugs simply because they did not have sufficient demand.[68] Others were quick to point out, however, that lack of demand is not the same as lack of need; rather, lack of demand might have reflected either lack of insurance to pay for the medications or the failure of physicians to prescribe painkillers to those who need them. Yet these explanations may mean little to the older adults suffering from untreated pain and dyspnea. Many may go without their pain medications, or their family members may need to devote considerable time and energy traveling to find medications. R. Sean Morrison, the lead author of the New York City study, recounted to the *New York Times* that he was treating a seventy-four-year-old Hispanic woman from the South Bronx with severe pain from a spinal disease, for whom he prescribed morphine. When he followed up with her the next day, she was still in agony. Although her daughter had gone to every pharmacy in their neighborhood, she could not locate the drug. It was only when the doctor intervened that the family located and obtained the medication they needed. The subtle and overt ways in which racism operates in everyday life are at the core of race disparities in pain management at the end of life.[69]

Hospice

The hallmarks of hospice care are the soothing of pain and the provision of comfort care. Hospice care is a comprehensive program that facilitates dying at home with one's family and emphasizes palliation (pain relief) and comfort rather than aggressive treatment at the end of life. Roughly 60 percent of hospice patients receive services in their own homes and the rest in institutions, although these rates vary based on the availability of services in different geographic areas.[70]

Hospice use has increased dramatically over the past two decades, with the number of sites in the United States increasing at about 3.5 percent a year from 2000 to 2010.[71] In 1997, 17 percent of all deaths in the United States occurred under the care of hospice; by 2011, this proportion had more than doubled, to 45 percent.[72] Roughly half of all Medicare decedents had been receiving hospice care.[73] The growing popularity of hospice among dying patients reflects shifting attitudes favoring quality of life over length of life. The movement toward hospice also is due to increased Medicare funding for hospice services as a way to reduce the costs associated with high-tech end-of-life care.

Medicare beneficiaries who are certified by a physician to have a terminal illness and less than six months to live are eligible for the Medicare hospice benefit. If the patient lives longer than six months, then hospice coverage may continue if the primary care provider and hospice team recertify the eligibility criteria.[74] This benefit provides services not covered under "traditional" Medicare such as nursing care, counseling, palliative medications, up to five days of respite care to assist family caregivers, and bereavement support for family members after the patient has died. Importantly, Medicare does not currently reimburse for hospice services until a patient has agreed to forgo curative care. (This may change, however. Medicare is currently conducting a pilot study that allows terminally ill patients to receive hospice care yet also see doctors and get medical treatments, like chemotherapy or hospitalization, intended to fight their illnesses.)[75]

Hospice is widely praised by the patients and caregivers who use its services, yet many Americans hold strong misconceptions that may frighten them away from hospice. Hospice care typically involves withholding or withdrawing medical treatments that may sustain a patient's life, but it is not a form of euthanasia or physician-assisted suicide (PAS), whereby patients are directly administered medications that may hasten their death. Despite this profound difference between hospice and PAS, many laypersons misunderstand precisely what hospice is and does. Patients and family caregivers may believe that hospice "starves" patients to death by depriving them of feeding tubes, or that hospice care means giving up all hope that the patient will live.[76] Even more dire, one study found that more than half of all palliative care physicians had been accused by a distraught family member of "committing murder."[77]

This misunderstanding is an obstacle to using hospice services and may contribute to poorer-quality deaths among some older adults. Clinical trials have found that patients receiving hospice services have fewer ICU admissions, greater satisfaction with their medical care, and reduced levels of pain, while surveys document significantly better mood and superior quality of life.[78] The family caregivers of hospice patients also report feeling supported and experiencing fewer symptoms of sadness and anxiety. The benefits of hospice linger even after the patient has died. Bereaved family members whose loved one received hospice care have reduced risks of mortality, depression, and traumatic grief. These positive outcomes are due partly to the fact that the death is less stressful for caregivers, as hospice provides support services to bereaved caregivers in the immediate aftermath of the death.[79]

Open-ended interviews, blogs, and personal essays by bereaved family members reveal a tremendous sense of gratitude to hospice for the care it delivers. For instance, Open to Hope Foundation, a nonprofit foundation with "the mission of helping people find hope after loss," regularly features on its webpages first-person essays and readers' reactions. The essays written by bereaved older persons who relied on hospice services are overwhelmingly positive. One widow wrote that "my husband of 42 years passed away in 2009. After a one-year fight to keep him alive, we brought in hospice to our home from which he transitioned ... I will be forever grateful for their tender care, responsiveness and for the bereavement counseling they provided after my husband's death." Another older widower shared that "my wife Patt was put under hospice care [in 2011], due to ovarian cancer. She fought a hard battle for about 2.5 years, but got to the point where her body couldn't take chemo anymore. We had hospice care at home. ... Patt only lived for one month. I couldn't have made it without our hospice people."[80]

The benefits of hospice are financial as well as physical and psychosocial. A hospice stay of two to four weeks has been found to save Medicare nearly $6,500 per patient.[81] Part of the cost savings results from hospice patients' reduced use of other costly life-sustaining treatments and services, including ER visits and hospital admissions in the last month of life and chemotherapy within the last two weeks of life.[82] However, some policy analysts worry that these savings are starting to erode—and will continue to do so—as growing numbers of for-profit hospice providers engage in practices that boost their corporate bottom line yet potentially hurt patients (and overwhelm the Medicare payment system).[83]

Despite its many benefits, experiences with hospice are not uniformly positive. Both scientific studies and personal narratives suggest that hospice is most beneficial to the patients and family members receiving services for fairly long periods. A well-documented limitation of hospice is that patients may receive these services only very late in their illness. One-third of hospice patients receive these services for one week or less; the median duration in hospice is nineteen days.[84] Patients who receive hospice care only at the very end of life—for three or fewer days—are more susceptible to major depression relative to those who receive longer-term care.[85] These statistics cohere with the laments of an Open to Hope blogger and widow, Paula, who had recently lost her husband of thirty-five years to cancer. After struggling with his illness for many years, Paula's husband died less than one week after he entered in-hospital hospice care. As Paula wrote: "If I could go back in time and make that decision [to place her husband in hospice] over again, I would have chosen not to have hospice care. I know that many people speak highly of hospice and the care that is given; this was not my experience. Perhaps if you are home and the care is being provided there it is different. But in-hospital hospice care seemed to be just another layer in

Figure 8.2 Medicare Hospice Enrollees, by Ownership of Hospice Provider, 2000–2011

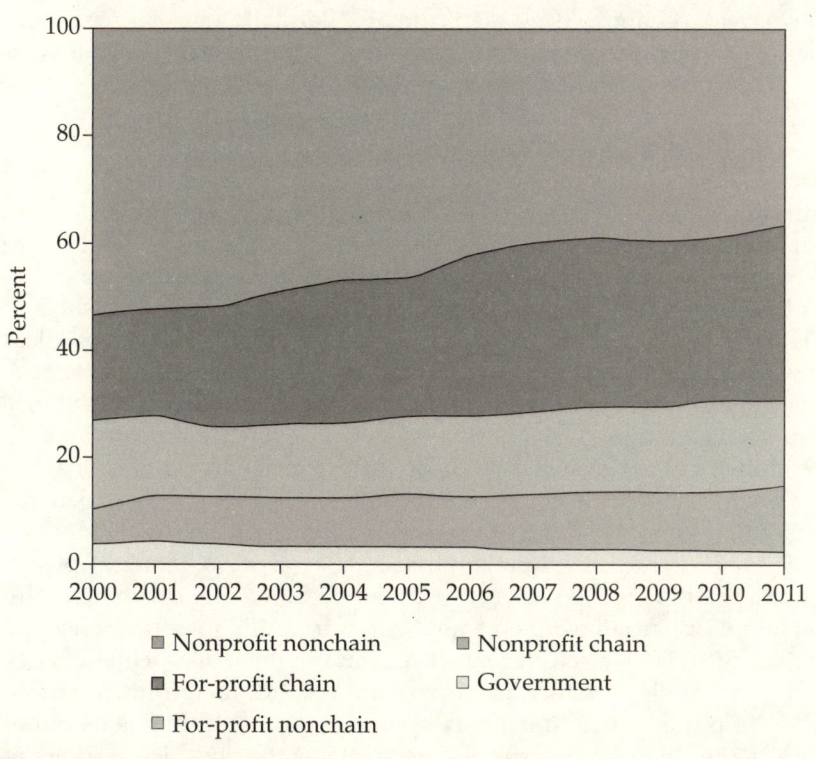

Source: Stevenson et al. 2015.
Note: Data are from Medicare cost reports, which must be submitted annually by all Medicare-certified hospice agencies and are publicly available from the Centers for Medicare and Medicaid Services.

the system. What could they have done differently? Perhaps, the hospital administration could have explained the process more thoroughly."[86] In general, hospice works best when patient and family members are told what to expect and they receive services for longer durations to help transition them toward the death.

Another potential threat to the quality of hospice care is the rapid increase in the number of for-profit hospice providers, who differ from nonprofit providers in important (and troubling) ways. While just 5 percent of hospice providers were for-profits in 1990, by 2000 this share had reached one-third, and by 2011 one-half (see figure 8.2).[87] This shift in the composition of hospice providers carries potential problems for patients and their families. In general, for-profit hospices exist within larger corporate systems and are motivated to run as efficiently as possible. Regardless of whether a hospice provider is for-profit or nonprofit, they are all reimbursed by Medicare at a flat daily rate. The daily per diems vary slightly by state, and by place and duration of care, but averaged around $160 to $200 per day in 2018.[88]

Federal watchdog groups like the Medicare Payment Advisory Commission (MedPAC) have cautioned that because of this flat-rate reimbursement system, some for-profit hospice providers may be selectively enrolling patients in an effort to maximize their profit margins. Patients who remain in hospice for a long time yet have less complex health care needs are the most profitable, whereas patients at the very end of life with short, service-intensive stays are the least profitable.[89] In short, if all hospice providers are going to receive roughly $180 a day, regardless of what services they provide, the "rational" decision would be to focus on patients whose needs are modest and avoid those patients whose care needs are time- or labor-intensive. Consequently, for-profits tend to fill their patient rosters with those suffering from conditions that are less onerous to treat, leaning toward dementia and heart disease patients rather than cancer patients, who require intensive pain treatments.[90]

These processes affect patient care in several ways. First, for-profits generally offer a narrower range of services, leaving out potentially valuable services like bereavement care for family members once the patient dies. They also offer fewer community benefits such as charity care or training sites for care providers. Second, for-profits are more likely to provide care to patients in nursing homes or hospitals rather than in their homes. It is simply more efficient for hospice workers to see multiple patients in a single institution, especially when basic routine tasks like bathing have already been taken care of by the nursing home staff. Home-based patients, by contrast, may require extensive travel to far-off homes and neighborhoods, and the caregiving tasks may be especially time-consuming, as the patient's family members cannot pick up the workload in the way that paid nursing home workers can. What that means is that more patients are dying in institutions, which betrays their desire to die at home.

Third, in an effort to run "mean and lean," for-profit hospice providers tend to maintain lower staff-to-patient ratios, and with less professionalized staff, care may be rushed or inadequate.[91] The dire consequences of understaffing were vividly recounted in Karen Brown's 2018 *New York Times* op-ed, where she details how her dying father's final night was marked by excruciating untreated pain because of a long delay in an overworked hospice provider arriving at his bedside. As Brown recalls, "At the end of life, things can fall apart quickly, and neither medical specialist nor hospice worker can guarantee a painless exit. But we were told a palliative expert would be at my father's bedside if he needed it. We were not told this was conditional on staffing levels." Individual hospice workers may be every bit as kind, compassionate, and dedicated to their patients in for-profit as nonprofit hospice organizations, yet organizational constraints prevent them from delivering the high-quality care they would like. Some experts believe that these gaps in quality of care may be particularly troublesome for black and Latino hospice patients, who are more likely than whites to be recruited by and enrolled in a for-profit hospice.[92]

Finally, for-profits are slightly more likely than nonprofits to disenroll patients at the very end of life, when they require more frequent visits and more intensive support.[93] The difference is quite small; 6 percent of nonprofits and 10 percent of for-profits disenroll hospice patients when they are still alive. In some cases, patients request it after having a change of heart about their care. In other cases, hospice providers have little incentive to care for the most challenging patients when they can receive the same per diem reimbursement for easier and less time-consuming patients, thus enabling larger (and more profitable) caseloads.[94] Yet when patients leave hospice, regardless of the reason, they may end up costing Medicare more money, as these patients may resort to high-cost medical treatments in emergency rooms and ICUs. As a result, they are more likely to die in hospitals, a setting that is widely considered part of a "bad death."[95]

Disparities in Hospice Use Hospice was designed as a program that should be available to all, although in practice, it may be out of reach for many who need it. In the preamble to its formal *Standards of Practice*, the National Hospice and Palliative Care Organization states that hospice "offers palliative care for all individuals and their families without regard to age, gender, nationality, race, creed, sexual orientation, disability, diagnosis, availability of a primary caregiver, or ability to pay."[96] Yet despite NHPCO's well-intended philosophy of egalitarianism, some individuals face obstacles to hospice use.

The first obstacle is hospice policies that disproportionately affect those with fewer social and economic resources, such as patients without a family caregiver at home. The first-ever national survey of enrollment policies at nearly six hundred hospices found that 78 percent of hospices had at least one enrollment policy that could restrict access to care. For example, 12 percent of hospices required that the patient have a family caregiver at home and would not provide services to those without a caregiver present.[97] On the one hand, this policy is defensible: the hospice philosophy emphasizes the importance of family in providing support and care to dying patients. On the other hand, this policy is implicitly biased against those who are unmarried, childless, or socially isolated, as well as those whose family members cannot afford to take time off work. Low-income and black older adults, being less likely to be married and thus more likely to lack a coresidential spouse caregiver, are particularly affected by such requirements.

For older adults living in urban or suburban areas with many hospices nearby, such a restriction may be of little consequence; they may choose another hospice program that does not have it. Yet older patients living in remote rural areas may have few if any alternatives. A case in point is ninety-five-year-old Wyoming rancher Bill Kolacny, who wanted to die peacefully at his log home with his wife Beverly by his side. After he suffered heart failure, Bill and his family looked into hospice services. The hospice closest to his four-hundred-acre ranch on the Clarks Fork River was located in Red Lodge, Montana, and was not licensed to care for patients over the state line in Wyoming. Yet the closest Wyoming hospice could not afford to send its staff to the Kolacny ranch, more than sixty miles away.[98] Ultimately, Bill's son and two daughters each traveled more than an hour each way to care for their ailing father.

A second obstacle is lack of awareness of what hospice does. This is one of the main reasons why blacks and Latinos are less likely than whites to use hospice and more likely, when they do, to enroll at more advanced disease stages and thus have shorter spells of care. Analyses of Medicare beneficiary records show that roughly half of white but only one-third of black older adults used hospice services in the last week of life.[99] Yet informational barriers to African Americans' use of hospice are potentially modifiable and can be minimized with patient education and outreach programs. One small study of two hundred community-dwelling older adults found that 19 percent of blacks yet just 4 percent of whites had never heard of hospice, while 72 percent of whites and fewer than half of blacks said that they knew a lot about hospice. Among both blacks and whites, greater knowledge about hospice is a predictor of holding favorable attitudes toward it.[100] Health care providers and institutions could develop targeted educational programs to increase knowledge of, preferences for, and ultimately enrollment in hospice among blacks.

A third barrier is fear or skepticism about what the program entails; these beliefs are particularly common among blacks and have deep roots in the historical mistreatment of blacks by the U.S. health care system.[101] As Maisha Robinson, a palliative care physician at the Mayo Clinic, told the *New York Times:* "You have people who've had a difficult time getting access to care throughout their lifetimes" because of poverty, lack of health insurance, or difficulty finding a medical provider, "and then you have a physician who's saying, 'I think that we need to transition your mother, father, grandmother to comfort care or palliative care.' People are skeptical of that."[102] This skepticism is compounded by the Medicare reimbursement rule that hospice patients must forgo curative treatments. Blacks who have had to fight and advocate for quality health care throughout their lives may not be comfortable actively forsaking these treatments.[103]

Some older adults believe that hospice is at odds with their religious beliefs. African Americans in particular may view hospice as a challenge to beliefs such as "God will decide when it's my time to die," or that miracles may occur if one is kept alive long enough.[104] The miracle might be a dying parent reuniting with an estranged child, a patient rediscovering his or her faith as death nears, or, on rare occasions, recovering from terminal illness and exiting hospice care. To withhold treatment, some African Americans believe, "would get in the way of God's will" or be antithetical to the belief that suffering can be redemptive or a "test from God."[105] Yet promising new interventions and educational programs conducted in partnerships between health care systems and religious leaders aim to increase rates of hospice among older blacks. The National Hospice and Palliative Care Organization has produced a guide for older African Americans and their community leaders, to explain what hospice does and challenge pervasive myths about the service.[106] One early example of success was the establishment of the Caring Touch Ministry, a church-based hospice education and coordination program started by Cassandra Cotton, a church leader, certified nursing assistant (CNA), and community relations coordinator at a local hospice. Cotton says, "Providers must find ways to educate faith communities and engage faith leaders in end-of-life care conversations. The congregation must have an informed, trained leader who has an understanding of the range of hospice services and how these services are delivered."[107] These programs have high potential to create a context in which blacks and whites alike may die with dignity.

Death with Dignity: Subjective End-of-Life Appraisals Surprisingly little research has explored subjective aspects of end-of-life experiences, in part because of the methodological challenges involved. Subjective end-of-life assessments must be provided retrospectively by a proxy because the decedent cannot report the care he or she received in the last few days of life. Yet proxy assessments are often of questionable validity. If they are obtained too soon after the death, the proxy reporter's assessments may by biased by symptoms of grief, depression, or anxiety. But if the assessments are done long after those initial symptoms have passed, the proxy may not recall all the details of the death.[108] The handful of studies done in this area suggest few race or socioeconomic differences in subjective aspects of death quality.

One of the richest resources for exploring proxy assessments of death quality is the NHATS, which asked survivors of older adults who died between 2011 and 2013 to rate the quality of nine objective and subjective aspects of death. Although these data reveal high levels of dissatisfaction with pain (67 percent) and shortness of breath (56 percent), the proportions reporting interpersonal or spiritual concerns are much lower: fewer than one in five recalled that the dying patient was treated without respect, decisions were made without enough input from the decedent or family, the decision went against what the decedent would have wanted, or the family was not always kept informed.[109] Also using NHATS data, the sociologist Elizabeth Luth found that blacks were more likely than whites to report unsatisfactory pain treatment.[110] She found no differences, however, regarding more subjective concerns, like being kept informed, being treated with respect, and having spiritual concerns met.

Similar patterns were detected in three other data sets: the Changing Lives of Older Couples, a prospective study of spousal bereavement in the 1980s and 1990s; the Wisconsin Longitudinal Study, a longitudinal study that tracked white Wisconsin high school graduates from their senior year in 1957 through old age in 2011; and the New Jersey End of Life Study, a sample of 305 black, white, and Hispanic terminally older adults.[111] Although blacks reported less satisfaction with pain management, no race differences emerged for other subjective measures of death quality, like the patient's awareness of and acceptance of death, positive family interactions at the end of life, and the survivor's belief that the decedent led a full life.[112] These results are consistent with a key theme of fundamental cause theory: social and economic resources are protective only in situations where they can be used to gain an advantage.[113] Although money, status, and power may help in advocating for appropriate medical care and pain medication, those resources may be of little value as family members prepare emotionally and spiritually for the death of their loved one.

Agency in Dying: Advance Care Planning

Death may be inevitable, but a bad death is not. In an effort to combat highly medicalized, costly, protracted bad deaths, policymakers and practitioners are working to give patients and their families greater latitude in decision-making. In 1990, the U.S. Congress passed the Patient Self-Determination Act (PSDA), which requires all health care facilities receiving federal funds "to ask patients whether they have advance directives, to provide information about advance directives, and to incorporate advance directives into the medical record."[114] An advance directive has two main components: a living will and a durable power of attorney for health care (DPAHC) designation. A living will is a legal document specifying the medical treatments a person would like to receive if he or she is not healthy or aware enough to make those decisions at the moment they are required. A DPAHC permits a person appointed by the patient to make decisions about health care if the patient is incapable of doing so.

The benefits of advance care planning are well documented. Older adults with advance directives in place are much more likely to experience several core components of a good death, including greater use of hospice or palliative care, reduced use of invasive or futile treatments such as feeding tubes or ventilators, a stronger belief that they have some control over the end-of-life process, a greater chance of dying at home rather than in an institution, and fewer instances of receiving treatments that are discrepant with their wishes.[115]

ACP also eases the experiences of family members. It reduces their decision-making burden, thus minimizing their anxiety and depressive symptoms. New findings from the Wisconsin Study of Families and Loss (WISTFL) reveal how ACP minimizes the decision-making burden.[116] The WISTFL is a study of 750 bereaved family members of recently deceased Wisconsin Longitudinal Study participants. The survivors were asked whether their loved one had done ACP, and whether it helped, hurt, or had no effect on the quality of the loved one's death. The survivors then described in their own words precisely how the ACP helped or hurt. Most noted that the decedent's planning had helped, and that the living will eased decision-making in five ways. First, it provided family members with knowledge of the end-of-life process. As one bereaved spouse recalled, "We had discussed how everything was supposed to work so when time got closer everyone knew where we stood."[117]

Second, it clarified family members' responsibilities. A bereaved son reported, "Us kids knew who it [the DPAHC] was so there was no bickering . . . it was never an issue as to who should make decisions." Third, survivors felt affirmed that the decedent's preferences were heeded. One daughter found comfort in the recognition that "we knew that my mom could make the decisions that she wanted." Fourth, the formal designation of power reduced ambiguity. A widower believed that the living will helped because it provided "the security in knowing you had that power ability." Finally, family members felt supported when making a difficult choice. A son responsible for making the decision regarding his elderly father's care recalled, "I was the one that said 'well, we will not prolong his life' and that was it. The nurses and the director knew the same thing; they are the ones that finally helped me let it go. . . . You have to make a decision and you have to do it rather quickly. If people are wishy-washy about it, the living will takes that away. At least it did for me."[118]

Despite the many positive consequences of ACP, it cannot guarantee a good death. The limitations of living wills are widely documented.[119] The treatment preferences stated may not be relevant to the patient's condition at the very end of life, especially for those who drafted their living wills years earlier. Physicians may not have access to the document at the critical decision-making moment. The living will might be stashed away in a safe deposit box, or it might be sitting in a desk drawer in a Wisconsin home when an older adult is unexpectedly hospitalized while wintering in Arizona. Many advance directives begin with the statement: "If I have a terminal condition, then . . ." This statement requires that a physician evaluate whether the patient's condition is terminal. Until that determination is made, the content of the advance directive does not hold, despite what the patient and family had hoped.

Physicians also may be reluctant to follow the orders stated in the living will for fear of legal liability; physicians believe that their liability risk is greater if they do not attempt resuscitation than if they provide it against patient wishes.[120] Family members may not know (or agree with) the document's content, or they may not know how to translate vague preferences into specific clinical practices. A statement like, "If I'm ever a vegetable, pull the plug," has no clinical meaning and provides no clear instructions for providing or withholding treatments. For these reasons, some states are encouraging the use of physician orders for life-sustaining treatment.[121] POLSTs are completed by a patient in consultation with health care providers during a clinical encounter. The document is signed by a physician and kept in the patient's record. Unlike a living will, a POLST is a formal "order," so health care providers are required to follow its content.[122]

DPAHC appointments also have practical limitations. The designated DPAHC is granted decision-making authority, yet may make decisions that create distress or disagreement among family members. The WISTFL data reveal that, according to some family members, the DPAHC designation created problems and conflict at the end of life.[123] Problems typically arise when the appointed decision-maker tries to carry out the patient's preferences and other family members disagree with that decision. One bereaved daughter recounted the difficulty of serving as DPAHC after her mother's recent death: "My father was unable to make the decision to pull life support, which fell to me. [I knew] it was the right thing to do, not letting her live like that, but my brothers wanted her alive. It helped that one person was responsible for the decision, but it caused issues with the family." In other cases, problems arose because aggrieved family members believed that they themselves should have been chosen for the job, rather than the person named as DPAHC. One widow recalled that her late husband's son from a prior marriage tried to contest her decision: "We had both been married before and had children. His oldest son felt that maybe he should make decisions for his dad instead of myself."[124]

A further difficulty is that the appointed decision-maker may not actually know what the patient wants; multiple studies document that the decision-maker's knowledge of the patient's preferences is usually no better than chance. Often believing (incorrectly) that they and the patient hold the same preferences, proxies often assume that their own preferences should guide the end-of-life decision.[125] As one study concluded, "surrogates are not perfect ambassadors of patient preferences."[126] Older adults themselves, in the mistaken belief that their loved ones intuitively understand their preferences, often do not see a need to explicitly inform the legal proxy of their views.

For some patients, their proxy's limited knowledge is unproblematic. Some older adults prefer to have a family member do what he or she feels is best, rather than abide by their own stated preferences.[127] Others may trust their physicians to make decisions for them. Still, the patient's deference to a specific decision-maker's wishes may create distress or conflict for concerned family members who do not hold legal decision-making power and who may also create additional problems and conflict. Clinicians often share anecdotes of what they call the "daughter in California" phenomenon. In this common scenario, a family member who resides far away from the dying patient and has had little involvement in the patient's end-of-life care jets into town at the eleventh hour, swoops in, and tries to redirect the family conversation and decision-making at the patient's final stage of life. These individuals may try to undo or undermine the decisions made by local family members who were engaged in the care and decision-making process from the start. These family disagreements, in turn, make it difficult for health care teams to provide quality end-of-life care.[128]

Given these limitations of formal ACP, some practitioners suggest that informal discussions with loved ones and care providers are the most critical component of end-of-life planning. Analyses of data from married couples in the WLS show that discussing end-of-life issues with one's spouse increases the chances of correctly identifying his or her end-of-life treatment preferences.[129] Even though these discussions are not formal or legally binding, they can help to facilitate care consistent with the patient's wishes; Laraine Winter and Susan Parks conclude that "those who avoid . . . end-of-life conversations are the least likely to have treatment wishes respected, because their proxies are unlikely to know their wishes."[130]

Conversations about an older adult's values also may be useful because very few of us know precisely how and of what cause we will die, making it difficult to specify particular medical interventions that we would want (or not want) at the end of life, such as feeding tubes or chemotherapy. A general conversation about values ("I don't want to be a vegetable") and global preferences ("I don't want to be hooked up to machines") may provide family members with a road map for representing their loved one's wishes even in the absence of a formal living will. Discussions may facilitate decision-making in cases where the patient has not legally appointed a DPAHC. Most states have established default systems for authorizing proxy decision-makers. State laws vary, but such lists prioritize the immediate family—starting with the spouse, followed by an adult child, a sibling, and other relatives.[131] Frank conversations about a patient's values may empower and inform state-authorized proxies when making difficult decisions about their loved one's care.

The timing of these discussions is crucial, however, as some discussions may be too little too late. Conversations regarding end-of-life issues often are triggered by a patient's health-related crisis, such as a heart attack or hospitalization. When discussions occur following such trigger events, the patient and family often are too distressed or frightened to make an informed or levelheaded decision about imminent care needs. Growing recognition of the importance of timely, in-depth conversations between dying patients and their family members and health care professionals was one impetus for the 2016 ruling by the Obama administration that clinicians are to be reimbursed for the time they spend discussing end-of-life issues with Medicare-beneficiary patients and their families. Although this benefit, provided as part of the Affordable Care Act, has an uncertain future under the current political administration, it has high potential to make advance care planning more common, especially among ethnic minorities, persons with fewer socioeconomic resources, and other older adults who face serious obstacles to ACP.

Advance Care Planning: Trends and Disparities

Professional recommendations from organizations like the American Medical Association, public awareness and education campaigns, popular books, and public policies like the PSDA—all aim to increase rates of ACP, yet these efforts have been met with only moderate success. Only one-third to one-half of all adults in the United States have completed an advance directive, although rates are as high as 70 percent among older adults.[132] ACP rates have increased sharply since 1990: the proportion with a written advance directive has more than doubled, from 16 percent in 1990 to 35 percent in 2013.[133] This trend is partly attributable to the passage of the PSDA in 1990; high-visibility cases of contested end-of-life decisions, such as the fifteen-year legal case of Terri Schiavo; public awareness campaigns like Respecting Choices and the "Five Wishes"; and media programs such as Bill Moyers's PBS series *On Our Own Terms*.[134] The Five Wishes, for example, is a user-friendly advance directive written in nontechnical language that includes identification of a proxy and preferences for medical and nonmedical treatment and comfort.[135]

Race Disparities Although ACP rates are steadily inching upward, stark racial disparities persist. Dozens of studies, based on national, regional, and clinical samples, all point to the same finding: blacks and Latinos are less likely than whites to do advance care planning, despite its well-documented positive consequences for death quality. Studies generally show that whites are two to three times as likely as blacks and Latinos to have an advance directive; the gap is much narrower for end-of-life discussions. These gaps persist even when education, income, health literacy, health, and other social factors are controlled.[136] Explanations for these differentials include: ethnic minorities' limited access to the medical and legal professionals who may provide assistance in preparing such documents; literacy or language barriers; cultural beliefs that such documents are unnecessary because family members will make decisions collectively on behalf of the patient; historically rooted distrust of physicians and medical institutions; and adherence to religious beliefs like "God will decide" when it is time for a patient to die and "those who believe in God do not have to plan for end-of-life care." Some research suggests that blacks and Latinos believe that they do not need a living will because they tend to want all possible interventions at the end of life and think that living wills limit their ability to request treatment.[137]

Blacks and Latinos may view ACP as unnecessary because they believe that their family members already know their end-of-life preferences. I analyzed open-ended data from the New Jersey End of Life Study, a study of ACP among a racially diverse sample of dying older adults. The most common reason given by blacks and Latinos for not having an advance directive was: "I don't need to, my family knows my preferences." This response, along with the explanation "I've never thought about it," were the top two reasons offered by ethnic minorities, with 69 percent of blacks and 78 percent of Latinos offering these two answers. Whites differed dramatically: only 18 percent said that ACP was unnecessary because their families knew their views. Rather, more than 50 percent attributed their lack of ACP to procrastination, saying things like, "I just haven't gotten around to it yet," and, "I know I need to do this, it's been on my to-do list for a long time."

Yet this lack of ACP among black and Hispanic older adults may prevent them from receiving the treatments they desire. One national study found that among older cancer patients who want aggressive treatments, blacks are one-third as likely as whites to receive such treatment.[138] Other research shows a substantial racial gap in end-of-life health care costs: in 2001, the average cost of care in the last six months of life ranged from $20,166 among whites to $26,704 among blacks and $31,702 among Latinos.[139] Fully 85 percent of the race gap in expenditures is accounted for by blacks' and Latinos' greater usage of costly and invasive treatments. Low rates of ACP, in turn, are a key mechanism contributing to a racial gap in quality of death, because lack of end-of-life planning is linked to the use of costly and intrusive treatments, the failure to receive desired treatments, more pain, fewer home-based deaths, and less use of palliative care services.

Socioeconomic Disparities Surprisingly few studies explore social class differences in ACP, yet recent work shows that older persons with lower levels of education, income, and assets and lower homeownership rates have lower rates of formal ACP relative to their wealthier counterparts, although SES is only weakly related to discussions of treatment preferences. Older adults with greater net worth and homeowners are nearly twice as likely as renters and those with no or few assets to do ACP.[140] Wealth may be linked to health care planning in an indirect way, in that older adults with more assets to protect are more likely to do estate and financial planning than are their less wealthy counterparts. A visit to a lawyer to do financial planning may trigger the completion of related documents, including living wills and DPAHC appointments. If a person or couple is completing their will, they may decide to draft their living will at the same time.

Planning is not linked to financial resources alone. Older adults with more education are more likely to plan, whereas those with lower levels of literacy are less likely to do so. One recent study of patients age fifty-five to seventy-four found that rates of ACP were 12.5, 25, and 50 percent for those with low, marginal, and adequate literacy, respectively.[141] Low literacy may be linked to limited knowledge about specific health conditions and possible treatments at the end of life. This lack of knowledge and uncertainty may impede ACP, as older adults often are reluctant to make decisions about treatments they do not understand.

Social Isolation or Integration   The bleak platitude that "we die alone" has been attributed to everyone from director Orson Welles to contemporary folk singer Loudon Wainwright, to seventeenth-century philosopher Blaise Pascal's *Pensées*. In reality, very few people die alone, and ACP helps to ensure that family members know, understand, and feel empowered to carry out the end-of-life treatment preferences of their loved one. Not surprisingly, both whether one does ACP and its effectiveness are tightly linked to one's social integration and connectedness. People with close-knit and harmonious relationships are more likely than those with troubled relationships to prepare an advance directive. Married older adults whose marriage is marked by high levels of warmth and low levels of conflict are more likely to appoint their spouse (versus an adult child or someone else) as their DPAHC.[142]

For older adults who do not have close family members, however, ACP is either left undone or delegated to individuals who have less intimate knowledge of their values and preferences. This is particularly the case for unmarried and childless older adults. Single, separated, and divorced people are much less likely than their married peers to discuss end-of-life issues with friends or extended family—presumably because they do not have a close confidant with whom to share such highly personal and potentially intimidating conversations. They also tend to name as proxies more distant family members who may not be as well informed about their preferences.[143] As figure 8.3 shows, among WLS respondents, nearly all married parents (96 percent) chose a spouse or child as their DPAHC; 69 percent selected their spouse, while 27 percent named a child. Fewer than 2 percent of married parents chose another relative, a friend, or a professional. Among married childless persons, the majority named their spouse (80 percent), while a similar proportion of unmarried parents named a child as DPAHC. Very different patterns emerge among unmarried, childless older adults. Equal proportions named a sibling or another relative (33 percent each), while another 16 percent chose a friend or coworker, and a handful named a romantic partner, such as an ex-spouse, or a professional, such as clergy, as their DPAHC designee.

At face value, these choices may not be problematic. Yet in practice, older adults have more frequent contact and meaningful communication with their spouses and children compared to other relatives, friends, and professionals. And given the very low rates of end-of-life discussions among unmarried older adults, it is likely that their DPAHC designees are not as well informed and thus less capable of effectively con-

Figure 8.3 Durable Power of Attorney for Health Care Appointments Among Wisconsin Longitudinal Study Respondents, by Marital and Parental Status, 2003–2004

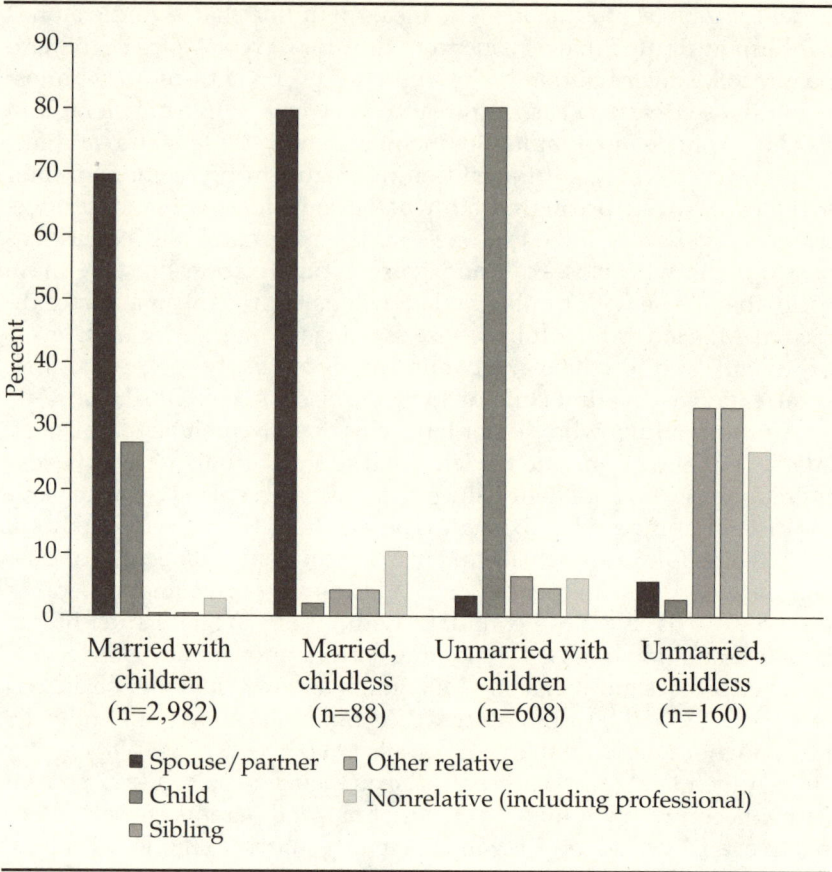

Source: Carr and Khodyakov 2007.

veying the older patient's preferences to health care providers. These results underscore the powerful ways in which social isolation undermines all aspects of older adults' experiences in both life and death.

Diverse obstacles—economic, informational, structural, and interpersonal, as well as public policies, including Medicare and Medicaid reimbursement structures—may impede older adults' access to pain medication, hospice care, the opportunity to die at home, and other benefits that accompany a good death. Given the large and growing numbers of older adults who will require end-of-life care in the coming decades, practitioners and policymakers have been especially intent on developing cost-effective strategies and policies to enhance the quality of end-of-life care. Placing decision-making responsibility in the hands of older patients and their families, regardless of their personal resources, has been facilitated by developments like increasing reliance on POLSTs and reimbursing physicians for conducting an ACP consultation session with their Medicare beneficiary patients. However, these practices require careful monitoring to ensure that they are effective. The Institute of Medicine has called for developing quality-of-care metrics and tying insurance reimbursement to these metrics.[144] Ideally, these indicators would capture an alignment of the patient's goals, values, and preferences, as articulated in a living will or POLST, the documented treatment plan, and the treatment ultimately delivered.

An equally important goal is raising awareness and utilization of hospice care, given its widely documented benefits. Yet experts recognize that the expansion of hospice care and the rapid growth of for-profit providers carry potentially negative consequences for patients and their families.[145] Innovative solutions include changes to how Medicare reimburses hospices; considerably higher reimbursements could be offered for those patients who have more complex medical conditions or who do not have family members or the support system necessary to help with less intensive daily care, which thus becomes the responsibility of hospice care workers.[146] Other approaches would be developing more refined measures of the quality of care delivered and keying Medicare reimbursements to quality as well as types of hospice services offered. These practices might allow older adults, regardless of their family ties, economic resources, or knowledge of end-of-life policies and procedures, to die comfortably, peacefully, and on their own terms.

= Chapter 9 =

Conclusion: Future Trends and Policy Considerations for the Twenty-First Century

Old age can be the best of times, marked by health and vigor, unprecedented longevity, emotional well-being, a comfortable home, a fulfilling romantic partnership, loving relationships with children and grandchildren, the support of dedicated caregivers, meaningful daily activities, and the equanimity, self-acceptance, and wisdom that comes from a lifetime of experience. But this gilded existence is not within the grasp of all older adults. Old age also can be the worst of times. Some older Americans are struggling with poor health, subpar housing, constant worries about how to pay for their next meal or prescription refill, and isolation or unreasonable demands from the friends and family who should be providing care and support. Although Medicare, Medicaid, and Social Security have played critical roles in providing health care, long-term care, and a minimum standard of living to older adults, these programs alone are not sufficient to erase the deep-seated disparities that have accumulated gradually over the life course. These programs also have well-documented shortcomings that limit their capacity to eradicate these disparities. Social Security disproportionately benefits older adults who have lived what sociologists characterize as a white middle-class life: a long-term marriage between a breadwinner and a homemaker. Medicare has important gaps in coverage, especially for older adults who are struggling with multiple health conditions or who cannot afford the costly out-of-pocket expenses of the medications or long-term care services they desperately need.

As we look to the future, two predictions are certain. The first is that the population of older adults will continue to grow dramatically, especially the oldest-old in their eighties and beyond. The second is that future cohorts of older adults will be very different from their parents or grandparents who are experiencing old age today. Yet precisely how baby boomers and the Generation X and millennial cohorts that follow will experience their later years is uncertain. There are many reasons for optimism. Birth cohorts that came of age in the 1960s and later have more education than their parents' generation, they have benefited from scientific innovations ranging from medical and pharmaceutical advances to environmental protections, and they are tech-savvy, capable of relying on virtual worlds for the information, advice, and social support that may help them manage some challenges of aging.[1] Growing up in the years since the civil rights, feminist, and LGBTQ pride movements, they have enjoyed rights, benefits, and opportunities that were unimaginable in earlier decades (although the dream of full equality remains elusive). These cohorts also tend to hold more flexible and equitable gender roles than their parents, so future cohorts of widows may be prepared to manage their household finances in ways their mothers were not, while widowers may be adept at preparing meals, ordering medications, and maintaining close social ties in ways that their fathers were not.

Yet other indications point to a less optimistic and more bifurcated future. Current social and economic trends suggest that future cohorts will witness an even greater gap between the haves and have-nots at every stage of the life course—with this divide reaching its most dramatic chasm in old age. For those on the very top rung of the economic ladder, old age might be characterized as the "platinum years," with top-notch concierge health care, luxurious housing, enjoyable leisure activities, and skilled assistants and state-of-the art technologies to help with daily life once their health starts to decline. Yet for those on lower rungs of the ladder, old age may be marked by daily struggle, physical health challenges, and economic scarcity. Just as we have seen for current generations of older adults, major advances in technology, health care, and education may disproportionately benefit those baby boomers and Generation Xers who have the means to best access and make use of these breakthroughs.[2]

In this chapter, I provide a glimpse into the future and suggest ways in which current social, economic, and political trends may be setting the stage for old age among those cohorts born since the late 1940s. Predictions are necessarily speculative, and mine are no exception. I draw on demographers' and economists' projections based on rigorous national data to help provide a reasonable foundation for these forecasts.[3] I then describe broad strategies that we as a society could undertake to elevate the well-being of current and future cohorts of older adults, with the particular goal of sustaining good health, happiness, social integration, and longevity for the most vulnerable.[4]

Looking into the Future: What Will Old Age Look Like for Baby Boomers and Beyond?

In many ways, members of the Greatest Generation born in the years surrounding the Great Depression enjoyed historical luck, and their lives exemplify the life-course theme that personal biographies are shaped by historical contexts. Many were beneficiaries of social policies that helped them launch careers, purchase homes, and start families when they were young adults. At least for whites, the GI Bill helped young men—even those of limited means—to establish a secure financial foundation for the future. They entered the labor market during the economic boom years of the 1950s, when lucrative and stable jobs were ample. When the Great Recession struck in the late 2000s, most already owned homes, had steady jobs, or were in the early years of retirement, and thus were relatively immune to the economic strains that have plagued their children's and grandchildren's lives.

Yet these aggregate-level snapshots of good fortune conceal vast disparities: African Americans, those with limited education, and women have been particularly vulnerable to economic downturns, poor health, substandard housing, and the blocked opportunities that accompany lives of cumulative disadvantage. Although Medicare, Medicaid, and Social Security have provided an unequivocal boost to the health and economic well-being of the nation's least advantaged, these policies have not fully eradicated the deep disparities that have emerged slowly over decades. And some experts predict that those disparities may widen even further for the 75 million baby boomers entering old age and the cohorts that follow. The combined forces of an unprecedented number of adults entering old age and a widening divide between the advantaged and disadvantaged will necessitate public policies, creative community-based initiatives and private ventures, and a collective shift in mind-set to help ensure that all Americans have an opportunity to age well.

I describe five contemporary social and economic realities that will lay the foundation for the aging experiences of the large baby boom cohort and the Generation X and millennial cohorts that follow: (1) rising levels of economic inequality; (2) lingering impacts of the Great Recession; (3) escalating rates of high-risk health behaviors; (4) increasing numbers of reconfigured and nontraditional families; and (5) the challenges presented by extreme longevity, including insufficient numbers of caregivers to meet the needs of an aging population.

Rising Levels of Economic Inequality

Levels of economic inequality in the United States have risen dramatically since the 1970s; in the early 2000s, economic inequality was at its most extreme since shortly before the Great Depression of the early 1930s. Similar patterns have been documented in other wealthy nations in the Global North, including Canada, France, Germany, and Japan, yet no nation has witnessed divides as dramatic as those in the United States.[5] Rising economic inequality refers to a widening gap between the income and wealth of the most elite, usually defined as those in the top 1 or 5 percent of the distribution, and that of everyone else. As figure 9.1 shows, since the late 1960s the income levels of the top 5 percent of earners in the United States have increased steeply, whereas income growth has been much more muted or even flat among those at the lower rungs of the earnings ladder. To give a concrete example, in 1980 Americans in the top 5 percent of the income distribution earned on average 6.7 times more than those in the bottom 20 percent of the distribution. By 2016, they earned about 9.4 times more.[6] Analyses by the Congressional Budget Office offer a slightly different portrait: the CBO finds that income inequality continued to rise between 2007 and 2015, but at a much slower pace compared with the three previous decades of widening.[7]

The reasons behind this high level of inequality are complex and far beyond the scope of this book.[8] Experts generally point to three driving factors: shifting human capital requirements, globalization, and public policies.[9] First, the United States has transitioned from a manufacturing to a white-collar, knowledge-based economy. As a result, substantial wage premiums have accrued for those with high levels of education and technological knowledge, but less-educated workers have not reaped the same benefits. A high school diploma was sufficient to secure a well-paying unionized job in a Detroit automobile factory in the early to mid-twentieth century. Today a high school diploma cannot guarantee the same career prospects, earnings, job stability, and pension wealth that a college degree typically delivers.

Second, with globalization, the United States has been importing more and more goods from overseas, especially from China. Heavy reliance on products manufactured abroad has led to the decline of U.S. industry and the loss of American jobs. The third and most compelling explanation is that economic, trade, and employment policies dating back to the late 1970s have favored the rich and hurt the working and

Figure 9.1 U.S. Income Inequality, 1967–2016

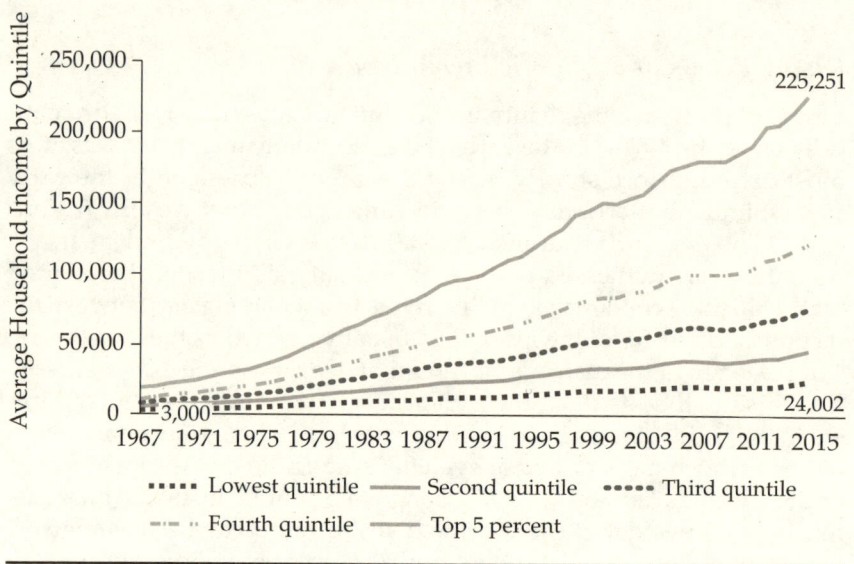

Source: U.S. Census Bureau 2017.
Note: Categories refer to the income limits for each fifth and to the top 5 percent of U.S. households.

middle classes. The deregulation of Wall Street, antilabor union policies, federal monetary policies, and regressive tax changes that favor the wealthy, including cuts to corporate, capital gains, estate, and gift taxes, have effectively reduced jobs, lowered wages, and weakened the national safety net. As the economist and *New York Times* columnist Paul Krugman has observed: "Soaring incomes at the top were achieved, in large part, by squeezing those below: by cutting wages, slashing benefits, crushing unions, and diverting a rising share of national resources to financial wheeling and dealing. . . . Perhaps more important still, the wealthy exert a vastly disproportionate effect on policy. And elite priorities—obsessive concern with budget deficits, with the supposed need to slash social programs—have done a lot to deepen [wage stagnation and income inequality]."[10]

Economic inequality has far-ranging consequences for the well-being of nations and their people. Multinational studies show that levels of social integration, trust, mental and physical health, and prospects for upward mobility are better in nations that have a more egalitarian distribution of resources, whereas nations in which income and wealth are clustered in the hands of relatively few fare worse on these dimensions.[11] In the United States, the psychic toll of economic inequality can be profound given widespread allegiance to the Protestant work ethic ideal, which views financial success as a product of hard work and talent and financial precarity as a consequence of laziness or personal deficiencies. Older adults who fall behind may suffer from compromised emotional well-being and even reduced political efficacy. Political scientists have observed that those at the top of the income distribution have the money and social connections to help elect candidates who represent their personal and political interests, whereas those at the bottom do not. As a result, those with low income may feel alienated and discouraged from voting or participating in other civic activities.[12]

Older adults may also suffer materially when levels of income inequality are high. The goods and services they need, whether housing, groceries, or home-health assistance, may be beyond their reach as their wealthier peers drive up demands and costs.[13] An even more serious concern is that public and private pension benefits contribute to an ever-widening gap in financial well-being during the retirement years because they are tied to workers' lifetime earnings. A recent study by the National Academies of Science, Engineering, and Medicine compared the experiences of older adults born in 1930 with projections of what old age might look like for baby boomers born in 1960.[14] One marker these researchers constructed was an indicator of lifetime benefits, or the total value of benefits a person might receive from Social Security, Medicare, and Medicaid. They found that for men born in 1930, those in the top and bottom lifetime earnings quintiles received roughly equal benefits. Among the late boomers, however, men in the top earning quintile were projected to receive $132,000 more in benefits over their lifetime than those in the bottom quintile, while the gap for women was $28,000.

Even more dire, rising income inequality throughout the late twentieth and early twenty-first centuries may further widen disparities in life expectancy among future cohorts of older adults. The National Academies of Science, Engineering, and Medicine analysis found that men in the lowest income quintile who were born in 1930 and who reached age fifty could expect to live another twenty-seven years, whereas life expectancy after fifty among those in the highest tier was thirty-two years—a five-year life expectancy gap.[15] By contrast, the projected life expectancy gap at age fifty for the cohort born in 1960 was an astounding twelve years. These trends suggest that the fortunes of aging baby boomers and the cohorts that follow will diverge even more dramatically than for current cohorts of older adults. For a growing share of older adults, the prospect of entering their golden years may remain elusive.

The Lingering Impacts of the Great Recession

The Great Recession struck in the late 2000s, following the heady decade of the 1990s, when housing prices skyrocketed and predatory lenders started doling out risky mortgages to millions of Americans eager to join in on the housing boom. Blacks and poorer adults who might have faced difficulty securing home loans in the past were particularly vulnerable to unscrupulous lenders offering subprime loans, which have much higher interest rates than traditional loans. By 2007, the housing bubble had burst, leaving many working-poor and middle-class Americans with homes in foreclosure and their already modest savings accounts depleted. As the financial crisis spiraled outward, home values plummeted and unemployment rates spiked. Although the Great Recession technically lasted just nineteen months, from December 2007 to June 2009, its impact was vast. More than eight million Americans lost their jobs, nearly four million homes were foreclosed each year, and more than two million businesses shut their doors.[16]

Older adults were largely spared the recession's harshest impacts. Most were already retired when the financial crisis struck, so they were relatively unaffected by job layoffs. Many had owned their homes for decades, so they were less likely to fall prey to foreclosure. For most Americans, their home is their largest asset, and it can serve as an important financial cushion in the face of threats like job loss or health care costs.[17] Current generations of older adults have had good fortune when it comes to homeownership: many purchased their homes at relatively modest prices in the 1950s, '60s, and '70s and have watched their home values soar through the decades.[18]

The consequences of the recession for younger and midlife adults have been more serious and long-lasting, especially for low-income and ethnic minority adults who were already in a precarious position with respect to employment or housing. According to a national survey by the Pew Research Center, more than half of all working adults said that during the recession they experienced a spell of unemployment, a pay cut, or reduced work hours, or that they were stuck with a part-time job when they would have preferred full-time work.[19] More than 60 percent of workers currently in their fifties said that they would probably need to delay their retirement because they did not have enough income or savings to support themselves. Fully 70 percent of workers without a college degree, yet just half of college grads, anticipated that they would need to delay retirement due to lingering effects of the recession. Yet those without a college degree and those working in strenuous manual and service industry jobs are precisely the people who experience earlier onset of health problems that may push them out of the labor force prematurely. Generation X and millennial cohorts also are more likely than their predecessors to be part of the "gig" economy, working on a contract or freelance basis. These nonstandard workers are less likely to have steady full-time work, health benefits, and pensions and thus may need to work longer than they would otherwise prefer.[20]

Economists estimate that Americans lost trillions of dollars in wealth and home equity during the recession, and declines in home values are linked to stress, depressive symptoms, and unhealthy behaviors, like delaying or forgoing doctors' appointments, not refilling pricey prescriptions, and eating cheaper, less nutritious foods.[21] And recent data from the Federal Reserve Board suggest that the short- and long-term wealth impacts of the Great Recession are especially harsh for each subsequent generation, with Generation X faring worse than boomers, and millennials faring the worst of all.[22] These generational disparities reflect key themes of life-course and cumulative disadvantage theories; the impact of an event depends on one's age at that moment, and relatively small differences in income and savings early in life beget ever-increasing gaps in the longer term. The recession struck when the millennials were just getting started with their careers and families, while the older generations were more established. The Federal Reserve study compared the 2016 wealth levels of households headed by persons born in the 1930s to those of later cohorts. Households headed by someone born after 1960 fared worse than those born earlier, and householders born in the 1980s, the youngest group in the study, fared worst of all. In 2016, the millennials' median net worth was 34 percent lower than what past trends would predict for their age group, while Gen Xers were 18 percent behind prior projections.

Curmudgeons have blamed the millennials' sparse savings on their wasteful spending on luxuries like avocado toast, gourmet coffee, and tickets to the pricey Coachella music festival, yet this is pure fiction. Federal Reserve data show that Americans born in the 1980s save their money at higher rates than boomers or Gen Xers did at their age. However, they are strapped with student debt, car loans, and hefty credit card balances. Fewer than half are homeowners, and few hold assets like stock; experts predict that millennials who are now in their thirties will never be able to amass wealth quickly enough to match prior generations. Although some economists point out some cause for optimism in the fact that millennials and Gen Xers are more highly educated than the cohorts that precede them—suggesting that they may eventually earn enough income to get out of debt and start amassing wealth—the less optimistic (and more realistic) prediction is that they will never accumulate the financial cushion sufficient to buffer late-life threats like high medical and long-term care bills and to bolster their retirement and pension earnings. Taken together, eroding housing wealth and savings, precarious employment, and the physical and emotional toll that the recession has taken on young and midlife adults bode poorly for the least-advantaged boomers and Generation Xers approaching old age.

Escalating Rates of High-Risk Health Behaviors

The United States witnessed steadily rising life expectancies over the past century, yet this trend turned around in 2015, when life expectancy dipped. It dipped once again in 2016, and preliminary data from the Centers for Disease Control show that another drop in 2017 is likely.[23] If the 2017 trend holds, it will mark the first time since the 1910s flu pandemic that the United States has had three consecutive years of declining life expectancy. Over this three-year period, death rates from multiple causes increased, including heart disease, stroke, diabetes, accidental deaths, and suicides. Although many factors contribute to death rates and, consequently, life expectancy, epidemiologists point to two serious public health crises that are playing an outsized role: obesity and rising rates of heroin and opioid addiction. Both of these crises disproportionately affect those already suffering from other social and economic disadvantages. Obesity rates are highest among those with fewer socioeconomic resources, blacks, and Latinos, while the opioid crisis has disproportionately affected whites with lower levels of education and income.[24]

Obesity strikes as early as young childhood. Epidemiologists document that one in five African American and Latino children age two to nineteen are obese. Low-income children across all racial and ethnic groups are especially vulnerable. An estimated 15 percent of toddlers (age two to four) whose mothers are receiving WIC are obese, compared to just 8.9 percent of toddlers overall.[25] The impact of obesity on educational and career prospects, mental and physical health, social relationships, and daily functioning is profound. Obesity is linked to poorer performance in school, lower rates of college attendance, more frequent workplace discrimination, and lower wages, as well as myriad health problems, including early-onset diabetes and metabolic syndrome, high blood pressure, heart disease, some cancers, sleep apnea, lower body impairments, and ultimately a hastened death.[26] In short, obesity is both a cause and consequence of social inequality and may undermine the health and economic well-being of future cohorts of older adults. At worst, it may prevent the most vulnerable from surviving until old age.[27]

The obesity crisis has evolved over the past four decades, but the ravages of the opioid epidemic are still fairly recent, with a gradual rise in addiction-related deaths since 2002 and a steep uptick since 2014. As

Figure 9.2 Opioid and Heroin Overdose Death, 2002–2015

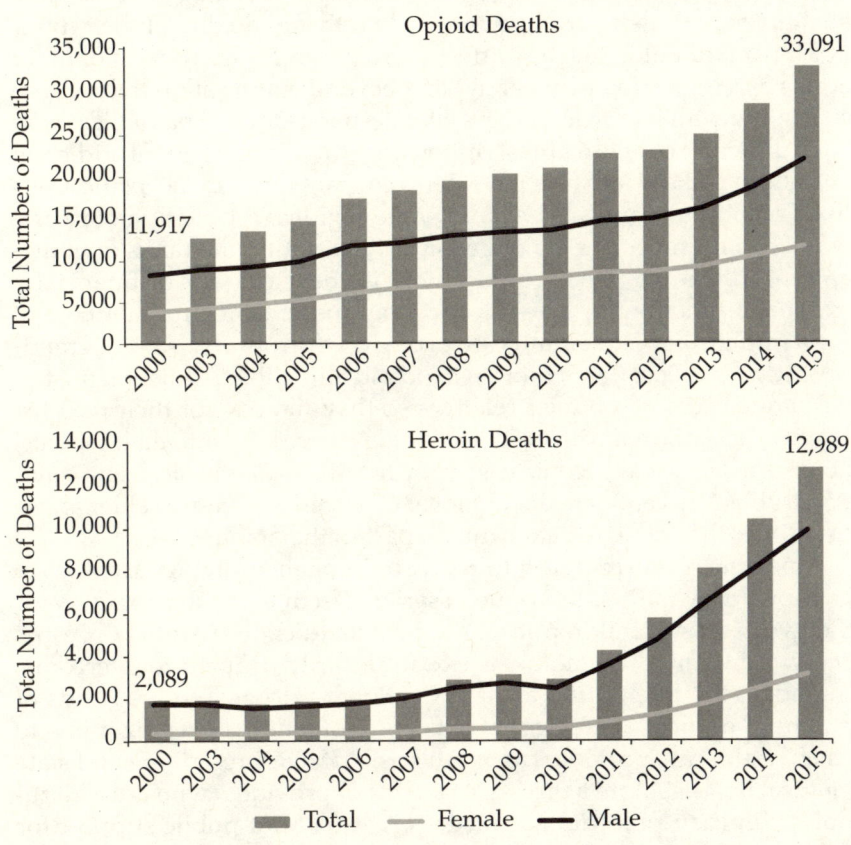

Source: National Institute on Drug Abuse 2018.

figure 9.2 shows, the number of deaths due to opioid overdose nearly tripled between 2002 and 2015, while heroin deaths more than quintupled.[28] In 2016, more than sixty-four thousand Americans died of drug overdoses, and roughly two-thirds of those overdoses were from prescription opioids, synthetic opioids, or heroin.[29] Blue Cross Blue Shield found that between 2010 and 2016 the number of people diagnosed with an addiction to opioids—including both legal prescription drugs like oxycodone and hydrocodone and illicit drugs—quintupled.[30] Yet during the same period the number of people getting treatment to manage their addiction increased by just 65 percent. The economists Anne Case and Angus Deaton find that lower-income whites are especially at risk of opioid addiction and death.[31] If these patterns continue, they could contribute to an even further bifurcation between advantaged versus disadvantaged adults with respect to the length and quality of their lives.

The opioid epidemic may affect current and future cohorts of older adults in far-reaching ways, above and beyond cutting short lives. Those struggling with injury and illness who desperately need painkillers may have difficulty obtaining prescriptions as growing fears about addiction and abuse make health care providers reluctant to prescribe medications like Percocet or Vicodin.[32] And in some regions, especially poor rural white communities, the opioid crisis is devastating the ranks of young and midlife adults who would otherwise be caring for or financially supporting their aging parents and grandparents. Rising numbers of rural midlife and older adults are taking on the role of custodial grandparent, having lost their children to opioid addiction. Addiction pushes desperate users to rob their relatives so they can pay for their next fix. When adult children with opioid addiction move back into their parents' home, the latter can become easy prey for financial, physical, and emotional abuse. Recent data document a 37 percent increase in elder abuse cases over the past five years, due in part to the opioid crisis.[33]

Moreover, some midlife adults are draining their savings accounts to pay for pricey (although not necessarily effective) rehab programs for their young adult children struggling with addiction.[34] Addiction, especially to heroin and opioids, is extraordinarily difficult to overcome. Initiatives are attempting to stem the flow of drugs into the hands of potential addicts, including efforts by professional organizations to teach health care providers about the risks of overprescribing and state medical boards' more aggressive pursuit of providers who are unscrupulous in their prescribing practices. Yet without public support for programs that increase drug education, encourage safe and healthy prescribing of painkillers, limit access to drugs before addiction starts, and treat addicts once they are hooked, the deadly epidemic will continue to affect both drug users and their family members who rely on them.

More Reconfigured and Nontraditional Families

Over the past six decades, unprecedented demographic changes have transformed family life in the United States. With increases in educational attainment, couples are marrying later than ever, delaying childbearing, and having fewer children than prior generations. Adult children who move away from their parents' homes to pursue career and educational opportunities are further shrinking the already small pool of offspring available to care for aging parents.[35] One-quarter of all baby boomers do not have children and, as a result, will need to turn to other sources of personal care when they reach old age.

Marriage has also changed dramatically over the past half-century, in terms of whether, when, how often, and whom one marries. Rising numbers of adults, especially black women, are not marrying at all. Marriage has arguably become an institution for the privileged and thus one that, in turn, perpetuates privilege. According to data from the American Community Survey (ACS), 56 percent of upper- or middle-class adults age eighteen to fifty-five are currently married, compared to just 39 percent of working-class and 26 percent of poor people.[36] LGBTQ adults, once prohibited from marrying legally, can now formalize their unions thanks to the 2015 Supreme Court decision guaranteeing the right to same-sex marriage. Marriages, whether same-sex or opposite-sex, are increasingly homogamous on the basis of socioeconomic status—that is, college graduates are marrying fellow college graduates and high school dropouts are marrying other high school dropouts, perpetuating the widening income and wealth gap between the haves and have-nots.[37]

Having only one marriage "till death do us part" is an outdated notion for many baby boomers and the cohorts that follow. Expanding opportunities for women's economic independence, coupled with cultural values promoting individualism over familism, were linked to a steep increase in the divorce rate between 1960 and 1990, with a leveling off in recent decades for all populations except for midlife and older adults. Rates of divorce among people in their fifties and older have outpaced all other age groups. Yet divorce does not mean a lifetime of romantic asceticism for older adults: 28 percent of all married men and 23 percent of married women age sixty and older are remarried.[38] Growing numbers of divorced and widowed older adults are choosing not to remarry, preferring instead to cohabit with a romantic partner or maintain a "living apart together" arrangement in which they date their partner exclusively but keep their finances separate and do not share a home.[39]

These shifts in family structure may affect the lives of future cohorts of older adults in many ways, some boosting well-being and others reducing it. Among the most serious concerns is that Social Security is structured for "traditional" family arrangements—that is, it favors those who have been married for life and who maintained a breadwinner-homemaker arrangement. Lifelong singles—a small yet rapidly growing group, especially among women of color—receive Social Security based solely on their own earnings, which typically have lagged behind those of their married counterparts. Those who had short-lived marriages—

lasting less than ten years—are not eligible for spouse benefits and must rely on retired worker benefits based on their earnings alone. Those who have divorced after being married for ten or more years are eligible for only half of their ex-spouse's benefits, provided the ex-spouse is eligible for retired worker benefits. Widow(er)s, by contrast, are entitled to 100 percent of their late spouse's benefits. Given black-white differences in rates of getting married and staying married, some researchers project that half of all black women born in 1960 (but just 10 percent of their white counterparts) will be ineligible for spouse or widow benefits, underscoring how early-life disparities can impede later-life well-being.[40]

Spouses in dual-earner marriages also are penalized by current benefit rules. This is a serious concern because 60 percent of married couples with dependent children today are dual-earner families, compared to just 25 percent in 1960.[41] The math behind benefit levels is complicated, but Pamela Herd and her colleagues provide a clear example to illustrate how the dual-earner couple penalty emerges.[42] Imagine two married couples, each of whom has an annual income of $60,000. One couple is a dual-earner family, and each spouse earns $30,000 per year. The other is a sole-breadwinner household: the husband earns $60,000 a year. When those marriages end, the wife in the sole-breadwinner household will receive a $1,200 widow benefit, whereas the wife in the dual-earner household will receive just $800. As a widow, she would have a survivor benefit of $800, and her retired worker benefit would also be $800. However, dual-eligibles—those eligible for benefits based on their own income as workers or on their former spouse's work record—must choose just one of the two options, whichever is larger. Unless Social Security alters its rules—such as reducing the ten-year marriage rule to a shorter duration or adjusting the entitlement levels for widow(er)s and divorcées who also are retired workers—the financial well-being of future cohorts of older women, and especially black women, will continue to lag substantially behind that of men.

Remarriage also will affect the daily lives of older adults in future decades. Remarriage and the stepchildren it brings do not necessarily provide an expanded pool of potential caregivers for older adults. To the contrary, negotiating caregiving duties can be a serious challenge in blended families.[43] Adult children often are reluctant to care for stepparents, while step- and biological children might not agree on an appropriate division of labor when caring for their "shared" parent, especially when the remarriage happened fairly late in their parents' lives. Remarried older men, in particular, often have strained relationships with adult children from their first marriage, a consequence of infrequent visits and inconsistent child support payments in earlier years and strained relationships with their ex-spouse.[44] Older adults' remarriages, cohabitations, or LAT relationships may not bring the same emotional and practical support as long-term marriages. The health benefits of remarriage and cohabitation are less than those reaped in a first marriage, owing in part to the stress of maintaining ties with ex-spouses and children from the new and old partnerships.[45]

As evolving family forms become more common, accepted, and legally validated, their benefits for older adults may flourish as well. Cross-national research shows that cohabitation is just as health-enhancing as marriage in nations where it is a culturally normative and legally protected institution. In Finland, France, the Netherlands, and other nations where cohabitation is widespread, married and cohabiting adults fare equally well with respect to their physical health, mental health, and longevity.[46] One reason is that cohabitors are granted many of the same rights and privileges as married couples. Such protection, predictability, and reassurance are especially important for older adults. For example, in the Netherlands, registered cohabitors have the same rights as married couples when it comes to inheritance and pension receipt following a partner's death, which may lessen older cohabitants' financial anxieties.[47] Likewise, research in the United States tracking the health of older LGBTQ adults finds that with the legalization of same-sex marriage, the protective effects of same-sex romantic partnerships increased. The legalization of same-sex marriage brought about reductions in discrimination and stigma, better access to health care through a partner's insurance, and higher levels of social integration and perceived support.[48]

Innovative social programs beyond U.S. borders provide promising models for helping those aging outside the traditional institution of marriage to have the social and institutional supports they need. For women and older LGBTQ persons in particular, who may grow old without a romantic partner or a child nearby, "families by choice" may be essential to well-being. Cohousing, which has started to flourish in the United Kingdom, the Netherlands, and other European nations, allows older adults to live with, share resources with, and rely on emotional and practical support from their friends.[49] For example, Older Women's Co-Housing (OWCH) in London is a groundbreaking project designed and managed by the women who live there. More than two dozen single women, ranging in age from their midfifties to their eighties, have their own apartments but share a common room, a community kitchen, guest rooms for visitors, and a garden. They also share cooking, cleaning, gardening, and home maintenance tasks. As Shirley Meredeen, the eighty-six-year-old cofounder of OWCH, told a British newspaper, "It's a way of retaining your independence and your dignity and being among people who can be supportive of you at the same time."[50] Fewer and fewer Americans will be growing old with their first and only spouse by their side or with their children living just across town. Baby boomers and Generation Xers have formed (and dissolved) relationships that have met their personal needs throughout the life course. With the right structural and cultural supports, these social ties can be every bit as protective for health and social integration as the more traditional family relationships maintained by the generations that came before them.

The Challenges of Extreme Longevity

Surviving until age one hundred is a rare accomplishment, achieved by fewer than two-tenths of 1 percent of all Americans. That is why we celebrate the lives of centenarians like Goldie Michelson and Susannah Mushatt Jones. For cohorts born in the very early twentieth century, surviving until one's eighties, nineties, or beyond was an anomaly, attained by those who had the hardiness or genetic good fortune to survive infancy and childhood in an era before vaccinations, antibiotics, and other life-saving medical advances were widely available. But for cohorts born in the 1930s, 1940s, and later, joining the ranks of the oldest-old will be an increasingly common milestone, especially for those from more advantaged backgrounds. The number of Americans age eighty-five and older will more than triple by 2030, from roughly 6 million today to more than 20 million, while the number of centenarians is projected to quintuple, from 72,000 to well over 300,000 during the same time period.[51] Extreme old age means that more young people will have the joy of knowing their grandparents and even great-grandparents. Those octogenarians and nonagenarians who are in good health often give back to their communities by volunteering in youth tutoring programs or meal delivery programs, or they inspire others to value their aging bodies, like yoga master Täo Porchon-Lynch. But extreme longevity also presents profound challenges to health care systems, the national safety net, the loved ones who care for their oldest-old kin, and the oldest-old themselves, who struggle with physical or cognitive declines.

As the population of the oldest-old Americans increases, the number who suffer from disablement and the diseases associated with extreme old age will increase as well, with earlier onset among those from more-disadvantaged backgrounds. One of the most daunting concerns is the number of older adults suffering from Alzheimer's disease. The good news is that researchers have documented that the overall rate of Alzheimer's among older adults dropped between 2000 and 2012, a credit to rising levels of education and the health benefits that education con-

Figure 9.3 Projected Number of Persons Age Sixty-Five and Older with Alzheimer's Disease, by Age Group, 2010–2050

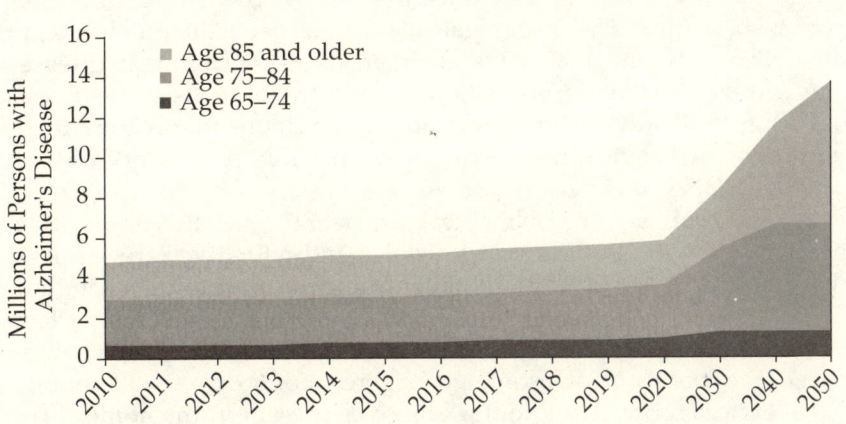

Source: Alzheimer's Association 2016, adapted from Hebert et al. 2013.

fers.[52] The bad news is that the sheer number of older adults in the United States means high and rising numbers of older adults with dementia. Roughly 5 million older adults today suffer from Alzheimer's, and this number is projected to reach 16 million by 2050, as shown in figure 9.3. Alzheimer's patients require intensive and long-term care, and these caregiving needs intensify with each passing year as the disease progresses. While the average Alzheimer's patient survives four to eight years after diagnosis, increasing numbers of patients are living as long as twenty years with the disease.[53] The investments of time, money, and emotional energy can be overwhelming, especially for older caregivers suffering physical health problems of their own. When family members are no longer capable of delivering this exhausting round-the-clock care at home, they may need to enlist costly long-term care assistance, whether at home or in a skilled nursing facility. Given that dementia risk is higher for ethnic minorities, those with lower levels of education, socially isolated older adults, and adults with strained or estranged social relationships, Alzheimer's disease and its caregiving burden may contribute to ever-widening disparities in the quality of life enjoyed by older adults.[54]

Extreme longevity and the diseases that accompany it will also strain health care systems and the federal budget. Older adults with Alzheimer's and other forms of dementia typically have twice as many hospital stays each year as those suffering from other chronic conditions. According to estimates from the Alzheimer's Association, annual medical and long-term care expenditures for all dementia patients total roughly $260 billion, yet Medicare and Medicaid cover only two-thirds of those costs—leaving family members to cover nearly $56 billion in out-of-pocket spending.[55] These aggregate costs are expected to quadruple, to more than $1 trillion, by 2050. Alzheimer's is just one of many diseases that will require long-term treatments and care. Millions of the oldest-old adults will suffer from other chronic conditions that require long-term care, including cancer, chronic obstructive pulmonary disease (COPD), diabetes, and heart disease.

An important advance in medical care over the past two decades has been the growing popularity of hospice and palliative care services, which provide comfort care to patients and support to their families. Despite the many benefits of hospice care, the program is not perfect. Because the program emphasizes the importance of family members as part of the care team, an estimated 12 percent of hospices will not provide services to those without a caregiver present in the home.[56] The rules are biased against those who are unmarried, childless, or socially isolated, as well as those whose family members cannot afford to take time off work. Because low-income and black older adults are less likely to be married (and thus lack a coresidential spouse caregiver), they are particularly hurt by such requirements.

A further challenge is that hospice care is cost-effective when its use is limited to relatively short spells at the very end of life. Dementia patients in particular tend to enter hospice early—that is, more than six months prior to their death. (Medicare will cover hospice payments for patients who are certified by a physician to have a terminal illness and a life expectancy of six months or less.) One reason for early entry into hospice for Alzheimer's patients is the difficulty of accurately projecting how long a dementia patient will survive. This is one reason why, with typically longer hospice stays for Alzheimer's patients, Medicare expenditures for care in the last year of life have increased over the past decade.[57] Over the past decade, this problem has been exacerbated by the rising numbers of for-profit hospices that load their rosters with dementia patients, incentivized by Medicare's flat reimbursement rates. Hospice care for dementia patients is less labor-intensive than cancer care, and their longer hospice spells make them more profitable.[58]

Long-term care experts also worry that the United States does not have enough young and midlife adults to provide informal care to their aging kin. AARP projects that an unprecedented shortage in caregivers may be imminent. As figure 9.4 shows, the ratio of potential caregivers to care recipients is estimated to plummet from seven-to-one today to just three-to-one by 2030. Other studies predict that as many as one in four baby boomers will be an "elder orphan"—without a spouse, child,

Figure 9.4 Projected Ratio of Caregivers to Care Recipients, 1990–2050

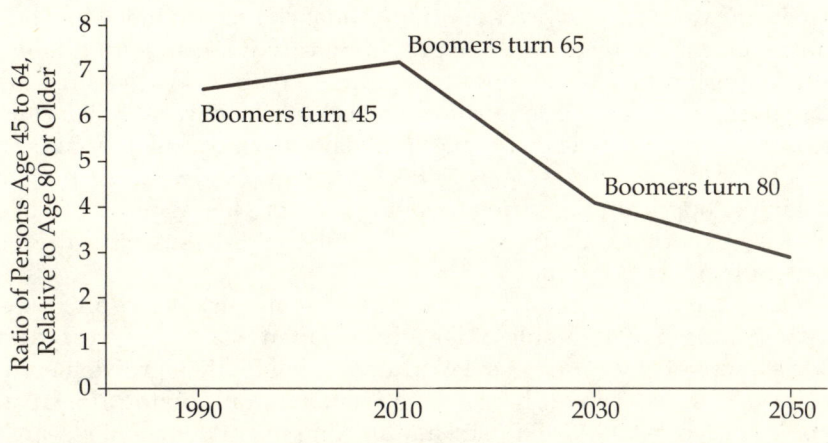

Source: Redfoot, Feinberg, and Houser 2013.
Note: The caregiver support ratio is defined as the population age 45 to 64 to the population age 80 or older.

or other family member to be their primary caregiver in old age.[59] Although some older adults have the means to pay a home health aide or visiting nurse, this option may be out of reach for those with limited financial resources, especially given Medicare's limited coverage of such services.[60]

Paid caregivers also will be in short supply. According to the Bureau of Labor Statistics, paid caregivers top the list of occupations expected to grow between 2012 and 2022.[61] Personal care aides rank first, with 580,800 new positions projected, followed closely by home health aides in fourth place (424,200 new jobs) and nursing assistants taking sixth place (312,200 jobs). This total estimate of 1.3 million jobs is low because it includes only those positions hired by companies. The Paraprofessional Healthcare Institute (PHI) calculated an alternate estimate that included caregivers hired directly by consumers, and it concluded that nearly 5 million direct care workers will be needed by 2020.[62] Frontline caregiver jobs are overwhelmingly filled by low-income and ethnic minority women, and one in five are immigrants. As a result, the pool of paid caregivers will shrink even further should national immigration policies grow more restrictive.[63]

The incentives to entice new paid caregivers are few, given their low wages. Some experts argue that increasing their wages simply is not realistic. Middle- and working-class families who pay their caregivers directly cannot afford higher wages. Home health agencies cover roughly three-quarters of their workers' wages through Medicaid and Medicare, which already face enormous financial constraints. More feasible enticements might include providing care workers with training and opportunities for advancement. Other creative solutions for the caregiver shortage include recruiting experienced family caregivers into paid caregiver jobs or encouraging retired health care providers, nurses, and other caring professionals to take part-time paid work or pursue volunteer opportunities caring for ailing seniors—just as programs like AARP's Experience Corps recruit older volunteers to share their skills with vulnerable children.[64]

Other nations are initiating innovative community-based programs to help care for vulnerable older adults. Japan has one of the oldest populations of any nation in the world, so caring for their growing numbers of dementia patients has become a national concern. In 2015, Japan implemented its ORANGE plan, a multicomponent dementia research and treatment program. Calling for a "total community" approach, the program engages ordinary citizens to help support dementia patients and their caregivers. Volunteers attend a ninety-minute dementia lecture and then receive a bright orange bib or bracelet signifying that they are a member of a neighborhood patrol. These volunteers—currently twenty-five thousand strong—walk around neighborhoods, check in on those in need of home visits, pass out flyers describing dementia support services, and assist older dementia patients who might have wandered off from their homes.[65] These street patrol members are not a substitute for highly trained round-the-clock caregivers, but they do fill an important and emerging need.

One of the most intriguing and hotly debated innovations for meeting the care needs of older adults is the use of robots. Although the word "robot" conjures up images of sci-fi characters like R2-D2 from *Star Wars*, in reality robots resemble more ordinary (and less futuristic) devices, like the Roomba vacuum cleaner or voice-activated assistants like Alexa. The use of robots for elder care has flourished in Japan. The Japanese government has invested in the development of devices like an electric-boosted mobility aid that an older adult can grab onto when walking around his or her neighborhood. The sensors detect whether the older adult is walking uphill; if so, a booster function is activated. Conversely, an automatic break kicks in when the person is walking downhill, as a protection against falls. Other innovations under development include simple robotic devices that help frail older adults get out of bed and into a wheelchair or that can help lift and then lower them into bathtubs.[66] These devices are hardly a replacement for personal care from a trusted and loved family member, yet they are helping to fill some gaps in the more straightforward and physical aspects of care, especially for socially isolated older adults who cannot turn to kin for support.

Americans show guarded optimism about using technology to help care for older adults. According to a recent Pew survey, 70 percent of adults believed that robot caregivers would help alleviate the burden of caring for aging relatives, although just 40 percent said that they would ever consider using them.[67] Openness to the idea increases across generations; nearly half of millennials but just 37 percent of older adults today would consider using robots. And blacks were only half as likely as whites, and high school graduates about half as likely as college graduates, to consider the use of automated caregiving supports. Despite the potential of assistive technologies in elder care, the use of these robots—like other scientific advances—may be limited only to those with the greater economic means.[68] While they may help meet caregiving demands among future cohorts of older adults in the aggregate, they may not help to stem disparities in the caregiving experiences.

Public and Private Strategies for Promoting "Golden Years" for U.S. Older Adults

The graying of America is in full swing, and this dramatic population shift brings unprecedented challenges that warrant creative solutions. But government programs alone, while essential to the well-being of older adults, will not be sufficient to meet the diverse and complex needs of older adults and the family and friends who care for them. Social programs that provide support early and often for education, health, nutrition, housing, and income security are a critical first step to provide all people, not just those born with a silver spoon in their mouth, the capacity to experience golden years in old age. But putting our collective faith in policymakers to do the right thing is unwise, especially during historical periods in which progressive values emphasizing equality and opportunity, social welfare, and a strong safety net are eclipsed by conservative values advocating for individual freedoms, personal responsibility, and a limited role of government in improving the lives of citizens. I describe four broad strategies for improving the quality of life of both current and future cohorts of older Americans, paying particular attention to the needs of those whose lives have been marked by limited opportunity, financial precariousness, social isolation, and other threats to well-being. I also underscore that older adults are not the passive and needy recipients of federal resources, volunteer services, and innovative public-private initiatives. Rather, older adults have a tremendous capacity to give back to their communities, to care for and nurture the generations that follow, and to develop creative strategies for living well—even when their health may be declining and their financial resources are sparse.

Expanding Access to and the Quality of Health Care

Delivering high-quality, respectful, and timely health care to older adults must remain one of our nation's top priorities. Access to care alone will not resolve late-life disparities in health and longevity; as James House and others have argued, health care accounts for just 10 to 20 percent of premature mortality in the United States.[69] That statistic notwithstanding, older adults need informed, sensitive, and timely care, especially those growing old with multiple conditions that reduce their quality of life. Structural and psychosocial obstacles ranging from insurance reimbursement policies to the implicit biases we hold may hamper the quality of care that older patients receive—especially those who are most disadvantaged and isolated.

Untreated geriatric depression provides a clear illustration. An estimated one in four older adults have depression that goes untreated, with even higher rates for older blacks and men.[70] This problem stems not only from lack of access to care but from inaccurate diagnoses even for those who do seek care. First, some depressed older adults cannot get an appointment with a mental health care provider. Ninety percent of physicians but just half of psychiatrists are willing to accept new Medicare patients, who are considered undesirable from a purely financial perspective owing to low reimbursement rates and the need for multiple and often long-lasting visits.[71] Second, even when older patients do get an appointment, their symptoms are sometimes misdiagnosed and treated inadequately (or not treated at all). Practitioners may incorrectly assume that sadness and sluggishness are "normal" aspects of aging and thus do not require medical attention.[72] Some care providers may not probe further when older blacks and men show symptoms of lethargy yet hide their symptoms of depression or anxiety for fear that they will be stigmatized, shamed, or judged.

These two obstacles, compromised access for Medicare patients and inadequate treatment once a patient does see a provider, are closely and subtly intertwined—the former is a cause and the latter a consequence of the dearth of geriatric specialists in the United States. Geriatricians—physicians with formal training in the complex physical, emotional, and social needs of older adults—are in woefully short supply. According to estimates from the American Geriatrics Society (AGS), only 7,500 physicians in the United States are certified geriatricians, although more than 17,000 are needed to care for the booming population of older patients. Formal training in geriatrics emphasizes important topics that are often given short shrift in traditional medical education, including a holistic approach to care that considers multiple organ systems and comorbidities and the psychosocial and cognitive aspects of health.[73]

This shortage partly reflects the fact that recent medical school graduates are reluctant to enter one of the profession's lowest-paid and most poorly reimbursed specialties. Geriatricians tend to treat patients who are covered by Medicare and Medicaid, which have lower reimbursement rates than private health insurance companies. This translates into lower lifetime earnings for geriatricians relative to their peers working in other specialties. Especially for recent medical school graduates who already have an average of $183,000 in debt, specializing in geriatrics may seem an unwise financial choice.[74] Roughly half of the geriatrics fellowship training slots go unfilled each year, especially at training programs in economically depressed regions with few amenities to entice young professionals.[75] Geriatrics fellowship candidates face little competition, so promising applicants can easily find positions at more prestigious programs in more cosmopolitan locations.

The American Geriatrics Society (AGS) recognizes that recruiting newly minted medical school graduates to geriatrics may be an uphill battle, so the organization has developed programs to bring geriatrics training to established practitioners in other areas of medicine. In 1994, AGS launched the Geriatrics-for-Specialists Initiative, which helps practitioners acquire the skills and knowledge needed to address older patients' complex needs. The initiative has developed guidelines on postoperative delirium for surgeons, recommendations for how emergency departments can be more accommodating to older adults, lessons on managing or consolidating multiple medications, and primers on geriatric psychiatric conditions.[76] The program's overarching vision is that every health care provider should have basic knowledge and skills in geriatric care. Medical schools and residencies also are starting to incorporate geriatrics education into their curricula, conveying the important message that a knowledge of geriatrics—like pediatrics—is essential to all care providers regardless of their specialty. And enlisting geriatrics specialists to teach occasional courses or provide guest lectures may convey the importance and complexity of the field, as well as the personal rewards of treating older patients; geriatricians consistently report the highest levels of job satisfaction of any medical specialty.[77]

Current and future cohorts of medical students may be particularly receptive to curricular approaches that directly address the complex social, cultural, economic, and even political factors that affect older adults' health, well-being, and quality of end-of-life care. In 2015, the

Association of American Medical Colleges (AAMC) introduced a new Medical College Admission Test (MCAT) that debuted sections evaluating knowledge of behavioral and social sciences. Among the topics covered are prejudice and discrimination, power and privilege, social institutions, and social stratification—phenomena that are at the very core of producing and sustaining late-life health disparities. Although it is too soon to tell whether this initiative will affect how health care providers treat older patients, it is an important effort in providing practitioners with an awareness of the ways in which social class, race, and gender shape patients' symptoms and how those symptoms present, ultimately affecting patient survival.

Increasing practitioners' knowledge of and sensitivity to the complex needs of diverse older adult populations is an important first step. Yet it is not a panacea; the most effective way to recruit more geriatric specialists and incentivize all health care providers to see Medicare beneficiaries as patients is to increase reimbursement rates, especially in geographic areas where payments are low. The politics and mechanics behind Medicare reimbursement are complex, although promising advances have been made in the past decade. In 2015, Congress passed the Medicare Access and CHIP Reauthorization Act (MACRA), which was widely viewed as an improvement over the former Sustainable Growth Rate (SGR) program. MACRA rescues physicians from what would have been a double-digit reduction in Medicare payment rates and instead provides five years of a 0.5 percent payment rate uptick, followed by five years of no increase (but also no decrease) in the payment rate.[78]

MACRA has not been perfect, and some policy analysts argue that it does not do enough to entice reluctant providers to take on Medicare patients. Yet even for the overwhelming majority of providers who do accept Medicare patients, the reimbursements may not be seen as an adequate incentive to dedicate the time and care needed to really understand older patients' health conditions and the life circumstances with which they may be struggling. Short visits may not be sufficient for physicians to build rapport and develop an understanding of the myriad factors shaping their older patients' health. After developing sophisticated projection models, the Center for Medicare and Medicaid Services concludes that current federal policies will not be sufficient for Medicare payments to keep pace with either general inflation or the costs of running a medical practice. According to CMS, there is "reason to expect that access to physician services for Medicare beneficiaries would be severely compromised . . . [and] the quality of care provided to Medicare beneficiaries would likely not keep pace with care furnished to other types of patients."[79]

Health policy experts agree that innovative solutions are necessary, or else more physicians will restrict the number of Medicare beneficiaries they see and stop accepting new Medicare patients—at precisely the time when more than 70 million baby boomers are marching into old age. Some providers will adapt by cramming more patient appointments into their already tight schedules, compromising the quality of care they can provide. Others may choose to treat only private-pay patients, or they will provide highly personalized, care-on-demand "concierge" services to those who can afford it.[80] Some practitioners may raise the prices for those patients who can afford to pay. All of these physician strategies, although wisely self-protective, are likely to compromise older adults' care, especially for those who cannot afford private insurance to supplement their Medicare, or the $1,500 to $2,000 per year annual retainer for concierge services.

Large expansions of social welfare programs, like dramatic increases in Medicare reimbursement payments, would no doubt be effective in reducing late-life inequalities, yet would incur vast costs. According to Congressional Budget Office projections, net Medicare spending is expected to nearly double, from $590 billion in 2017 to $1.2 trillion in 2027.[81] Recognizing these costs, policy experts propose alternative solutions that could uphold the quality and reach of care while also containing spending. These proposals include tying Medicare payments to the quality of care received by the patient; using strategic "global-based" payments for patients with particularly complex and costly medical needs; adjusting payments to reflect regional variation in the costs of providing care; and paying a slight margin to "high-value providers," or those providers delivering high-quality and effective care at the lowest possible cost.[82]

Addressing the Roots of Late-Life Inequalities

High-quality, accessible, and affordable health care delivered to older adults is critical to their quality of life. Yet this may be too little too late for the most disadvantaged. For those who live on the streets or in prisons, or whose lives are marked by persistent poverty, social isolation, physical or mental illness, interpersonal mistreatment, or emotional desolation, reaching one's sixty-fifth birthday (and the federal health benefits bestowed at that time) is an elusive milestone. Early onset of health problems may reduce the capacity to earn a living, enjoy satisfying social relationships, maintain independence, and live a long and well-rounded life.

Efforts to improve the life chances of young and midlife Americans will benefit them directly as they grow old and also may bolster the well-being of their families, their communities, and the nation. Policies and practices that support one generation necessarily benefit their kin and communities. Efforts to eradicate health disparities, especially those rooted in early life, may reap broader societal benefits. Experts estimate that premature onset of disease costs the nation $35 billion in excess health care expenditures, $10 billion in illness-related lost productivity, and nearly $200 billion in premature deaths annually.[83]

The most obvious (and hotly debated) strategy for improving Americans' health at all ages is to provide affordable health insurance for all. The Affordable Care Act, enacted into law in 2010 under President Barack Obama, reduced the number of uninsured Americans by 20 million, including more than 2 million people age fifty-five to sixty-four who are nearing retirement. The ACA also increased coverage for children and young adults. It authorized increased funding for the Children's Health Insurance Program (CHIP), a public insurance program for children in families that earn too much to qualify for Medicaid. Another ACA provision allows parents (or more specifically, those parents with employer-provided or ACA marketplace insurance) to cover their children up until age twenty-six.

The most vulnerable—especially low-income and unhealthy Americans—also have benefited tremendously. The ACA removed barriers to insurance coverage for those with preexisting conditions and offered states the opportunity to expand Medicaid.[84]

The impact of these two provisions has been remarkable. Prior to ACA, nearly half of all adults with preexisting conditions who tried to purchase health insurance were denied coverage, charged a higher premium, or found that their condition was excluded from coverage. Preexisting conditions are far-ranging and encompass alcoholism, cancer, diabetes, drug addiction, heart attack and stroke, HIV/AIDS, rheumatoid arthritis, and myriad other conditions. Yet even healthy people with nondisease conditions that are considered a threat to health, like obesity, could be denied coverage. The ACA forbids this differential treatment, so it has been particularly beneficial for poor and ethnic minorities, who are more likely to suffer from these conditions and to do so at younger ages than their more-advantaged peers.[85]

The expansion of Medicaid also has increased coverage among low-income, working-age adults. As part of the ACA, the federal government pays for the total cost of the expanded Medicaid coverage through 2020, and then 90 percent of the coverage thereafter, leaving the states to provide the remainder of funds. To date, thirty-one states and the District of Columbia have bought in, and they have witnessed significant drops in the ranks of their uninsured. One review of 108 studies on the impact of Medicaid expansion, published between January 2014 and January 2017, showed unequivocal increases in access to care, utilization, and affordability, especially for the most vulnerable patients.[86] For instance, one analysis by the Urban Institute and the Robert Wood Johnson Foundation found that blacks, Hispanics, and adults with less than a high school degree were especially likely to gain coverage between 2010 and 2015.[87] Medicaid expansion also was linked with desirable economic outcomes, including reduced out-of-pocket spending on medications, fewer unpaid medical bills, reduced medical debt, higher rates of employment among those whose health had previously limited their work, and even reduced reliance on high-interest payday loans.[88]

The ACA is far from perfect, and its limitations are well known. Premiums can be pricey. As many as one million workers were dropped from their employer-provided insurance, either because employers wanted to save money or they presumed that their workers could find cheaper plans on the exchanges. Yet the overwhelming majority of policy analysts, health care providers, and major organizations, including AARP, the American Medical Association (AMA), and the American Hospital Association (AHA), have urged the continuation of ACA and protested vehemently against its replacement with Republican-designed plans, whether the American Health Care Act or the Graham-Cassidy bill introduced in 2017, which would leave 23 million Americans uninsured over the next ten years.[89]

The Trump administration's efforts to repeal the ACA have failed, yet several executive orders have undermined key aspects of the program, leading to higher premiums and rising numbers of uninsured Americans.[90] Republicans are calling for replacement plans that rely heavily on block grants to the states—up until 2027, when the federal funds will disappear. Protection for the 130 million working-age Americans with preexisting conditions also would disappear. Proponents of these proposals say that they provide options for consumers and would allow insurers to provide lower-cost, stripped-down insurance plans. However, policy analysts caution that these low-cost plans could cause premiums to skyrocket for sicker people if healthy people move to the less costly options.

Yet the most punitive component of the Republican proposals is the call to repeal Medicaid expansion, which would be devastating for low-income adults and their families. Not only does Medicaid provide access to health care for low-income Americans, but roughly half of federal and state Medicaid funding in 2015 went for long-term care services—an obligation that could fall back upon burdened family members.[91] The Medicaid directors of all fifty states have urged against these draconian proposals, which the renowned surgeon and *New Yorker* essayist Atul Gawande has described as "mass suicide" for Americans.[92]

In sharp contrast, some liberal Democrats are enthusiastic about Senator Bernie Sanders (I-VT) call for "Medicare for all," a shorthand label for a single-payer system. Even Sanders himself has said that he does not believe such a bill will pass, but Democratic support is coalescing for bills that would allow Americans age fifty-five and older (the Senate's Medicare at 55 Act) or age fifty and older (the House's Medicare Buy-In and Health Care Stabilization Act) to buy into Medicare at a reasonable cost.[93] The enactment of such plans could be life-altering for the 52 percent of near-retirement-age Americans who suffer from high blood pressure, the 15 percent with diabetes, or the millions suffering from depression, anxiety, or substance use.[94] It would also relieve their financial burden, as adults age fifty-five to sixty-four pay an average of $1,200 each year on out-of-pocket medical expenditures, along with insurance rates that are roughly three times higher than younger adults'.[95] Surveys show that most Americans would support expanding Medicare to those in their fifties; this public support, amplified by the sheer size of the baby boom electorate, could impel policymakers from both sides of the aisle to support the initiative.[96]

Health care reform has been at the center of impassioned and drawn-out political debates, yet access to health care is just one step toward ensuring that Americans from all backgrounds have the opportunity to grow old with good health, dignity, and physical comfort.[97] As the United Kingdom's *Black Report* showed in the 1980s, access to medical care is not enough—additional education, employment, and tax policies also are necessary.[98] Investments in public education, beginning in early childhood with programs like Head Start and universal prekindergarten, can enhance children's cognitive development, physical health, chances of graduating from high school, and ultimately their prospects for upward mobility.[99] Affirmative action programs can open up educational and career opportunities for blacks, Latinos, and Native Americans, who still face daunting structural obstacles. Expanded job training programs and low-interest college loans could bring promising opportunities to young adults of limited financial means. Given the strong gradient between education and health, such that higher levels of education reap better health and longer lives, support for education may be among the most effective strategies for enhancing population health and mitigating disparities on the basis of socioeconomic status and race.[100]

Income support programs also may mitigate disparities in health and well-being, although the most effective approaches would target those at the lower end of the income distribution. Increasing income among the poor and near-poor brings substantial short- and longer-term health benefits, although increasing income among those at the middle and higher levels of the income distribution does little to bolster population health.[101] Sustained and increased investment in the Earned Income Tax

Credit program targeting poor and near-poor working-age adults and in Supplemental Security Income for low-income older adults may be especially effective in reducing economic and health disparities.

Another promising approach for boosting the economic well-being of low-income older adults is the development of a minimum benefit plan (MBP). This proposal, recently developed by the sociologist Pamela Herd and her colleagues, incorporates components from EITC and Canada's Guaranteed Income Supplement (GIS) program, which provides a minimum income to older adults.[102] The centerpiece of the proposed MBP is providing older adults with a minimum benefit guaranteed at 100 percent of the poverty line. Poverty-line cutpoints would be adjusted to reflect the recipient's marital status, recognizing the ways in which women and especially women of color are disadvantaged by current Social Security guidelines. The program would also tweak some of the current Social Security eligibility criteria so that MBP recipients would not be penalized for their receipt of other income sources. Likewise, poor older adults' receipt of Medicaid benefits would not be penalized because of their participation in the MBP program. The details of the program are complex, but the upshot is that by targeting older adults at the lower end of the distribution and having stringent yet reasonable eligibility criteria, the incomes of the poorest older adults would be bolstered in a cost-effective way.[103]

Policies that help poor families save for the future over the longer term also could help future cohorts of older adults age well. This is especially important given declining numbers of workers (especially lower-income workers) who have private pensions and the transition from defined-benefit to defined-contribution plans, which shifts financial risks from employers to employees. Researchers at the University of California at Berkeley's Haas Institute argue that raising the savings rates and facilitating working- and middle-class households' capacity for accumulating wealth are essential to their long-term well-being.[104] Automatically enrolling workers in retirement plans or providing a savings credit or a federal match for retirement savings accounts could help financially precarious households amass at least modest levels of wealth, which is an essential source of financial protection in later life.

Facilitating and Supporting Family Caregiving and Decision-Making

Most Americans grow old, manage illness, and make decisions about life-and-death medical treatments with their family members—whether by blood, law, or choice—by their side. An estimated 40 million Americans age fifteen and older are now providing care to their aging loved ones. Public policies, community programs, and private ventures that target the well-being of family caregivers are essential, especially for low-income and ethnic minority caregivers, who often cannot afford paid assistance or feel that it is their duty to care for the aging parents or grandparents who once looked after them.

Nearly all Americans will spend some time as a family caregiver. Caregivers find purpose and meaning when helping their aging spouse, parents, grandparents, siblings, or other loved ones, yet most will also withstand some hardships in providing that care, including lost wages, exhaustion from juggling elder care with other demands like paid work or child care, sadness from watching their loved one suffer, and compromised health as they neglect their own symptoms or suffer bodily harm from physically grueling caregiving tasks. Some of these strains can be mitigated through well-thought-out policy. The Family and Medical Leave Act (FMLA), enacted in 1993, could be expanded to better meet the needs of caregivers, especially low-income caregivers. FMLA offers up to twelve weeks of unpaid leave to workers who need to care for a family member, whether a newborn infant or an ailing parent. However, only half of all workers are covered by FMLA; those who work for smaller businesses (fewer than fifty employees) or have not been on the job long enough to qualify are not eligible for leave. More importantly, unpaid leave threatens the economic security of the poorest Americans and those with precarious employment; they simply cannot afford to forsake their paycheck.[105] Paid leave could make a world of difference for financially strapped caregivers, who are often caught between a rock and a hard place: give up paid work to care for their loved one, or use up their few savings to pay for assistance.

Three states now offer more generous policies on their own: California, New Jersey, and Rhode Island offer paid family leave public insurance programs. Evaluations of these programs suggest that they have been effective in helping workers balance work and family demands and in providing a financial cushion for them to do so. For example, before California implemented its paid family leave (PFL) program, black new mothers averaged just one week of leave, while white mothers averaged one month. After the policy's implementation, both black and white mothers increased their leave times substantially, and the racial gap was virtually eliminated.[106]

Corporations are stepping up, although only 12 percent of private-sector workers currently receive paid family leave.[107] Companies like Deloitte, Facebook, and Microsoft, as well as other tech firms now offer paid leave (typically four or six weeks) to employees caring for family members.[108] Lucrative tech firms competing to retain their most-skilled workers may need to provide these benefits, yet low-income workers in less competitive professions are unlikely to receive such perks. The Bureau of Labor Statistics estimates that just 5 percent of workers in the lowest 25 percent of earners receive paid family leave benefits, compared to more than 22 percent of workers in the top 10 percent of earners.[109] The United States stands out as the only wealthy nation to lack a coordinated system of providing paid caregiving leave.[110] In this way, current family leave benefits disproportionately benefit those who already possess the greatest social and economic advantages.

Several innovative policies are currently being proposed and debated as ways to fill this gap. The Family and Medical Insurance Leave (FAMILY) Act would create a shared fund that makes paid leave affordable for employers of all sizes and for workers and their families. The Social Security Caregiver Credit Act would offset lost contributions during those spells when workers take their unpaid family care leave. Workers would receive a credit so that caregiving hours are included in the final calculation of their Social Security benefits. Other innovative proposals move beyond the family as a pool of potential caregivers. The Caregiver Corps Act would follow in the footsteps of successful programs like the Peace Corps and AmeriCorps, which place energetic, community-minded young people in settings where they can help those in need. Incentives like college scholarships, loan forgiveness programs, new job skills acquired in a formal elder care training program, and impressive work experience on their résumé might entice young volunteers to assist frail older adults who have no family of their own.[111]

Nonprofit organizations also offer structured programs for ensuring that older adults, especially the most socially isolated, are looked after. One of the most effective is the Meals on Wheels Association of America (MOWAA). The program does not provide direct care but instead focuses on one important care need: meal provision. Not only does this service benefit older adults directly, but it relieves their caregivers of the daily burden of preparing three nutritious meals. In 2016, Meals on Wheels delivered roughly 218 million meals to the homes of 2.5 million older adults, including a half-million veterans. The meal recipients are among the most vulnerable; many cannot afford food on their own or cannot leave their homes to shop for food because of their ailing health or fears about neighborhood safety. The organization provides a vivid illustration of the power of community generosity to provide for those in need. The drivers and assistants who deliver meals are a largely volunteer force, many of them retirees themselves. The organization is funded almost wholly through private contributions and private grants; government funds make up just 3 percent of the total budget.[112] The organization's coffers had an unexpected boost in March 2017 when President Donald Trump announced that he would abolish the community development block grant (CDBG), which was the source of a small amount of the organization's funding. In the days following the announcement of the anticipated funding cut, Meals on Wheels witnessed a remarkable 500 percent increase in its private donations and a surge in volunteer sign-ups.

Family caregivers need more than assistance with direct care tasks. They also need support as they help their aging relatives plan for end-of-life medical care. Despite melodramatic claims that "we die alone," the truth is that we make life-and-death decisions surrounded by family and loved ones. Most older adults designate their spouse or an adult child to serve as their durable power of attorney for health care, and most say that they prefer either to make medical decisions in consultation with a family member or to delegate the decision entirely to family.[113] However, family members cannot make informed decisions that meet their loved one's needs unless they are engaged in this planning from start to finish. Family conversations help to ensure that the aging patient's preferences are met and that surviving family members can carry out those preferences without fear of guilt, conflict, or distress.

An important advance in end-of-life planning was the introduction of one doctor-patient consultation for all Medicare beneficiaries, many of whom relay these conversations to their loved ones or DPAHCs. Yet this Medicare benefit, included as part of the ACA, is available only to those age sixty-five and older; health care providers also should encourage young and midlife adults to broach these sensitive yet essential topics with their kin. Other simple ways to put the topic of end-of-life planning on the radar of families include making standard advance care planning documents available when a person registers to vote, renews his or her driver's license, or signs up for benefits like Social Security, Medicare, or Medicaid. Given high and rising rates of gray divorce and remarriage, living wills and DPAHC designations also could be encouraged by attorneys processing divorce papers.[114] As families change, end-of-life plans need to change accordingly, and all family members engaged in decision-making must be kept informed and engaged.

Recognizing Older Adults as Valuable Equals, Partners, and Contributors

Public and private investment in health and welfare programs is a necessary step toward promoting comfort, dignity, and an acceptable standard of living for older adults and their families. Yet broader cultural shifts, including a more nuanced and realistic view of older adults and their capacity to contribute to society, are also essential to promoting healthy aging. Societal views of older adults have waxed and waned throughout history, and these attitudes can play an important, albeit indirect, role in shaping popular and political support for them.

In colonial America, older adults were respected, holding prestigious religious and political positions and other perks of high status, such as seats at the front of their church congregation.[115] Puritan teachings instructed young people to behave respectfully and even obsequiously toward older adults. Popular fashions of the day, from clothing styles that appeared to make men's backs look slightly hunched over, to white powdered wigs, helped younger people look older and more respectable. Historical analyses of census data from the eighteenth century show a slight bias toward age *over*-reporting, a stark contrast from the contemporary trend of celebrities (and job applicants who fear ageism) strategically shaving a decade off their lives. Yet this veneration of older adults was not due simply to religious and ideological teachings that encouraged respect for elders; it had cold, hard financial roots. Older men owned and controlled their land and properties, and their sons would inherit these assets only when their father died—so the young had selfish reasons for deferring to their elders. Or more precisely, deferring to their white male landowning elders. Blacks, women, and immigrants, who could not own land, were not afforded the same status as their white male peers.

In the decades that followed, the cultural tides turned and youthful vigor replaced sage wisdom as a status symbol, driven in part by nineteenth-century industrialization and urbanization, which provided ambitious young men with economic opportunities far away from their father's farmland. Throughout the twentieth and early twenty-first centuries, attitudes toward older adults have once again shifted. For much of the twentieth century, older adults were seen as dependent, incapable of making productive contributions to society, and in desperate need of public support. Factory work in the early twentieth century required young, strong bodies. Technical jobs that emerged at midcentury, following the 1946 debut of the first modern computer, were believed to require nimble fingers and quick minds that could easily master the latest technical innovation. These pervasive beliefs were generally consistent with mid-twentieth-century gerontological theories promoting older adults' disengagement from society as a path to their well-being. Yet these intertwined forces of paternalism and pity also helped impel two of the most important and successful policy reforms of the twentieth century: the establishment of Social Security in the 1930s, and the expansion of Social Security and the birth of Medicare in the 1960s.

In contemporary U.S. society, attitudes toward old age are optimistic, perhaps unrealistically so. The media and business community exalt healthy and vigorous older adults like nonagenarian yoga master Täo Porchon-Lynch and hardworking moguls who still show up at the office every day, like octogenarian billionaire and former Berkshire Hathaway chair Warren Buffett. At age eighty-five, Buffett famously told *Fortune* magazine that it would be "crazy" for him to stop working. Retirement, he said, "is not my idea of living."[116] Widespread recognition that most older adults are mentally sharp and physically vigorous well into their seventies and eighties is one reason why (along with concerns about the financial sustainability of the public pension system) the age at which older adults can retire with full benefits is creeping up from sixty-five to sixty-seven, with some legislators calling for a further bump to age seventy.

These inspiring and aspirational images of successful, strong, and influential older adults may help to conquer ageist beliefs and boost the self-esteem and happiness of older adults. Yet these idealized images of old age also have potentially damaging consequences. The most obvious is that the focus on "optimal agers" detracts attention from and potential support for the millions of older adults who are poor, physically or cognitively compromised, and socially isolated—not to mention those Americans who die in midlife and do not have the luxury of surviving until old age. Yet another unintended consequence of celebrating vigorous old age is that images of wealthy octogenarians like Warren Buffett reveling in their golden years may fortify and fuel the belief that older adults are doing just fine and do not need public pensions and health insurance. Legislators have proposed several policies motivated precisely by the perception that older adults are doing fine, including not only efforts to raise the age at which people can start collecting Social Security benefits but also reducing cost-of-living increases to monthly Social Security checks and increasing the eligibility age for Medicare.

Simplistic perceptions that older adults are doing just fine also contribute to long-simmering intergenerational conflicts whereby some young adults who are struggling financially view older adults as grabbing government resources that they do not need or as clinging to coveted jobs that could otherwise go to Generation Xers or millennials looking for a professional foothold.[117] These feelings of resentment may intensify as the demographic and ideological characteristics of the generations diverge, with current cohorts of older adults more likely to be white and politically conservative and millennials (who actually surpass baby boomers in sheer numbers) more likely to be black, Latino, or Asian and politically liberal.[118]

Yet despite popular media articles and blogs inveighing that the large cohort of aging boomers is to blame for the millennial generation's bleak employment and financial prospects, researchers find the exact opposite to be the case.[119] Empirical studies find no support for the "lump of labor" theory—the proposition that older adults' delayed retirement will crowd out younger workers, keeping them either underemployed or unemployed. To the contrary, greater employment of older persons leads to better outcomes for young people, including reduced unemployment rates, increased employment, and higher average wages. Economists point out that the total number of available jobs is dynamic, not fixed. The more people there are who hold jobs, the more the economy expands, creating more new jobs and putting more people to work.[120] And workplace studies show that older workers benefit their younger colleagues by mentoring them on skills like juggling tasks, taking control over their work duties, setting workplace boundaries, and managing their personal finances.[121]

Given how interconnected human lives are, policies and practices that benefit one generation generally benefit the others. Few scenarios are zero-sum. Public investments in national service programs like those supported by the Edward M. Kennedy Serve America Act of 2009 enhance the well-being of older and younger Americans alike. The Serve America Act reauthorized and expanded national service programs administered by the Corporation for National and Community Service (CNCS). Among the service programs administered under CNCS are AmeriCorps and SeniorCorps, which encompasses the Foster Grandparent Program, Retired and Senior Volunteer Programs (RSVPs), and the Encore Fellowships Program. These federally funded initiatives enable older adults of all socioeconomic strata to put their skills to work helping younger Americans. AmeriCorps, for instance, places volunteers in schools and other community settings. The Serve America Act stipulates that 10 percent of AmeriCorps slots be earmarked for volunteers age fifty-five and older. The Foster Grandparent Program assigns older volunteers to serve as friends and mentors to disadvantaged youth, while the Encore Fellowship Program places people age fifty-five and older in management or leadership positions to work with nonprofits and government in areas of "national need" like education, health, and energy.

Investment in these programs has clear payoffs for young people, who receive support, mentorship, and even unpaid child care from program volunteers. Yet these initiatives also provide productive opportunities for older adults who may not be physically able to work full-time or who cannot afford other postretirement leisure activities like traveling or golf. As part of the Serve America Act, the minimum age for Foster Grandparent volunteers was reduced from sixty to fifty-five, and stipend eligibility was raised from 125 percent up to 200 percent of the poverty line, opening up rewarding opportunities for near-poor older adults.[122] Volunteers who are particularly active also are eligible for other financial perks. The CNCS-supported Silver Scholarship Grant Program provides $1,000 scholarships to volunteers age fifty-five and older who have completed at least 350 hours of service. These funds, in turn, can be transferred to the older volunteer's child, grandchild, or stepchild.

Volunteering provides benefits to older adults and the youth they are serving. More than two thousand older volunteers in more than twenty cities participate in the AARP Foundation Experience Corps, a volunteer-based literacy tutoring program serving more than thirty thousand children in struggling elementary schools. Volunteers put in an average of six to fifteen hours per week, and their efforts pay off: program assessments find a 60 percent improvement in the children's critical literacy skills. The older adult volunteers also showed improved social integration, sense of achievement, physical activity, cognitive functioning, and physical health. These benefits were largest for lower-SES and black older adults, a boost that the program designers attribute both to the uplifting feeling of giving back to the community and to more tangible benefits like the monthly stipend (about $250 taxable dollars a month) and the lunches, social engagement, and structured routine that the program provides.[123]

Older adults are one of the country's most valuable yet arguably unsung resources. A recent CNCS study documented that more than 21 million adults age fifty-five and older contributed more than 3 billion hours of service to their communities in 2015.[124] The study valued the cost of this service at roughly $77 billion per year. The tasks that older volunteers perform range from collecting and distributing food donations for local food drives to more skilled tasks like fund-raising or providing professional and managerial assistance to nonprofits. Older adults—wealthy or low-income, healthy or frail—give back to the community to the extent that their resources allow, and in the process they are helping younger generations while also enhancing their own well-being.[125]

Conclusion

The graying of the U.S. population is one of the most profound social changes occurring in the twenty-first century. By 2050, more than one in five Americans will be age sixty-five or older. Popular press coverage of population aging veers toward the dramatic and foreboding, using language like "tsunami," "explosion," or "avalanche" to characterize the rapidly growing numbers of men and women reaching their seventies, eighties, and beyond. Yet older adults are neither a problem to be solved nor a population to be either pitied or glorified. Rather, people age sixty-five and older are just as diverse, complex, multifaceted, and difficult to characterize as young people. Whether older adults are frail or vigorous, socially engaged or isolated, prosperous or poor, varies widely based on factors as idiosyncratic as their personality, the good or bad decisions they have made, or the genetic good fortune or risks they inherit. Powerful structural factors—like the historical period in which they grew up, the financial security or precariousness they experienced as a child, whether they live in a state with generous or sparse social welfare programs, whether they have worked in a satisfying profession with generous benefits or toiled at an unpleasant part-time job, and the opportunities they have been afforded or denied, often on the basis of race, sex, or social class—have a profound influence on how older adults have lived, how they have aged, and how they will die. Biology certainly plays a role in the aging process, including the kinds of diseases we inherit or contract, when those diseases strike, how we respond to treatment, and when and how we die. But these biological processes are powerfully shaped by the social contexts in which we live. Stressors ranging from racism to persistent financial insecurity to mistreatment at the hands of caregivers can weaken our immune systems, intensify oxidative damage, and hasten how quickly our cells age.

Yet, while biology is inevitable, social stress, adversity, and structural inequalities are not. Public policies, community initiatives, creative collaborations between public and private ventures, and innovative professional training programs can alter or ameliorate many of the factors that set us on a course toward a satisfying or distressing old age. Social Security provides a minimum standard of living to older adults, while EITC programs provide economic security to millions of working poor and SSI provides an income boost to the poorest older adults. Medicare, Medicaid, and the Affordable Care Act have made tremendous strides in bringing affordable health care to Americans of all ages. Innovative professional training programs have alerted law enforcement officials and social workers to the subtle signs of elder abuse and mistreatment and taught health care providers to abandon ageist practices like "elderspeak." Advocacy organizations like AARP have designed creative programs that enlist older adults from all walks of life to offer their wisdom and skills in stipend-based volunteer programs like ExperienceCorps. Charitable organizations like Meals on Wheels, largely supported by private donors, provide meals and social support to vulnerable older adults and at the same time provide some reprieve for exhausted caregivers who would otherwise be preparing meals. None of these programs is a cure-all. Social inequalities in the United States are deep, persistent, and widening over time. Creative solutions must continue to evolve and garner public support. Yet widespread recognition that human lives are intertwined and that initiatives that benefit older adults also benefit all members of society is a critical first step toward helping future generations enjoy physical comfort, good health, meaningful social relations, dignity, and a sense of purpose in old age.

Notes

Chapter 1: Golden Years? An Introduction

1. Ducharme 2016.
2. For further information on the data, methods, and findings from the Georgia Centenarian Study, see Poon et al. (1992). Regularly updated information on the New England Centenarian Study can be found at http://www.bumc.bu.edu/centenarian/ (accessed September 24, 2018).
3. Hummer and Hernandez 2013.
4. Henry J. Kaiser Family Foundation 2018. An analysis of National Longitudinal Mortality Study data found that state characteristics like economic environment, social cohesion, sociopolitical orientation, physical infrastructure, and tobacco environment accounted for 60 percent of state-level variation in women's mortality rates, whereas women's personal characteristics accounted for just one-third of the variance (Montez, Zajacova, and Hayward 2016). For regular updates on state-level life expectancies, see Henry J. Kaiser Family Foundation (2018).
5. Culhane et al. 2013.
6. Thompson 2014.
7. Chetty et al. 2016.
8. Galea et al. 2011.
9. Pew Research Center 2015.
10. Each of these statistics will be elaborated more fully in subsequent chapters. Estimates based on Federal Bureau of Prisons data suggest that 165,000 inmates in state and local prisons in 2018 were age fifty-five and older (Jaquad 2018). The U.S. Department of Housing and Urban Development estimates that slightly more than 300,000 persons age fifty and older currently live on the streets or in shelters (Henry et al. 2016). An analysis of National Health and Aging Trends (NHATS) data showed that 6 percent of all older adults (roughly 2 million persons age sixty-five and older) living in their own homes are homebound (Ornstein et al. 2015).

11. Estimates of poverty vary based on the definition used. Based on data from the 2017 Current Population Survey Annual Social and Economic Supplements (CPS ASEC), the U.S. Census Bureau estimates that 4.6 million (or 9.3 percent of) persons age sixty-five and older lived beneath the federal poverty line in 2016 (Semega, Fontenot, and Kollar 2017). However, when the Census Bureau's newer Supplemental Poverty Measure (SPM) is used, these numbers spike up to an estimated 7.1 million (or 14.5 percent of) persons age sixty-five and older. See note 7.
12. Choi et al. 2015.
13. Nyce and Schieber 2005.
14. Weintraub 2010.
15. For further information and regular updates on the National Academy of Medicine's Grand Challenge, see https://nam.edu/initiatives/grand-challenge-healthy-longevity/ (accessed September 24, 2018).
16. Friend 2017.
17. Hilary Hoynes and Diane Schanzenbach (2018) estimate that in 2015 the federal government spent roughly $35,000 per person age sixty-five or older, mostly through Social Security and Medicare, yet just $5,000 per child through programs like food stamps, Medicaid and tax credits. Even when public spending on elementary and secondary education is considered, estimated at just over $11,000 per child, the per capita age gap in public spending persists, although it narrows considerably.
18. For a fuller description of precisely how the SPM is calculated, see Bridges and Gesumaria (2015). The SPM estimates are considered a more accurate snapshot than the CPS measure because they reflect a broader set of older adults' financial resources and liabilities, especially out-of-pocket medical spending, which is disproportionately high among older adults, and the inapplicability to older adults of social programs that disproportionately benefit youth, such as the National School Lunch Program (NSLP), the Supplemental Nutrition Assistance Program (SNAP), and the Special Supplemental Nutrition Program for Women, Infants, and Children (WIC) (Cubanski et al. 2018).The higher SPM estimates also reflect the fact that official poverty rates use lower household income thresholds for older adults, based on the assumption that older adults spend less on food than younger households. (The poverty threshold is set at the point at which a family would have to spend more than one-third of its income on food.)
19. Medicare benefits exclude dental, vision, hearing, and long-term services and contain no ceiling on out-of-pocket costs for covered services. As a result, beneficiaries often bear high costs, which may be prohibitive to the most disadvantaged older adults. More than 25 percent of Medicare beneficiaries spend at least one-fifth of their incomes on premiums plus medical care (Schoen, Davis, and Willink 2017).
20. For an excellent in-depth analysis of the limits of health care policy and ac-

cess to care as solutions to health disparities in the United States, see House (2015).

21. A fascinating qualitative study of thirty job-seekers age forty-five to sixty revealed the efforts made by applicants to conceal their age, including dying their hair, getting toupees (men), and exercising to look "in shape" (Berger 2009).

22. Cubanski et al. 2018. Under the official poverty measure, 9.3 percent of older adults (4.6 million persons) lived beneath the poverty line in 2016; this figure is 14.5 percent (7.1 million older adults) when the alternative measure, the SPM, is used. Regardless of the measure used, estimates show that late-life poverty rates are consistently higher for women, blacks and Hispanics, and people in relatively poor health. These trends will be elaborated in chapter 2 (Cubanski et al. 2018).

23. Life expectancy at birth increased steadily for most of the late twentieth and early twenty-first centuries, despite dipping downward in 2016 for the second consecutive year. Life expectancy declined from 78.7 to 78.6 years overall during this period, and from 76.3 to 76.1 among men, although women's life expectancy held steady at 81.1. This recent trend is due to rising death rates among younger men, especially those age twenty-five to thirty-four, who were especially vulnerable to opioid-related deaths during this period. In sharp contrast, death rates among adults age sixty-five and older have continued to decline steadily (Kochanek et al. 2017).

Chapter 2: Older Adults in the Contemporary United States: A Snapshot

1. Federal Interagency Forum on Aging-Related Statistics 2016.
2. Steinhorn 2006.
3. Cutler and Meara 2004.
4. U.S. Census Bureau 2017.
5. Olshansky and Ault 1986.
6. Levy et al. 2002.
7. Jha et al. 2011.
8. Centers for Disease Control 1999.
9. Centers for Disease Control 2018a.
10. Centers for Disease Control 1999.
11. Hughes 1945.
12. The Fair Treatment for Experienced Pilots Act (Public Law 110-135) went into effect on December 13, 2007, raising the age to sixty-five from the previous sixty. In 2014, a federal court ruled that this mandatory retirement age did not constitute age discrimination because age was considered "a bona fide

occupational qualification (BFOQ)" of being a commercial pilot, on the grounds that the risk of sudden incapacitation in-flight significantly increased with age (Ripple 2014).

13. Roy and Harwood 1997.
14. Barrett and Cantwell 2007.
15. Mather, Jacobsen, and Pollard 2015.
16. Read and Gorman 2010.
17. Springer and Mouzon 2011.
18. Mather, Jacobsen, and Pollard 2015.
19. Roy and Harwood 1997.
20. Abdul-Malak and Wang 2016.
21. OECD 2011.
22. U.S. Census Bureau 2010.
23. Schmitt 2008.
24. Pampel, Krueger, and Denney 2010.
25. Wray et al. 1998.
26. Raley, Sweeney, and Wondra 2015.
27. Bennett, Hughes, and Smith 2003.
28. Brown and Lin 2012.
29. Cahill, Giandrea, and Quinn 2015.
30. Zoeckler and Silverstein 2016.
31. Federal Reserve 2015.
32. Moen 2016.
33. Johnson 2012.
34. Hurd and Rohwedder 2015.
35. Weil 2014.
36. For example, workers who start receiving Social Security checks up to thirty-six months before their full retirement age will see their benefits permanently reduced by five-ninths of 1 percent for each month of premature retirement. Those who retire even earlier—more than thirty-six months before full retirement age—see their benefits further reduced by five-twelfths of 1 percent per month. In more concrete terms, a person who starts receiving benefits at age sixty-two rather than sixty-six will see a permanent benefit reduction of 25 percent, whereas a person who delays from age sixty-six to age seventy ultimately receives a benefit 16 percent higher than what he or she would have received at age sixty-six. For complete details on precisely how benefits are allocated based on age at retirement, see Social Security Administration, "Benefits Planner: Retirement," https://www.ssa.gov/planners/retire/1943.html (accessed September 24, 2018).

37. Stoltzfus 2016. As recently as 1979, 28 percent of private-sector workers participated in DB plans, but by 2014 this proportion had plummeted to just 2 percent. Conversely, the proportion participating in DC plans more than quadrupled, from 7 to 34 percent, in the same period. For complete data, see Employee Benefit Research Institute, "FAWs about Benefits—Retirement Issues," https://www.ebri.org/publications/benfaq/index.cfm?fa=retfaq14 (accessed September 24, 2018).

38. Zoeckler and Silverstein 2016.

39. West et al. 2014.

40. Renwick and Fox 2016. Some economists counter that the 10 percent elderly poverty rate is misleading. They point out that using alternative measures, the SPM and an even newer measure proposed by the National Academy of Sciences, raises the rate to 15 or 18 percent, respectively.

41. Nyce and Schieber 2005.

42. Historical trend data on older adults' poverty rates are based on official poverty rates that used the CPS measure rather than the adjusted SPM.

43. Romig and Sherman 2016.

44. National Council on Aging 2015.

45. Thorne et al. 2018.

46. The Social Security program, including its eligibility rules and payment schedules, is highly complex. For a detailed and in-depth analysis of the program's history, structure, benefits, and limitations, see Harrington-Meyer and Herd (2007) or Hardy and Hazelrigg (2010).

47. Herd et al. 2018.

48. For data on historical changes in older women's eligibility basis for Social Security retirement benefits, see Social Security Administration (2013) and Iams and Tamborini (2012).

49. Recent estimates show how cumulative lifetime earnings (the basis for Social Security benefits) vary dramatically by race and gender, reflecting disparities in the kinds of work people do, how many hours a week they work, and the number of years they invest in paid work versus child-rearing. Consequently, white women earn about 83 percent as much as white men, black women earn about 90 percent of what black men earn, and Latino women earn about 89 percent of Hispanic men's lifetime earnings. Given that black and Latino older men earn considerably less than their white counterparts, women of color lag dramatically behind all other groups when it comes to lifetime earnings (Herd 2005).

50. Gifts, veterans' payments, and other sources make up a fifth income source, although just 5 percent of older adults rely on these (Federal Interagency Forum on Aging-Related Statistics 2016).

51. Rhee 2013. Data from the 2012 Current Population Survey (CPS) show that

57 percent of wage and salary workers work for an employer that sponsors a retirement plan and that just 48 percent participate in the plan. The proportion with access to such plans varies from 62 percent among whites to 54 percent among blacks and Asians, to just 38 percent among Latinos (Rhee 2013).

52. U.S. Census Bureau 2015.
53. Traub et al. 2017.
54. Shapiro, Meschede, and Osoro 2013.
55. For a detailed explication of why race gaps in lifetime earnings and assets widen over the life course, see Urban Institute (2015).
56. Social Security Administration 2018.

Chapter 3: Life-Course Perspectives on Social Inequalities in Later Life: A Brief Overview

1. National Research Council 2013.
2. Cumming and Henry 1961.
3. Cumming and Henry 1961.
4. Friend 2017; Rowe and Kahn 2015.
5. Extensive research, including one recent meta-analysis, shows that poor health—whether measured through self-assessed measures, illness checklists, or biomarkers—is a powerful predictor of early retirement, unemployment, and the receipt of disability pensions (van Rijn et al. 2013; see also Chatterji et al. 2017).
6. One recent analysis of HRS data explored occupational differences in the likelihood that a worker would retire by age sixty-two and by age sixty-five, controlling for other risk factors, including education, health, and family statuses (Helppie-McFall et al. 2015). In general, they found that workers remained in the workforce longer if their jobs entailed less physical effort, less stress, and the flexibility to reduce their hours. Workers in white-collar professions like law, finance, and engineering tended to retire later, whereas workers in physically challenging jobs like construction, manufacturing, and nursing retired earlier.
7. Havighurst 1963.
8. The expansion of community programs and activities for older adults also was spurred on by the Older Americans Act (OAA) in 1965. Congress implemented this program in response to policymakers' concerns regarding the limited availability of community social services for older individuals. The OAA has played a critical role in providing public services to older adults, including senior support centers and community centers (Colello and Napili 2016).

9. Anderson et al. 2014.
10. Li and Ferraro 2005, 2006.
11. Atchley 1971.
12. Rowe and Kahn 1998.
13. In response to these and other criticisms, Rowe and Kahn (2015) have reformulated their argument, placing greater emphasis on social factors that were not explicit in its initial formulation. In their essay "Successful Aging 2.0," they more explicitly emphasize that a person's capacity to age successfully is shaped by personal characteristics, such as race, gender, sexual orientation, and socioeconomic status; interpersonal and social factors, including family and friendships; and more distal macrosocial influences, including economic conditions, access to care, public transportation, and physical aspects of his or her neighborhoods.
14. For instance, researchers exploring whether blacks' heightened risk of childhood poverty accounts for racial disparities in later-life health need a sample large enough to compare older whites with older blacks, who account for just 9 percent of the sixty-five-and-older population today. That is why many of the studies cited in this book are based on large national longitudinal studies that include thousands of participants. For example, the Health and Retirement Study has tracked a racially and ethnically diverse cohort of roughly thirteen thousand men and women born in the 1930s and 1940s from their fifties (in the 1990s) through their eighties (in the 2010s). Other studies take an even longer view. The Wisconsin Longitudinal Study (WLS) began as a study of ten thousand Wisconsin high school seniors in 1957 and has followed them for more than sixty years to show how childhood experiences affect health and well-being in old age.
15. Elder 1994.
16. Mills 1959.
17. Wang and Parker 2011.
18. George 1993.
19. Elder 1999. Elder and his colleagues (Elder, Shanahan, and Clipp 1994; Pavalko and Elder 1990) compared the work, family, and health outcomes of three subgroups of World War II veterans based on their time of entry into the service: early (age eighteen to twenty-nine), middle (age thirty to thirty-two), and late (age thirty-three to forty-one years) entrants. The researchers found that service was more disruptive to the lives of the late entrants than it was for earlier entrants, as evidenced by more rapid declines in their physical health and their greater risk of marital dissolution. They attributed these findings to the greater "life course disruption" experienced by the later entrants.
20. MacLean and Elder 2007.
21. Barker and Osmond 1986.

254   Notes

22. Extensive research by Barker and his colleagues has prospectively linked prenatal and neonatal conditions with an offspring's health outcomes as many as seven decades later. For instance, when they tracked a sample of infants born between 1935 and 1943, they found that both placental weight and birth weight affected systolic and diastolic blood pressure when respondents were age forty-six to fifty-four, net of controls for adult BMI (body mass index) and health behaviors (Barker 1990). Similarly, when they tracked a cohort of men born between 1920 and 1930 through their early sixties, they found that low birth weight was linked with glucose tolerance and non-insulin-dependent diabetes, net of controls (Hales et al. 1991).

23. Ben-Shlomo, Cooper, and Kuh 2016.

24. See Duncan and Brooks-Gunn (1999) for empirical studies delineating the pathways linking early-life poverty with adolescent, midlife, and later-life physical, emotional, and economic well-being.

25. Sewell and Hauser 1975.

26. Warren 2009.

27. Ben-Shlomo, Cooper, and Kuh 2016.

28. Isaacs 2013.

29. Evans and Cassell 2014.

30. Bound and Turner 2002, 5.

31. Rothstein 2017. Multiple studies have documented that whites benefited considerably more than blacks from the GI Bill, despite its ostensibly "race-neutral" goal. John Bound and Sarah Turner (2002) attribute the race disparity to the geographic locations where veterans lived. Blacks disproportionately lived in the South, where there were fewer colleges and opportunities for attendance and more restrictive admissions practices than was the case in the North. Historians have further argued that the adherence of the Veterans Administration (established under the GI Bill) resulted in few home loans for blacks. Practices like redlining and failure to insure home loans made to blacks made banks far less likely to offer loans to black versus white would-be homeowners (Rothstein 2017).

32. Chen and Miller 2013.

33. Dannefer 1987; O'Rand 1996.

34. Merton 1968.

35. Crystal and Shea 1990; Ferraro and Shippee 2009.

36. Quadagno and Reid 1999.

37. *Newsweek* 1946, 79.

38. Carr 2004.

39. Hout and Cumberworth 2012.

40. Pearlin et al. 2005, 205.

Chapter 4: The Fit and the Frail: Physical Health Among Older Adults

1. Burroughs 2013.
2. Centers for Disease Control 2018b.
3. Neikrug and Ancoli-Israel 2009.
4. Brokaw 2001.
5. Mendes De Leon, Glass, and Berkman 2003.
6. Although socioeconomic disparities in health are present at every stage in the life course, they tend to be narrowest at those ages when people are most biologically robust (adolescence and early adulthood) or most vulnerable (infancy and very late life). Disparities are most pronounced during midlife and early old age (House, Lantz, and Herd 2005).
7. House 2015.
8. Link and Phelan 1995.
9. Research uniformly shows that some or all of black-white health disparities are explained away by socioeconomic resources, although the precise amount varies based on the specific health outcome and specific SES indicator considered. For example, Robert Hummer and Juanita Chinn (2011) estimate that about 0.5 percent of the black-white gap in adult mortality is accounted for by adult socioeconomic and marital statuses, with explanatory power slightly different based on age, sex, and cause of death. Raynard Kington and James Smith (1997) find that black-white gaps in later-life functional limitations are fully explained by SES, while Eileen Crimmins, Mark Hayward, and Teresa Seeman (2004) find that race gaps in hypertension and diabetes decline yet persist when SES is controlled.
10. Hummer and Chinn 2011.
11. Schroeder 2007. For a detailed explication of the limits of health care access and the importance of other psychosocial and environmental factors as an explanation for health disparities, see House (2015).
12. House 2015, xvi.
13. The study of social disparities in physical health and mortality is one of the most vibrant areas of research in the social sciences, public health, and medicine in recent years. The literature is too voluminous to discuss in-depth in this chapter. For excellent overviews of the field, see Adler et al. (2016); House (2015); Marmot (2005); or Rogers, Hummer, and Nam (1999).
14. Shanahan and Hofer 2005.
15. For a straightforward review of biological theories of aging, see Hayflick (1994).
16. Epel et al. 2004.

17. Needham et al. 2013.
18. Needham et al. 2012.
19. Romano et al. 2010.
20. Janicki-Deverts et al. 2009.
21. Dowd and Aiello 2009.
22. Alzheimer's Association 2016.
23. Johnson, Penke, and Spinath 2011.
24. Bostock, Soiza, and Whalley 2009.
25. Khera et al. 2016.
26. Barker and Osmond 1986.
27. Kuh and Ben-Shlomo 1997.
28. National Cancer Institute, "Malignant Mesothelioma: Patient Version," https://www.cancer.gov/types/mesothelioma (accessed July 6, 2017).
29. Lantz et al. 1998.
30. Zeng et al. 2015.
31. Hunt, Whitman, and Hurlbert 2014. Access to care alone does not explain the race gap in women's breast cancer mortality. Other factors, like health behaviors, obesity, and comorbid conditions, also contribute, although researchers disagree about the precise contribution of each explanatory mechanism. A lively debate in the *Journal of the American Medical Association* underscores how data quality issues and the statistical modeling technique used may lead to very different conclusions. Jeffrey Silber and his colleagues (2013) conclude that access to care accounts for less than 1 percent of the race gap in breast cancer survival, but Jeanne Mandelblatt, Vanessa Sheppard, and Alfred Neugut (2013) argue that the contribution of access to care is much more substantial, noting that adjuvant therapy and screening can account for anywhere from 18 to 30 percent of the black-white gap in breast cancer mortality.
32. Feinglass et al. 2007.
33. Nelson et al. 1990.
34. Schade and Swanson 1988; Steenland and Beaumont 1984.
35. Duncan et al. 2002.
36. Arias et al. 2008.
37. Noymer, Penner, and Saperstein 2011.
38. Ferraro and Farmer 1999.
39. Idler and Angel 1990.
40. Mora et al. 2013.

41. Salive 2013.
42. Katz and Akpom 1976.
43. Manton, Gu, and Lowrimore 2008.
44. House, Lantz, and Herd 2005.
45. In one of the most comprehensive studies to date, Stephanie Studenski and her colleagues (2011) used pooled data from nine cohort studies comprising nearly thirty-five thousand adults age sixty-five and older. These researchers found a strong inverse association between gait speed and survival, even after controlling for sociodemographics, health, and health behavior.
46. Friedman and Herd 2010.
47. Karlamangla, Singer, and Seeman 2006.
48. While death rates among older adults have declined steadily, life expectancy at birth declined slightly in 2015 and 2016 primarily because of an increase in death rates among young and midlife adults, a consequence of the opioid epidemic (Kochanek et al. 2017).
49. Schoeni et al. 2005.
50. Kontis et al. 2017.
51. A recent analysis of data primarily from 2013 to 2016 from key international organizations, including the Organization for Economic Cooperation and Development (OECD), shows that in 2016 the United States spent nearly 18 percent of its gross domestic product on health care, while comparable spending in the other wealthy nations ranged from 9.6 percent in Australia to 12.4 percent in Switzerland (Papanicolas, Woskie, and Jha 2018).
52. Link and Phelan 1995, S29.
53. Krieger, Chen, and Waterman 2010.
54. Omran 1971. This historic change in the leading causes of death, referred to as the "epidemiologic transition," will be discussed in greater depth in chapter 9.
55. Among current cohorts of older adults, Latinos tend to live as long as or longer than whites in the United States, despite their lower socioeconomic status—a phenomenon commonly referred to as the "Hispanic Paradox." The main explanations for the superior longevity of Latinos are selective migration (or the relatively good health of Hispanic migrants who move to the United States), lower rates of smoking, and supportive social networks that promote good health. However, emerging evidence suggests that this disadvantage may decline or even reverse among future cohorts of older adults, given relatively high rates of obesity and diabetes among current cohorts of midlife and young adult Latinos (Goldman 2016).
56. Heron 2016.
57. Xu et al. 2016.

58. Lines and Wiener 2014.
59. Langa et al. 2017.
60. Sharp and Gatz 2011.
61. Marmot 2006.
62. Dowd et al. 2011. Researchers have debated whether the association between income and health is linear, or whether the effects level off at higher levels of income. Recent studies in both Europe and the United States generally confirm that there are diminishing returns at the higher end of the income distribution, suggesting that while income can boost the health and survival of the poor and near-poor, income does not translate into better health for those with sufficient income to live on. Jennifer Dowd and her colleagues (2011), using data from the Panel Study of Income Dynamics (PSID), found a linear association between income and mortality risk at age thirty-five to sixty-four only at the lower levels of the income distribution; they concluded that a focus on the bottom 30 percent of distribution would bring the greatest benefits in reducing health disparities. By contrast, a study tracking a Swedish population cohort of more than eight hundred thousand older adults found a strong linear association between disposable household income and mortality risk among those in the bottom half of the income distribution, a diminishing effect for those between the fiftieth and ninetieth income percentiles, and no association among those in the top 10 percent of the income distribution (Rehnberg and Fritzell 2016).
63. Kawachi, Daniels, and Robinson 2005.
64. Fuchs 2011.
65. Roberts 2001.
66. Kawachi, Daniels, and Robinson 2005.
67. Cooper et al. 1997; Gravlee 2009.
68. National Research Council 2004; Quinn 2011.
69. Northcutt 2008.
70. Mathews and MacDorman 2013.
71. National Research Council 2011a.
72. Springer and Mouzon 2011.
73. Case and Deaton 2015.
74. Warren 2009. The selection-causation debate does not apply solely to education, jobs, and income. As subsequent chapters will show, researchers also debate whether social strains like loneliness, elder abuse, or living in a dangerous neighborhood undermine older adults' health or whether poor health, by leaving them especially vulnerable to social isolation and abuse, renders them incapable of moving out of an unhealthy neighborhood.
75. Montez, Hayward, and Wolf 2017.

76. Sapolsky 2005.
77. Turner and Avison 2003.
78. Meyer 1995.
79. Williams et al. 1997.
80. Geronimus et al. 2006.
81. Geronimus et al. 2006, 826.
82. Pearlin and Schooler 1978.
83. National Academies of Sciences, Engineering, and Medicine 2016.
84. Cornwell 2015.
85. Taylor and Seeman 1999.
86. Freeman 1989.
87. James 1994.
88. Thomas et al. 1997.
89. Jackson and Stewart 2003.
90. Hummer and Chinn 2011.
91. The American Psychological Association has conducted the annual Stress in America survey for more than a decade and has consistently found that "money problems" are the most common source of worry to Americans. "Money problems" was bumped from the top spot for the first time ever in 2017, when the greatest source of concern was "the future of the nation"; 62 and 63 percent named each as a significant source of stress. For complete surveys, see American Psychological Association, "Stress in America Press Room™," http://www.apa.org/news/press/releases/stress/index.aspx?tab=10 (accessed September 24, 2018).
92. Center on Budget and Policy Priorities 2016.
93. Montez, Hayward, and Wolf 2017.
94. Multiple studies document that the EITC is linked with better self-rated health and biomarker indicators of health among young mothers (Evans and Garthwaite 2014), increased infant birth weight (Hoynes, Miller, and Simon 2015), and reduced maternal smoking (Strully, Rehkopf, and Xuan 2010). These positive effects may have long-term benefits for mothers and children themselves and may indirectly benefit their older family members by providing a healthier group of potential caregivers.
95. Herd, Schoeni, and House 2008.
96. For a review of the effects of health behaviors on disease and mortality risks, see Pampel, Krueger, and Denney (2010).
97. Schroeder 2007.
98. Janssen and Mark 2007.
99. Hermanson et al. 1998.

100. Analyses of data from the Midlife in the United States survey found that adults with a body mass index of 35 or higher reported significantly more interpersonal and institutional discrimination (Carr and Friedman 2005) and received more criticism from family members (Carr and Friedman 2006) than those with a "normal" body weight. Such social and interpersonal strains, in turn, heighten obese persons' risk of other negative effects of their weight.

101. Shaw and Agahi 2012.

102. Hagger-Johnson et al. 2013.

103. Babb et al. 2017.

104. Pampel, Krueger, and Denney 2010.

105. Ford et al. 2011.

106. Pampel, Krueger, and Denney 2010.

107. Cruz 2015.

108. Drewnowski and Bellisle 2007.

109. Daniel 2016.

110. Darmon and Drewnowski 2008.

111. For further information on the impact of SNAP on older adults' health and nutrition, see Center on Budget and Policy Priorities (2017).

112. Hoynes, Schanzenbach, and Almond 2016.

113. Van Hasselt et al. 2015.

114. Link and Phelan 1995.

115. Schroeder 2007.

116. Whitehead 1992.

117. House 2015.

118. Kaiser Commission on Medicaid and the Uninsured 2017.

119. Link and Phelan 1995.

120. Decker 2012.

121. Henry J. Kaiser Family Foundation 2015.

122. Stuber et al. 2000.

123. Spevick 2003.

124. Tweedy 2015.

125. Decker 2012.

126. Gerontological Society of America 2017.

127. Schoen, Davis, and Willink 2017.

128. For full details on the range and costs of supplemental programs, see Medi-

care.gov, https://www.medicare.gov/what-medicare-covers/index.html (accessed September 24, 2018).
129. Jacobson, Damico, and Neuman 2017.
130. Hebert et al. 2005.
131. Whedon et al. 2015; Bian et al. 2016; Jha et al. 2005.
132. House 2015, xvii.

Chapter 5: The Satisfied and the Sorrowful: The Mental Health of Older Adults

1. Blanchflower and Oswald 2008. David Blanchflower and Andrew Oswald (2017) analyzed data from seven recent surveys covering fifty-one countries and more than 1.3 million randomly sampled participants. They consistently found that happiness and life satisfaction levels were lower among middle-aged persons relative to younger and older adults. Although the magnitude of the difference and the absolute levels of well-being varied across countries and data sets, the data consistently showed that people's level of well-being climbed through their sixties and seventies, then plateaued or dropped only slightly among people in their eighties and nineties.
2. Kessler et al. 2005.
3. Conwell, Van Orden, and Caine 2011.
4. I do not consider major mental disorders with a strong genetic basis, such as schizophrenia, which are beyond the scope of this book. For a helpful overview of more serious mental illnesses and disorders in later life, see Zarit and Zarit (2011).
5. World Health Organization 2016.
6. Data from the National Comorbidity Survey, considered one of the most rigorous population-based assessments of mental health conditions in the United States, show that the most prevalent mental illnesses include major depressive disorder (16.6 percent), alcohol abuse (13.2 percent), and phobias (12 percent) (Kessler et al. 2005).
7. Some researchers have suggested that survey-based methods focused on community samples are preferable to clinical samples, especially when studying African Americans and, to a lesser extent, persons from disadvantaged economic backgrounds. Clinical samples, by design, include people who are currently seeking medical care or who have been successfully recruited into a clinical study. Blacks in particular are underrepresented in clinical samples owing to lack of access to care, insurance issues, and fear or distrust, so clinical studies might provide downwardly biased reports of depression among older blacks (Graham, Scharlach, and Kurtovich 2018).
8. Radloff 1977.

9. Research by the eminent Stanford University psychologist Laura Carstensen shows that as we age we develop a greater capacity to manage or regulate our emotions—the highs are not as euphoric as those experienced during our hormonal teen years, but the lows are not as devastating (Carstensen, Fung, and Charles 2003). This muted and more balanced emotional response to life's ups and downs reflects biological and cognitive aspects of aging. Neuroscientists who study the human brain have found that the amygdala in older adults responds less to stressful or negative images relative to younger persons, and that older adults also experience a decrease in autonomic arousal. As a result, they are better able to ignore negative words and images that are irrelevant to their daily lives, and they have a greater capacity to recall more positive than negative memories. These processes may contribute to older adults' lower rates of depressive symptoms relative to younger persons.

10. Mechanic and McAlpine 2011.

11. The harmful and far-reaching consequences of depression for older adults are widely documented. One meta-analysis examined twenty-five studies with 106,628 subjects, 6,416 of whom were depressed. The overall relative risk of dying in depressed subjects was 1.81 compared to their nondepressed subjects (Cuijpers and Smit 2002). In another meta-analysis, Edward Chesney, Guy Goodwin, and Seena Fazel (2014) explored linkages between depression and life expectancy by examining 407 studies that totaled more than 1.7 million subjects; they found that persons with depression lived seven to ten fewer years on average than their counterparts without depression. A recent study of more than 10,000 older adults enrolled in the Chicago Health and Aging Project (CHAP) found that those in the highest tertile of depressive symptoms were at twice the risk of elder abuse relative to those with fewer symptoms (Roepke-Buehler, Simon, and Dong 2015).

12. Radloff 1977.

13. Charney et al. 2003.

14. Evans and Mottram 2000.

15. Sarkisian, Lee-Henderson, and Mangione 2003.

16. Federal Interagency Forum on Aging-Related Statistics 2016. Biological researchers attribute part of the gender gap to hormonal differences and older women's estrogen depletion, a topic that is beyond the scope of this book. For a fuller discussion of biological explanations, see Grigoriadis and Robinson (2007).

17. Several population-based studies explore race and gender differences in the factor structure and factor loadings of the CES-D in an effort to identify whether particular symptoms are more or less consequential for an individual's overall mental health (Kroenke and Spitzer 1998). Analyses of data from the more than four thousand black and white adults in the National Survey of American Life (NSAL) showed that motivational symptoms such

as "everything felt like an effort" and cognitive items like "people were unfriendly" are less central to the depressive symptoms of blacks versus whites—a finding that probably reflects experiences of discrimination rather than depression. (Assari and Moazen-Zadeh 2016; see also the analysis of the New Haven Established Populations for Epidemiologic Studies of the Elderly [EPESE] and the five-state Hispanic EPESE by Cole et al. 2000; Kim, Chiriboga, and Jang 2009). Evidence regarding gender differences in the factor structure of CES-D is more mixed, although multiple studies show that women are more likely to endorse symptoms of sadness such as "crying," which may upwardly bias women's overall symptom scores (Carleton et al. 2013).

18. Fiske, Wetherell, and Gatz 2009.
19. Conwell, Van Orden, and Caine 2011.
20. Mouzon 2013.
21. Conner et al. 2010. Other researchers suggest that the so-called mental health paradox among older ethnic minority adults reflects selective survival. Adults who have managed to survive until older age, despite the challenges of economic disadvantage, discrimination, and elevated risk of early-onset illness, are especially emotionally resilient. Those who survive until later life (and who complete time-intensive health surveys) may have better mental health than their peers who died earlier, who may have succumbed to earlier disadvantages (Beckett 2000).
22. Shellman, Granara, and Rosengarten 2011.
23. Cooper-Patrick, Crum, and Ford 1994.
24. Blazer et al. 2000.
25. Alegría et al. 2008. This disparity is particularly acute in the southern United States. One recent analysis of data from the Collaborative Psychiatric Epidemiology Surveys (CPES) found that black older adults living in the South were half as likely as their white counterparts to have used mental health services in the past year; comparable gaps were not detected in the Northeast, West, or Midwest (Kim et al. 2013).
26. Saraceno, Levav, and Kohn 2005.
27. See, for example, Kessler et al. 1995.
28. Reynolds et al. 2015.
29. Wolitzky-Taylor et al. 2010.
30. Byers et al. 2010. A recent analysis of data from older adults in the National Comorbidity Survey found that high school dropouts are at greater risk of anxiety than college graduates (14.4 versus 8.7 percent), while women are roughly twice as likely as men (15 versus 7.6 percent) to suffer an anxiety disorder (Byers et al. 2010).
31. Kwan and Wijeratne 2016.

32. Carstensen et al. 2000; Chipperfield, Perry, and Weiner 2003.
33. Taylor and Risman 2006. One longitudinal analysis of adults age forty and older from the Americans' Changing Lives (ACL) study found that African Americans reported higher levels of anger-in than whites; the race gap narrowed yet remained significant over a ten-year observation period. However, the black-white gap was largely accounted for by blacks' more frequent experiences with discrimination (Magee and Louie 2016).
34. Both population-based longitudinal surveys and experimental research document the impact of suppressed anger on older adults' risk of cardiovascular disease (for example, Anderson et al. 2006), sleep quality (Caska et al. 2009), and both all-cause and cardiovascular mortality (Harburg et al. 2003).
35. Rosenfield and Mouzon 2013.
36. National Institute on Alcohol Abuse and Addiction 2010.
37. Merrick et al. 2008.
38. Centers for Disease Control and Prevention 2015.
39. For complete age breakdowns of leading causes of death, see National Center for Health Statistics 2017.
40. Crosby, Ortega, and Stevens 2013.
41. Fiske, Wetherall, and Gatz 2009.
42. Siegel and Rothman 2016.
43. Siegel and Rothman 2016.
44. Carr 2014.
45. Pearlin et al. 2005.
46. Gill et al. 2006.
47. Vickers 2000.
48. Mutchler and Somerville 2016.
49. Abdul-Malak and Wang 2016.
50. Baum, Garofalo, and Yali 1999.
51. Leland 2008.
52. Butler 1969, 243.
53. Butler 1969, 12.
54. Nelson 2005.
55. Palmore 2005.
56. Holstein 2015, 71.
57. Levy and Banaji 2004.
58. Yuan 2007.

59. Kessler, Mickelson, and Williams 1999.
60. Pasupathi and Löckenhoff 2002.
61. Karel, Gatz, and Smyer 2012.
62. Neumark, Burn, and Button 2017.
63. David Neumark, Ian Burn, and Patrick Button (2017) submitted more than forty thousand mock applications for four different jobs that were advertised online in twelve cities: office administration, retail sales, security guard, and janitor. The "applicants" comprised three age groups—younger (twenty-nine to thirty-one); middle-aged (forty-nine to fifty-one) and older (sixty-four to sixty-six)—and all the "older" résumés were for people with more than five years of work experience. Overall, callback rates were 35 percent lower for older workers than for younger workers, although the gap was much more pronounced among women applicants. For sales jobs, older men were twice as likely as older women to be called back.
64. Rexbye et al. 2006.
65. Gunn et al. 2009. Participants in the Longitudinal Study of Aging Danish Twins provided detailed life-course information on their socioeconomic status, physical and mental health, health behaviors, body mass index, and family factors and also agreed to have a facial photograph taken. Trained raters assigned an "age" to the photo based on physical traits like wrinkles, age spots, and other visible aspects of aging (Rexbye et al. 2006). Multivariate analyses showed that more than 40 percent of facial age variation was attributable to nongenetic factors, and that social class was a significant predictor for how men and women aged, even after multiple measures of physical and mental health were controlled.
66. Few studies explore the demographic or socioeconomic characteristics of cosmetic surgery patients, although one recent survey of a dermatological practice found that patients using anti-aging treatments like fillers and Botox had significantly higher levels of education and employment than indicated by census data for the immediate geographic region (Schlessinger, Schlessinger, and Schlessinger 2010).
67. Fiske, Wetherell, and Gatz 2009.
68. Druss and Walker 2011, 4.
69. Druss and Walker 2011.
70. Mather 2012.
71. Fiske, Wetherall, and Gatz 2009.
72. Jonas, Ibuka, and Russell 2011.
73. Carr, Ibuka, and Russell 2010.
74. Ray et al. 2015.
75. Clark et al. 1991.

76. Iezzoni and Freedman 2008.
77. Wolf 2016.
78. McPherson et al. 2007.
79. Horowitz et al. 2006.
80. Proulx and Aldwin 2016.
81. Taylor and Seeman 1999.
82. Yaffe et al. 2009.
83. Karlamangla et al. 2009.
84. Seery 2011.
85. Levenson et al. 1991.
86. Charles and Carstensen 2007.
87. Berkman et al. 2000.
88. Langford et al. 1997.
89. Ajrouch, Blandon, and Antonucci 2005.
90. Koenig, King, and Carson 2012.
91. Krause 2006.
92. Kahneman and Deaton 2010.
93. Kahneman and Deaton 2010.
94. Smith et al. 2005.
95. Sullivan, Neale, and Kendler 2000.
96. For a thoughtful review and critique of emerging research on gene-environment interactions and their implications for mental health, see Dick et al. (2015).
97. Schnittker 2015.
98. Graham 2013.
99. Bartels, Gill, and Naslund 2015.
100. Bishop et al. 2014.
101. World Health Organization 2016.

Chapter 6: The Loved and the Lonely: Social Relationships and Isolation in Later Life

1. Cherlin 2014.
2. Harrington-Meyer and Herd 2007.
3. Durkheim 1897.
4. Carr, Springer, and Williams 2014.

5. Bookwala 2012.
6. Raley, Sweeney, and Wondra 2015. The structural and cultural explanations for divergent marriage patterns among blacks and whites and lower- versus higher-SES adults are vast and intricate. A full discussion is beyond the scope of this chapter; see Raley et al. (2015) for a detailed analysis.
7. Cherlin 2014, 857.
8. Amato and Previti 2003.
9. Livingston, Parker, and Rohal 2014.
10. Idler, Boulifard, and Contrada 2012.
11. Umberson 1992.
12. Martikainen and Valkonen 1996.
13. Shapiro, Meschede, and Osoro 2013.
14. Angel, Montez, and Angel 2011.
15. Harrington-Meyer and Herd 2007.
16. Harrington-Meyer and Herd 2007.
17. Carr et al. 2001.
18. Tach and Eads 2015.
19. Brown and Lin 2012.
20. Carr, Freedman, and Cornman 2018.
21. De Jong Gierveld 2004.
22. Goldman 1993.
23. Dickens 1861.
24. Newport and Wilkie 2013.
25. DePaulo 2013.
26. Tamborini 2007.
27. Lin, Brown, and Hammersmith 2017.
28. Pudrovska, Schieman, and Carr 2006.
29. Koropeckyj-Cox 2005
30. Wilson 1987.
31. Barrett 1999.
32. Cwikel, Gramotnev, and Lee 2006.
33. Pudrovska, Schieman, and Carr 2006.
34. An analysis of Wisconsin Longitudinal Study data found that by age sixty-five only 5 percent of white high school graduates had a living father, 20 percent had a living mother, and 2.5 percent had two living parents (Carr 2016c). Analyses of National Longitudinal Survey (NLS) and Health and

Retirement Study data further showed that blacks have a significantly higher risk than whites of losing both their mother and father by age sixty (Umberson et al. 2017).

35. Umberson, Pudrovska, and Reczek 2010.
36. Suitor, Gilligan, and Pillemer 2016.
37. Sarkisian and Gerstel 2008.
38. Lye 1996.
39. Carr and Boerner 2013; Ha 2008.
40. Kaufman and Uhlenberg 1998.
41. Greenfield and Marks 2006.
42. White, Labouvie, and Papadaratsakis 2005.
43. Greenfield and Marks 2006.
44. Seltzer and Bianchi 2013.
45. Davies and Williams 2002.
46. Hayslip and Blumenthal 2016.
47. Connidis 2010.
48. Kaufman and Elder 2003.
49. Bruno Arpino and Valeria Bordone (2014) examined data from more than ten thousand older adult participants in the Survey of Health, Ageing, and Retirement in Europe (SHARE) and found that providing grandchild care had a positive effect on verbal fluency, suggesting that grandparenting may be a cognitively stimulating activity.
50. Davies and Williams 2002.
51. Davies and Williams 2002.
52. Hughes et al. 2007.
53. Another analysis of HRS data found that the arrival of a grandchild increases by 8.5 percent the likelihood that a woman will retire, with a further 1.5 percent increase for each new grandchild. Among near-retirement-age women age fifty-eight to sixty-one, the percentage working full-time was 43 percent for those with no grandchildren, 37 percent for grandmothers not caring for kids, and just 29 percent for those who were caring for children (Lumsdaine and Vermeer 2015).
54. Harrington-Meyer 2014.
55. Harrington-Meyer 2014, 21.
56. Skopek and Leopold 2017.
57. Hayslip and Blumenthal 2016.
58. One-quarter of Asians, blacks, and Latinos currently reside in multigenerational households, compared to just 13 percent of whites. The total propor-

tion of Americans living in skip-generation households is small, although the rate is more than twice as high among blacks (2.2 percent) than other racial groups (less than 1 percent). For full statistics, see Pew Research Center (2011).

59. Ellis and Simmons 2014.
60. Hayslip and Blumenthal 2016.
61. Turney 2014.
62. Seelye 2016.
63. Generations United 2014.
64. Hayslip and Page 2012.
65. Scommegna 2012.
66. Scommegna 2012.
67. Generations United 2014.
68. Ellis and Simmons 2014.
69. Hayslip et al. 2009.
70. Generations United 2014.
71. Sampson and Hertlein 2015, 87.
72. Blau and Fingerman 2010.
73. Carstensen 1992.
74. Cornwell and Laumann 2015.
75. Cotten et al. 2014.
76. Cornwell, Laumann, and Schumm 2008.
77. Cornwell 2015.
78. Rohe and Stewart 1996.
79. Desmond 2012.
80. Fiori and Denckla 2012.
81. Granovetter 1973.
82. Rainie and Wellman 2012.
83. Carr 2004.
84. Van den Hoonaard 2012.
85. Van den Hoonaard 2012, 111.
86. Van den Hoonaard 2012, 108.
87. Ajrouch, Antonucci, and Janevic 2001.
88. Roschelle 1997.
89. Carr 2004.

90. National Council on Aging 2015.
91. Klinenberg 2015.
92. Wilson and Moulton 2010.
93. Luhmann and Hawkley 2016.
94. Russell, Peplau, and Cutrona 1980.
95. Weiss 1973, 21.
96. Dykstra 1995.
97. De Jong Gierveld and Havens 2004.
98. De Jong Gierveld et al. 2009.
99. Luhmann and Hawkley 2016.
100. Hawkley and Cacioppo 2010.
101. Carr and Moorman 2011.
102. Manning and Brown 2011.
103. Carney et al. 2016.
104. Shadel and Pak 2017.
105. Ornstein and Huseman 2016.
106. Ornstein and Huseman 2016.
107. Lachs et al. 2016.
108. Roberto 2016.
109. Pham 2011.
110. For more information, see National Center on Elder Abuse, "Frequently Asked Questions: Types of Abuse," https://ncea.acl.gov/faq/abusetypes.html (accessed September 24, 2018).
111. Acierno et al. 2010.
112. Fredriksen-Goldsen 2016.
113. Acierno et al. 2010.
114. Anetzberger 2012.
115. Acierno et al. 2010.
116. Lachs and Berman 2011.
117. Acierno et al. 2010.
118. Acierno et al. 2010.
119. Roberto 2016, 377.
120. Hernandez-Tejada et al. 2013.
121. Acierno et al. 2010.
122. Metlife Mature Market Institute 2011.

123. Wiglesworth et al. 2010.
124. Cooper et al. 2009.
125. Brandl and Raymond 2012.
126. Acierno et al. 2010.
127. Schafer and Koltai 2014.
128. Williams et al. 2016.
129. Dimah and Dimah 2004.
130. Teaster, Roberto, and Dugar 2006.
131. According to 2015 data from the Federal Communications Commission (FCC), 53 percent of rural older adults lacked high-speed internet access (25 Mbps/3 Mbps of bandwidth), compared with 4 percent of those living in urban areas. For full data, see FCC (2015).
132. Lachs et al. 1998.
133. Pillemer et al. 2015.
134. For regular updates on the status of SSBG funding, see U.S. Department of Health and Human Services, Administration for Children and Families, Office of Community Services, "Social Services Block Grant Program (SSBG)," https://www.acf.hhs.gov/ocs/programs/ssbg (accessed September 24, 2018).
135. Steiger 2017.
136. National Academies of Sciences, Engineering, and Medicine 2016.
137. Julie Lima and her colleagues (2008) examined HRS data from 1,218 married adults age fifty-two and older who received impairment-related help with at least one activity of daily living. More than 80 percent of older adults, regardless of whether they were late middle-aged, young-old, or oldest-old, received most of their care from their spouse. Of these, more than three-quarters indicated that they were the only member of their network providing care.
138. Sayer 2005.
139. National Academies of Sciences, Engineering, and Medicine 2016.
140. Miller and Cafasso 1992.
141. Harrington-Meyer and Herd 2007.
142. Pinquart and Sörensen 2005.
143. Laditka and Laditka 2001.
144. Dilworth-Anderson et al. 2005.
145. Pinquart and Sörensen 2005.
146. Angel et al. 2014.
147. Mendez-Luck and Anthony 2016.

148. Nápoles et al. 2010.
149. National Alliance for Caregiving and American Association of Retired Persons 2015.
150. Bianchi et al. 2012.
151. National Academies of Sciences, Engineering, and Medicine 2016.
152. Spillman et al. 2014.
153. Perkins et al. 2013.
154. Collins and Swartz 2011.
155. Wang, Robinson, and Hardin 2015.
156. National Research Council 2011b.
157. Schulz and Sherwood 2008.
158. National Academies of Sciences, Engineering, and Medicine 2016.
159. Lin, Fee, and Wu 2012.
160. National Alliance for Caregiving, American Association of Retired Persons, and Public Police Institute 2015.
161. Family Caregiving Alliance 2001.
162. National Academies of Sciences, Engineering, and Medicine 2016.
163. Kong and Moorman 2015.
164. Span 2013a.
165. Span 2011b.
166. Span 2013b.
167. Richardson et al. 2013.
168. Alzheimer's Association 2016.
169. Rose, Noelker, and Kagan 2015.
170. For updated information on the bill's status, see ARCH National Respite Network, "Legislative Alerts," https://archrespite.org/national-respite-coalition/legislative-alerts (accessed September 24, 2018).
171. Another promising, although not yet fulfilled, initiative is the Recognize, Assist, Include, Support, and Engage (RAISE) Family Caregivers Act, which was signed into law in January 2018. The act requires the secretary of the Department of Health and Human Services (HHS) to develop a strategy to support family caregivers within eighteen months of enactment. The law also establishes an advisory council of experts to guide the development of this strategy. However, the act has no directives, no policies, and no budget. For a June 2018 letter from several dozen caregiver and health advocacy groups to HHS secretary Alex Azar, urging him to follow through and implement the act, see https://archrespite.org/images/RAISE_ACT

/RAISE_Family_Caregivers_Act_HHS_Implementation_Group_Letter_June_2018_Final.pdf (accessed September 24, 2018).

172. For updates on the bill's status, see "H.R.2505—Credit for Caring Act of 2017," https://www.congress.gov/bill/115th-congress/house-bill/2505 (accessed September 24, 2018).

Chapter 7: The Home Front: Residential and Community Experiences of Older Adults

1. Severson 2014.
2. Klinenberg 2015.
3. Federal Interagency Forum on Aging-Related Statistics 2016.
4. Scharlach 2012.
5. Federal Interagency Forum on Aging-Related Statistics 2016.
6. A survey by the AARP found that 88 percent of respondents over age sixty-five want to remain in their home for as long as possible, and 92 percent would like to remain in their community.
7. Joint Center for Housing Studies 2014.
8. Joint Center for Housing Studies 2014..
9. Brody 2016.
10. Centers for Disease Control 2017.
11. According to the Centers for Disease Control (2017), 2.8 million older adults require treatment in emergency rooms each year for falls, and more than 800,000 older adults are hospitalized at least one night. An estimated 300,000 of these hospitalizations are specifically for hip fractures, 95 percent of which are attributable to falls, especially sideways falls. The risk of fracture increases with age, and women with osteoporosis are especially vulnerable.
12. Giddan and Cole 2015.
13. Ornstein et al. 2015.
14. Musich et al. 2015.
15. Joint Center for Housing Studies 2014.
16. Freedman and Spillman 2014.
17. Tilly 2016. In 2014, fully 53 percent of national Medicaid spending for long-term services and supports (LTSS) was dedicated to HCBS, a near-tripling from the 18 percent figure in 1995. Evidence strongly suggests that providing HCBS helps to keep Medicaid beneficiaries in their own homes and out of skilled nursing and long-term care facilities. For instance, Nancy A. Miller (2011) examined the association between the proportion of Medicaid LTSS

funds dedicated to HCBS and older adults' use of nursing homes, adjusting for residents' health status and states' nursing home capacity. Between 2000 and 2007, greater investment in HCBS predicted lower use of nursing homes. Likewise, an analysis of data from older adults eligible for both Medicare and Medicaid (dual-eligibles) found that long-term nursing home use decreased by 0.17 percent for each one-percentage-point increase in the proportion of the state's Medicaid LTSS budget allocated to HCBS (Blackburn et al. 2016).

18. An important distinction between nursing home Medicaid and Medicaid waivers is that nursing home Medicaid is considered an entitlement, whereas waivers are not. In short, entitlement means that if older adults meet the eligibility requirements, they will automatically receive services. In sharp contrast, an older adult with a Medicaid waiver may meet the eligibility requirements but be unable to enroll in the program because waivers limit the number of individuals who are able to receive services. Some older adults may then be placed on a waiting list to receive benefits. Medicaid waivers may limit their services to specific geographic regions within a state, as well as to particular medical conditions, such as Alzheimer's disease (American Council on Aging 2018).

19. The Village-to-Village Network maintains a website showing where the current and under-development sites are located, as well as providing applications for older adults to start one in their community. See the Village-to-Village Network site at: http://www.vtvnetwork.org/content.aspx?page_id=22&club_id=691012&module_id=248578 (accessed September 24, 2018).

20. Butler and Diaz 2015.

21. AARP 2010.

22. Graham et al. 2017.

23. Jaffe 2017.

24. Graham et al. 2017.

25. Jaffe 2017.

26. Ball et al. 2009.

27. Span 2011a.

28. Brown and Finkelstein 2011.

29. National Opinion Research Center and the Associated Press 2015.

30. Henry J. Kaiser Family Foundation 2016.

31. For a review, see Gaugler 2016.

32. Henry J. Kaiser Family Foundation 2015.

33. Rau 2017.

34. Henry J. Kaiser Family Foundation 2015.

35. Cavan 1983.

36. Choi et al. 2015.
37. Glass and Balfour 2003.
38. Grafova et al. 2008, 2014.
39. Golant 2015.
40. Kaiser et al. 2016.
41. Scharlach 2012.
42. Housing Assistance Council 2014.
43. Federal Interagency Forum on Aging-Related Statistics 2016.
44. Estes 1979, 5.
45. Moorman, Stokes, and Morelock 2016.
46. Subramanian et al. 2008.
47. Golant 2015.
48. For more information, see the AARP webpage, "The AARP Network of Age-Friendly States and Communities," http://www.aarp.org/livable-communities/network-age-friendly-communities/ (accessed March 13, 2017).
49. Clarke and George 2005.
50. Gibbs et al. 2012.
51. Clarke and Gallagher 2013.
52. Ailshire and Clarke 2015; Ailshire and Crimmins 2014.
53. Weuve 2014.
54. Halonen et al. 2015.
55. Martin and McDade 2017.
56. Morgan and Mason 2014.
57. Latham and Clarke 2013; Latham and Williams 2015.
58. Needham et al. 2013.
59. Klinenberg 2015.
60. Herring et al. 2016.
61. Brunkard, Namulanda, and Ratard 2008.
62. Jenkins et al. 2014.
63. Freudenberg et al. 2009.
64. Centers for Disease Control and Prevention 2013.
65. *New York Times* 2012.
66. Gabler, Fink, and Yee 2017.
67. Gibson and Hayunga 2006.

68. For the American Red Cross policy on pets in shelters, see "Pets: Your Plan Should Include All Family Members," http://www.redcross.org/prepare/location/home-family/pets (accessed April 19, 2017).
69. Petrolia and Bhattacharjee 2010.
70. Gibson and Hayunga 2006.
71. Gibson and Hayunga 2006.
72. Jenkins et al. 2014.
73. Sanko 2014.
74. Bucsko 2003.
75. Waxman and Giannarelli 2017.
76. Savage 2016.
77. Kushel 2016.
78. Joint Center for Housing Studies 2014.
79. Kushel 2016.
80. Molinari et al. 2013.
81. Joint Center for Housing Studies 2014.
82. Kushel 2016.
83. Recognizing the difficulty of tracking the mortality of homeless adults, studies in the United States and Europe have estimated that homeless adults die ten to twenty years younger, on average, than their age-peers with stable housing. Data from Rotterdam in the Netherlands found that homeless men and women lived eleven and sixteen years less than their non-homeless counterparts, respectively (Nusselder et al. 2013), while data from New York City find a comparable gap of sixteen years (Culhane et al. 2013).
84. Jaquad 2018.
85. Chen 2017.
86. Belluck 2012.
87. Chiu 2010.
88. Carson and Sabol 2016.
89. Drucker 2002.
90. Aday 2003.
91. Human Rights Watch 2012.
92. Chiu 2010.
93. Marshall Project 2018.
94. Williams et al. 2011.
95. Marshall Project 2018.
96. Chen 2017.

Chapter 8: Is Death the Great Equalizer? Disparities in Dying

1. Moodie 1853.
2. Shirley 1919.
3. Carr and Luth 2015.
4. National Center for Health Statistics 2016.
5. Gruenberg 1977.
6. Omran 1971.
7. Gawande 2014.
8. Older adults who rely on hospice services are more likely to die at home compared to those who do not use hospice, as shown later in this chapter (Gruneir et al. 2007). However, as the balance of hospice care shifts from nonprofit to for-profit providers, growing numbers of hospice patients will die in hospitals or nursing homes. For-profit hospice providers are more likely than nonprofits to care for patients in nursing homes and also are more likely to disenroll their patients, ultimately sending them back to hospitals to die (Aldridge et al. 2014).
9. Steinhauser et al. 2000.
10. Starr 1982.
11. Institute of Medicine 2015, 3–5.
12. Malloy-Weir et al. 2015.
13. Lenzer 2012, 2.
14. Groopman and Prichard 2007.
15. Christakis 2001.
16. Pew Research Center 2013.
17. Institute of Medicine 2015.
18. Huynh et al. 2013.
19. Mitchell et al. 2016.
20. Cubanski and Newman 2017. Economists have debated precisely how much of total health care expenditures are channeled into end-of-life care. Estimates vary based on the methods and data sources used, with recent estimates ranging from 8.5 percent (French et al. 2017) to 10 to 12 percent (Emanuel and Emanuel 1994), to 13 percent (Aldridge and Kelley 2015). The proportion of total Medicare expenditures spent on care in the last year of life has remained at roughly one-quarter for the past three decades (Riley and Lubitz 2010).
21. Steinhauser et al. 2000.
22. Institute of Medicine 1997, 24.

23. Carr 2003.
24. Teno et al. 2015.
25. Carr 2009.
26. McPherson and Addington-Hall 2003.
27. Smith, Earle, and McCarthy 2009.
28. Joanne Lewis and her colleagues (2011) conducted an extensive database search of articles published between 1996 and 2010, using paired terms capturing socioeconomic status, such as "class" and "poverty," and end-of-life indicators, such as "dying" and "end-of-life care." This search detected only thirty-three articles focused on the United States. Nearly all thirty-three focused on race differences and used SES indicators such as education only as control variables.
29. Carr 2016a.
30. National Center for Health Statistics 2011; see also the Dartmouth Institute for Health Policy and Clinical Practice website for "The Dartmouth Atlas of Health Care," http://www.dartmouthatlas.org (accessed August 30, 2016).
31. The remaining few died in transit between care sites.
32. Teno et al. 2013.
33. Brazil et al. 2005.
34. Wright et al. 2010.
35. Teno et al. 2013.
36. Gozalo et al. 2011.
37. Coleman 2003.
38. Skolnick 1998.
39. Teno et al. 2013.
40. Gomes et al. 2015.
41. Gomes and Higginson 2006.
42. Gruneir et al. 2007.
43. Dartmouth Institute for Health Policy and Clinical Practice website for "The Dartmouth Atlas of Health Care," http://www.dartmouthatlas.org (accessed August 30, 2016).
44. Span 2016a.
45. Flory et al. 2004.
46. DeNavas-Walt, Proctor, and Smith 2004.
47. National Alliance for Caregiving and American Association of Retired Persons 2015.
48. Manning and Brown 2011.

49. Travis 1995.
50. Rhodes and Teno 2009.
51. Rhodes, Teno, and Welch 2006.
52. Patel et al. 2013.
53. Van den Beuken–van Everdingen et al. 2007.
54. Sawyer et al. 2006.
55. Teno et al. 2015.
56. Zimmer and Rubin 2016.
57. Chi and Demiris 2016.
58. Moorman and Macdonald 2012.
59. National Institutes of Health 2016.
60. Teno et al. 2015. Some experts believe that, against the backdrop of the current opioid epidemic, the number of older adults whose pain goes untreated will only increase; worries about fueling addiction may prevent even well-intended health care providers from giving patients the treatments they need to maintain comfort and functioning (National Academies of Science, Engineering, and Medicine 2017).
61. Meghani, Byun, and Gallagher 2012.
62. Tait and Chibhall 2014.
63. Cintron and Morrison 2006.
64. Hoffman et al. 2016.
65. National Academy of Science 2016.
66. Green et al. 2003.
67. Morrison et al. 2000.
68. Grady 2000.
69. Grady 2000.
70. National Hospice and Palliative Care Organization 2016.
71. National Hospice and Palliative Care Organization 2012.
72. National Hospice and Palliative Care Organization 2012.
73. Aldridge et al. 2014.
74. Center for Medicare and Medicaid Services 2013.
75. This pilot program started in 2016 and was focused on 150,000 Medicare patients with terminal illness who could receive hospice care to manage their symptoms and offer counseling to them and their families, but also could receive standard medical procedures like chemotherapy or hospitalization. Although it is too soon to tell what the pilot found, practitioners are optimistic—especially because several small clinical studies found that this

dual-prong approach is linked with longer life spans of terminally ill patients (see, for example, Temel et al. 2010).

76. Rogers 2009.
77. Goldstein et al. 2012.
78. Meier 2010.
79. National Hospice and Palliative Care Organization 2015.
80. Laurel, May 20, 2011, and Bill Gard, May 21, 2011, comments on Paula Ezop, "My Experience with Hospice Care," Open to Hope, http://www.opentohope.com/my-experience-with-hospice-care/ (accessed September 8, 2016).
81. Kelley et al. 2013.
82. Teno et al. 2010.
83. Other evidence suggests that hospice use does not reduce aggregate medical expenditures among dying adults. For instance, between 2000 and 2012, the percentage of Medicare decedents who were using hospice care doubled from one-quarter to one-half, yet total hospice expenditures quintupled, from roughly $3 billion to $15 billion (Gozalo et al. 2015). These patterns may reflect the influx of for-profit hospice providers, whose enrollment and disenrollment practices ultimately lead to costly traditional care for some patients.
84. National Hospice and Palliative Care Organization 2015.
85. Kris et al. 2006.
86. Ezop 2011.
87. Stevenson et al. 2015.
88. Hospice is reimbursed at a daily rate based on which one of four levels of care is provided: routine home care, continuous home care, inpatient respite care, and general inpatient care. Home-based care and short-term stays (less than sixty days) receive slightly higher reimbursements to reflect the intensity of care required, although these differentials are modest. For a complete schedule of 2018 annual rates, see Kristin Fan, Director, CMS financial Management Group, HHS, "Annual Change in Medicaid Hospice Payment Rates—ACTION," memo to associate regional administrators, September 8, 2017, https://www.medicaid.gov/medicaid/benefits/downloads/medicaid-hospice-rates-ffy-2018.pdf (accessed September 24, 2018).
89. For the full report, see Medicare Payment Advisory Commission 2017.
90. Because for-profits tend to provide low-intensity care for these patients for longer durations of time, they are five times as likely as nonprofit providers (22 versus 4 percent) to have exceeded the Medicare cap at least once in the past five years (Aldridge et al. 2014). The salary cap refers to an organization's average cost of caring for their patients; the 2018 cap was set at $28,689.

91. For a review, see Aldridge et al. 2014.
92. Price et al. 2017. A recent analysis of data from 292,516 respondents for 2015–2016 from the Consumer Assessment of Healthcare Providers and Systems (CAHPS) hospice survey found that caregivers of black and Hispanic hospice patients reported less satisfaction than whites with the emotional and religious support they received (Price et al. 2017). The investigators suggest that one reason why is that black and Latino hospice patients are more likely than whites to be in for-profit hospice (48 and 52 percent, versus 39 percent).
93. Aldridge et al. 2014.
94. Stark differences in the quality and nature of care have been detected in samples focused both on the hospice providers themselves and on hospice patients. Melissa Aldridge and her colleagues (2014) obtained survey data from 591 U.S. hospices and identified significant differences in the provision of community benefits and quality of care based on hospice ownership. Melissa Wachterman and her colleagues (2011) drew similar conclusions from their analysis of data from the 2007 National Home and Hospice Care Survey, a nationally representative sample of 4,705 patients discharged from hospice.
95. Aldridge et al. 2014.
96. National Hospice and Palliative Care Organization 2010.
97. Carlson et al. 2012.
98. Span 2016a.
99. Johnson 2013.
100. Johnson, Kuchibhatla, and Tulsky 2009.
101. Johnson 2013.
102. Varney 2015.
103. Johnson 2013.
104. Carr 2011.
105. Varney 2015.
106. National Hospice and Palliative Care Organization 2016.
107. National Hospice and Palliative Care Organization 2016.
108. Carr and Luth 2015.
109. Teno et al. 2015.
110. Luth 2017.
111. Carr 2016a.
112. Carr 2003.
113. Phelan, Link, and Tehranifar 2010.

114. U.S. Department of Health and Human Services 2008, x.
115. Detering et al. 2010; Nicholas et al. 2011.
116. Carr 2016b.
117. Carr 2016b.
118. Carr 2016b. The impact of ACP on end-of-life medical costs is less clear. Most studies based on large population-based samples show no significant effect, whereas studies focused on specific disease groups, such as advanced cancer patients, suggest that ACP is linked to reduced medical expenditures in the last six months of life. For example, Lauren Nicholas and her colleagues (2011) found that median fee-for-service Medicare spending in the last six months of life did not differ based on whether a patient had a treatment-limiting advance directive. By contrast, among patients with advanced cancer, end-of-life medical costs were roughly one-third less for persons who had a treatment-limiting advance directive (Zhang et al. 2009). These patterns are largely explained by high costs of ICU use; the average cost of a terminal hospitalization with an ICU stay is roughly three times higher than a comparable stay without ICU use (Zilberberg and Shorr 2012).
119. Ditto et al. 2001.
120. Burkle et al. 2012.
121. For regular updates on which states use POLSTs, see National POLST Paradigm, "National POLST Paradigm Program Designations," http://polst.org/programs-in-your-state/ (accessed September 21, 2018).
122. For further information on POLSTs, see National POLST Paradigm, "Patient FAQs," http://polst.org/faq/ (accessed September 21, 2018).
123. Carr 2016b.
124. Carr 2016b.
125. Moorman and Inoue 2013.
126. Vig et al. 2006, 1688.
127. Moorman 2011.
128. Kramer and Yonker 2011.
129. Moorman and Carr 2008.
130. Winter and Parks 2012, 741.
131. American Bar Association 2018.
132. U.S. Department of Health and Human Services 2008; Carr and Moorman 2009.
133. Pew Research Center 2013.
134. On Respecting Choices, see Hammes 2003.
135. For information on the Five Wishes, see Aging with Dignity, "Five Wishes

Resources," http://www.agingwithdignity.org/five-wishes.php (accessed August 31, 2016).

136. Carr 2011.
137. Barnato et al. 2009.
138. Loggers et al. 2009.
139. Hanchate et al. 2009.
140. Carr 2012.
141. Waite et al. 2013.
142. Carr, Moorman, and Boerner 2013.
143. Carr and Khodyakov 2007.
144. Institute of Medicine 2015.
145. Kenen 2017.
146. Kenen 2017.

Chapter 9: Conclusion: Future Trends and Policy Considerations for the Twenty-First Century

1. Rogers and Mitzner 2017.
2. Link and Phelan 1995.
3. Projections about the future vary based on assumptions about current and future levels of economic growth and demographic processes like mortality, fertility, and migration. A full discussion of the assumptions guiding the broad predictions included here is beyond the scope of this chapter. However, further information on population projections with respect to outcomes like the number, health, family statuses, and income of the U.S. population is available from the U.S. Census Bureau as well as from think tanks like the Urban Institute. Many projections specifically focused on older adults' health and economic well-being are developed by the Social Security Administration. For further information, see https://www.census.gov/programs-surveys/popproj/about.html (accessed September 21, 2018); Urban Institute (2017); and Social Security Administration, "Disability Projects," https://www.ssa.gov/disabilityresearch/projects.htm (accessed September 21, 2018).
4. Public investment in one social program or initiative is necessarily at the expense of investment in another perhaps equally desirable initiative. A full cost-benefit analysis of the policy recommendations described in this chapter is beyond the scope of this book. However, readers interested in a thorough economic analysis should consult the website of the Congressional Budget Office (CBO), which provides nonpartisan economic analyses of

current and proposed policy initiatives (https://www.cbo.gov/topics/reports-policy-options, accessed September 24, 2018).

5. Piketty 2014.
6. Semega, Fontenot, and Kollar 2016.
7. The CBO (2018) estimates that inequality increased much more slowly between 2007 and 2014 than it did in the previous twenty-eight years. When inequality is measured using after-tax rather than pre-tax incomes, including government benefits, inequality actually declined slightly between 2007 and 2014. However, the "good news" of this stabilization of inequality is dampened by the CBO's finding that income growth flattened during this period.
8. For a detailed historical analysis, see Piketty (2014), and for a statistical analysis, see Congressional Budget Office (2018).
9. Noah 2012.
10. Krugman 2015. For a more thorough economic analysis of the implications for income inequality of tax rates on pre-tax income versus income after taxes and transfers, see Congressional Budget Office (2018).
11. Wilkinson and Pickett 2009.
12. Solt 2008.
13. Piketty 2014.
14. National Academies of Science, Engineering, and Medicine 2015.
15. National Academies of Science, Engineering, and Medicine 2015.
16. Shierholz 2014.
17. Glaeser and Gyourko 2018.
18. A recent analysis of Survey of Consumer Finance data calculated the average level of homeowner equity for households, by age of household head. Mean equity was calculated by multiplying the homeownership rate by the mean level of home equity for homeowners in each age group. Home equity equals the difference between home value and outstanding mortgage debt on principal residences. Researchers found that the average homeowner equity today (in 2016 dollars) is around $150,000 for older adults, but just a fraction of that ($55,000) for adults in their thirties and forties (Cortright 2018).
19. Pew Research Center 2010.
20. Weil 2014.
21. Yilmazer, Babiarz, and Liu 2015.
22. Emmons, Kent, and Ricketts 2018.
23. Centers for Disease Control 2018c. The CDC issues quarterly provisional estimates for specific mortality outcomes. At the end of 2017, it documented

an uptick in suicide and overdose deaths and speculated that its final 2017 life expectancy calculations would show a declining life span for the third year in a row.

24. Case and Deaton 2015.
25. Pan et al. 2012.
26. Carr and Tsenkova 2018.
27. An analysis of National Health and Nutrition Examination Survey data from 1988 through 2011 finds that rising body mass index in the United States has reduced the annual rate of improvement in death rates by more than half a percentage point—equal to a 23 percent relative reduction in the rate of mortality decline. Rising BMI had reduced life expectancy at age forty by 0.9 years in 2011 and accounted for 186,000 excess deaths that year (Preston, Vierboom, and Stokes 2018).
28. National Institute on Drug Abuse 2018.
29. Centers for Disease Control and Prevention 2018c.
30. Blue Cross Blue Shield 2017.
31. Case and Deaton 2015.
32. Span 2016b.
33. Grantmakers in Aging 2017.
34. Whalen 2018.
35. Manning and Brown 2011.
36. Wilcox and Wang 2017.
37. Schwartz 2013.
38. Kreider and Ellis 2011.
39. Brown and Wright 2017.
40. Harrington-Meyer, Wolf, and Himes 2006.
41. Pew Research Center 2015.
42. Herd et al. 2018.
43. Sherman, Webster, and Antonucci 2013.
44. Noël-Miller 2013.
45. Noël-Miller 2011.
46. Joutsenniemi et al. 2006.
47. Perelli-Harris and Gassen 2012.
48. Goldsen et al. 2017.
49. Baker 2014.
50. Williams 2016.

51. Federal Interagency Forum on Aging-Related Statistics 2016.
52. Kenneth Langa and his colleagues (2017) examined data from the 2000 and 2012 waves of the HRS and found that dementia prevalence rates dropped from 11.6 percent in 2000 to 8.8 percent in 2012.
53. For more information, see Alzheimer's Association, "Alzheimer's Disease Facts and Figures," http://www.alz.org/facts/ (accessed October 6, 2017).
54. National Academies of Science, Engineering, and Medicine 2016.
55. Alzheimer's Association, "Alzheimer's Disease Facts and Figures."
56. Carlson et al. 2012.
57. Gozalo et al. 2015.
58. Stevenson et al. 2015.
59. Carney et al. 2016.
60. Other nations are developing promising approaches to financing the long-term care needs of their aging populations. Both Germany and Japan recently implemented public universal long-term care insurance systems. Everyone contributes a fraction of their income and is eligible for care benefits, regardless of how much money they have or whether they have relatives nearby to provide them with care. The prices of home- and community-based services are set by the government and are the same in each region, so service providers compete for their customers on the basis of how convenient and high-quality their services are (Campbell, Ikegami, and Gibson 2010).
61. U.S. Bureau of Labor Statistics 2015.
62. Graham 2014.
63. Osterman 2017.
64. Graham 2014.
65. McCurry 2018.
66. Foster 2018.
67. Smith and Anderson 2017.
68. Link and Phelan 1995.
69. House 2015.
70. Mojtabai 2009.
71. Bishop et al. 2014.
72. Evans and Mottram 2000.
73. American Geriatrics Society 2013.
74. Olivero 2015.
75. For instance, West Virginia has the third-oldest population in the United States, yet only thirty-six geriatricians practiced there in 2016 (Lofton 2016).

That amounts to roughly one geriatrician per every 100,000 older adults in the state. Although West Virginia is home to four geriatric fellowship programs, they did not receive a single placement between 2013 and 2016. For complete data on the National Resident Matching Program results for 2018, see National Resident Matching Program (2018).

76. Burton, Lee, and Potter 2017.
77. Leigh, Tancredi, and Kravitz 2009.
78. Smoldt et al. 2017.
79. Center for Medicare and Medicaid Services 2015.
80. Luthra 2016.
81. Cubanski and Neuman 2017.
82. Smoldt et al. 2017.
83. Ayanian 2016.
84. Sykes 2017.
85. Long et al. 2016.
86. Antonisse et al. 2017.
87. Garrett and Gangopadhyaya 2016.
88. Allen et al. 2017; Antonisse et al. 2017.
89. Congressional Budget Office 2017.
90. Amadeo 2018.
91. Reaves and Musumeci 2015.
92. Gawande 2017.
93. Marans 2017.
94. Federal Interagency Forum on Aging-Related Statistics 2016.
95. Health Care Cost Institute 2016.
96. Brodie, Hamel, and Norton 2015.
97. House 2015.
98. Whitehead 1992.
99. Schanzenbach and Bauer 2016.
100. House 2015.
101. Dowd et al. 2011; Herd, Schoeni, and House 2008.
102. Herd et al. 2018.
103. The MBP would be payable at full retirement age (sixty-six or sixty-seven) and would be available to workers with at least twenty years of U.S. residency and ten years of payroll tax contributions and whose income fell below 100 percent of the poverty level. For further detail on the program's requirements and proposed benefit structures, see Herd et al. (2018).

104. Haas Institute, n.d.

105. Analyses of FMLA show that roughly equal proportions of black, white, and Latino workers meet the eligibility criteria (51, 45, and 41 percent, respectively), although these differences vary widely by state. However, Latinos are less likely to be able to afford to take leave; only 28 percent do so, compared with 40 percent of white and 38 percent of black workers. For complete data, see Brandeis University, Heller School for Social Policy and Management, diversitydatakids.org, "Working Adults Who Are Eligible for and Can Afford FMLA Unpaid Leave (Share) by Race/Ethnicity," http://www.diversitydatakids.org/data/ranking/530/working-adults-who-are-eligible-for-and-can-afford-fmla-unpaid-leave-share-by-ra (accessed September 24, 2018).

106. Rossin-Slater, Ruhm, and Waldfogel 2013.

107. U.S. Department of Labor 2015.

108. Darrow 2017.

109. For more detailed data on the characteristics of U.S. workers who are eligible for paid versus unpaid family leave benefits, see U.S. Bureau of Labor Statistics (2014).

110. Osterman 2017.

111. Ziettlow and Cahn 2017.

112. MOWAA 2016.

113. Carr and Khodyakov 2007; Moorman 2011.

114. Ziettlow and Cahn 2017.

115. Fischer 1978.

116. La Roche 2015.

117. North and Fiske 2013.

118. Maniam and Smith 2017.

119. Duke 2016.

120. Berkman, Boersch-Supan, and Avendano 2015.

121. Gratton and Scott 2016.

122. Generations United 2017.

123. Carr 2016b.

124. Corporation for National Community and Service 2016.

125. Carr 2016b.

References

Abdul-Malak, Ynesse, and Rebecca Wang. 2016. "Immigration, Life Course, and Aging." In *Gerontology: Changes, Challenges, and Solutions,* edited by Madonna Harrington Meyer and Elizabeth A. Daniele. Santa Barbara, Calif.: Praeger Publishers.

Acierno, Ron, Melba A. Hernandez, Ananda B. Amstadter, Heidi S. Resnick, Kenneth Steve, Wendy Muzzy, and Dean G. Kilpatrick. 2010. "Prevalence and Correlates of Emotional, Physical, Sexual, and Financial Abuse and Potential Neglect in the United States: The National Elder Mistreatment Study." *American Journal of Public Health* 100(2): 292–97.

Aday, Ronald H. 2003. *Aging Prisoners: Crisis in American Corrections.* Westport, Conn.: Praeger Publishers.

Adler, Nancy E., David M. Cutler, Jonathan E. Fielding, Sandro Galea, M. Maria Glymour, Howard K. Koh, and David Satcher. 2016. "Addressing Social Determinants of Health and Health Disparities." Vital Directions for Health and Health Care Series Discussion Paper. Washington, D.C.: National Academy of Medicine (September 19). https://nam.edu/wp-content/uploads/2016/09/addressing-social-determinantsof-health-and-health-disparities.pdf (accessed September 24, 2018).

Ailshire, Jennifer A., and Philippa Clarke. 2015. "Fine Particulate Matter Air Pollution and Cognitive Function Among U.S. Older Adults." *Journals of Gerontology Series B: Psychological Sciences and Social Sciences* 70(2): 322–28.

Ailshire, Jennifer A., and Eileen M. Crimmins. 2014. "Fine Particulate Matter Air Pollution and Cognitive Function Among Older U.S. Adults." *American Journal of Epidemiology* 180(4): 359–66.

Ajrouch, Kristine J., Toni C. Antonucci, and Mary R. Janevic. 2001. "Social Networks Among Blacks and Whites: The Interaction Between Race and Age." *Journals of Gerontology Series B: Psychological Sciences and Social Sciences* 56(2): S112–18.

Ajrouch, Kristine J., Alysia Y. Blandon, and Toni C. Antonucci. 2005. "Social Networks Among Men and Women: The Effects of Age and Socioeconomic

Status." *Journals of Gerontology Series B: Psychological Sciences and Social Sciences* 60(6): S311–17.

Aldridge, Melissa D., and Amy S. Kelley. 2015. "The Myth Regarding the High Cost of End-of-Life Care." *American Journal of Public Health* 105(12): 2411–15.

Aldridge, Melissa D., Mark Schlesinger, Colleen L. Barry, R. Sean Morrison, Ruth McCorkle, Rosemary Hürzeler, and Elizabeth H. Bradley. 2014. "National Hospice Survey Results: For-Profit Status, Community Engagement, and Service." *JAMA Internal Medicine* 174(4): 500–06.

Alegría, Margarita, Pinka Chatterji, Kenneth Wells, Zhun Cao, Chih-nan Chen, David Takeuchi, James Jackson, and Xiao-Li Meng. 2008. "Disparity in Depression Treatment Among Racial and Ethnic Minority Populations in the United States." *Psychiatric Services* 59(11): 1264–72. doi:10.1176/ps.2008.59.11.1264.

Allen, Heidi, Ashley Swanson, Jialan Wang, and Tal Gross. 2017. "Early Medicaid Expansion Associated with Reduced Payday Borrowing in California." *Health Affairs* 36(10): 1769–76.

Alzheimer's Association. 2016. "2016 Alzheimer's Disease Facts and Figures." *Alzheimer's and Dementia* 12(4): 459–509.

Amadeo, Kimberly. 2018. "Donald Trump on Health Care: How Trump's Health Care Policies Will Raise Premium Prices for You." *The Balance,* August 25. https://www.thebalance.com/how-could-trump-change-health-care-in-america-4111422 (accessed August 7, 2018).

Amato, Paul R., and Denise Previti. 2003. "People's Reasons for Divorcing: Gender, Social Class, the Life Course, and Adjustment." *Journal of Family Issues* 24(5): 602–26.

American Association of Retired Persons (AARP). 2010. "The Village: A Growing Option for Aging in Place." *Fact Sheet* 177(March). Washington, D.C.: AARP Public Policy Institute. http://www.aarp.org/content/dam/aarp/livable-communities/act/housing/the-village-a-growing-option-for-aging-in-place-2010-aarp.pdf (accessed March 12, 2017).

American Bar Association (ABA). 2018. "Default Surrogate Consent Statutes." Washington, D.C.: ABA (January 1). http://www.americanbar.org/content/dam/aba/administrative/law_aging/2014_default_surrogate_consent_statutes.authcheckdam.pdf (accessed September 24, 2018).

American Council on Aging. 2018. "What Counts as Income for Medicaid Long Term Care? Definitions, Exceptions, and Limits." Washington, D.C.: American Council on Aging (updated July 5, 2018). https://www.medicaidplanningassistance.org/how-medicaid-counts-income (accessed August 8, 2018).

American Geriatrics Society (AGS). 2013. "The Demand for Geriatric Care and the Evident Shortage of Geriatrics Healthcare Providers." Washington, D.C.: AGS (March). http://www.americangeriatrics.org/files/documents/Adv_Resources/demand_for_geriatric_care.pdf (accessed September 1, 2017).

Anderson, David E., E. Jeffrey Metter, Hidetaka Hougaku, and Samer S. Najjar.

2006. "Suppressed Anger Is Associated with Increased Carotid Arterial Stiffness in Older Adults." *American Journal of Hypertension* 19: 1129–34.

Anderson, Nicole D., Thecla Damianakis, Edeltraut Kröger, Laura M. Wagner, Deirdre R. Dawson, Malcolm A. Binns, Syrelle Bernstein, Eilon Caspi, and Suzanne L. Cook. 2014. "The Benefits Associated with Volunteering Among Seniors: A Critical Review and Recommendations for Future Research." *Psychological Bulletin* 140(6): 1505–33.

Anetzberger, Georgia. 2012. "An Update on the Nature and Scope of Elder Abuse." *Generations* 36(3): 12–20.

Angel, Jacqueline L., Jennifer Karas Montez, and Ronald J. Angel. 2011. "A Window of Vulnerability: Health Insurance Coverage Among Women 55 to 64 Years of Age." *Women's Health Issues* 21(1): 6–11.

Angel, Jacqueline L., Sunshine M. Rote, Dustin C. Brown, Ronald J. Angel, and Kyriakos S. Markides. 2014. "Nativity Status and Sources of Care Assistance Among Elderly Mexican-Origin Adults." *Journal of Cross-Cultural Gerontology* 29(3): 243–58.

Antonisse, Larissa, Rachel Garfield, Robin Rudowitz, and Samantha Artiga. 2017. "The Effects of Medicaid Expansion under the ACA: Updated Findings from a Literature Review." Issue brief. San Francisco: Henry J. Kaiser Family Foundation (March). http://files.kff.org/attachment/Issue-Brief-The-Effects-of-Medicaid-Expansion-Under-the-ACA-Updated-Findings (accessed September 23, 2017).

Arias, Elizabeth, William S. Schauman, Karl Eschbach, Paul D. Sorlie, and Eric Backlund. 2008. "The Validity of Race and Hispanic Origin Reporting on Death Certificates in the United States." *Vital and Health Statistics: Series 2, Data Evaluation and Methods Research* 148: 1–23.

Arpino, Bruno, and Valeria Bordone. 2014. "Does Grandparenting Pay Off? The Effect of Child Care on Grandparents' Cognitive Functioning." *Journal of Marriage and Family* 76(2): 337–51.

Assari, Shervin, and Ehsan Moazen-Zadeh. 2016. "Confirmatory Factor Analysis of the 12-Item Center for Epidemiologic Studies Depression Scale Among Blacks and Whites." *Frontiers in Psychiatry* 7(2): 1–13.

Atchley, Robert C. 1971. "Retirement and Leisure Participation: Continuity or Crisis?" *Gerontologist* 11(1): 13–17.

Ayanian, John Z. 2016. "The Costs of Racial Disparities in Health Care." *New England Journal of Medicine: Catalyst*, February 15. http://catalyst.nejm.org/the-costs-of-racial-disparities-in-health-care/ (accessed September 23, 2017).

Babb, Stephen, Ann Malarcher, Gillian Schauer, Kat Asman, and Ahmed Jamal. 2017. "Quitting Smoking Among Adults—United States, 2000–2015." *MMWR Morbidity and Mortality Weekly Report* 65(52): 1457–64.

Baker, Beth. 2014. *With a Little Help from Our Friends: Creating Community as We Grow Older*. Nashville, Tenn.: Vanderbilt University Press.

Ball, Mary M., Molly M. Perkins, Carole Hollingsworth, Frank J. Whittington, and Sharon V. King. 2009. "Pathways to Assisted Living: The Influence of Race and Class." *Journal of Applied Gerontology* 28(1): 81–108.

Barker, David J. 1990. "The Fetal and Infant Origins of Adult Disease." *BMJ: British Medical Journal* 301(6761): 1111.

Barker, David J. P., and Clive Osmond. 1986. "Infant Mortality, Childhood Nutrition, and Ischaemic Heart Disease in England and Wales." *Lancet* 327(8489): 1077–81.

Barnato, Amber E., Denise L. Anthony, Jonathan Skinner, Patricia M. Gallagher, and Elliott S. Fisher. 2009. "Racial and Ethnic Differences in Preferences for End-of-Life Treatment." *Journal of General Internal Medicine* 24(6): 695–701.

Barrett, Anne E. 1999. "Social Support and Life Satisfaction Among the Never Married." *Research on Aging* 21(1): 46–72.

Barrett, Anne E., and Laura E. Cantwell. 2007. "Drawing on Stereotypes: Using Undergraduates' Sketches of Elders as a Teaching Tool." *Educational Gerontology* 33(4): 327–48.

Bartels, Stephen J., Lydia Gill, and John A. Naslund. 2015. "The Affordable Care Act, Accountable Care Organizations, and Mental Health Care for Older Adults: Implications and Opportunities." *Harvard Review of Psychiatry* 23(5): 304–19.

Baum, Andrew, J. P. Garofalo, and Ann Marie Yali. 1999. "Socioeconomic Status and Chronic Stress: Does Stress Account for SES Effects on Health?" *Annals of the New York Academy of Sciences* 896(1): 131–44.

Beckett, Megan. 2000. "Converging Health Inequalities in Later Life—An Artifact of Mortality Selection?" *Journal of Health and Social Behavior* 41(1): 106–19.

Belluck, Pam. 2012. "Life, with Dementia." *New York Times*, February 25. http://www.nytimes.com/2012/02/26/health/dealing-with-dementia-among-aging-criminals.html (accessed February 20, 2017).

Ben-Shlomo, Yoav, Rachel Cooper, and Diana Kuh. 2016. "The Last Two Decades of Life Course Epidemiology, and Its Relevance for Research on Ageing." *International Journal of Epidemiology* 45(4): 973–88.

Bennett, Kate M., Georgina M. Hughes, and Philip T. Smith. 2003. "'I Think a Woman Can Take It': Widowed Men's Views and Experiences of Gender Differences in Bereavement." *Ageing International* 28(4): 408–24.

Berger, Ellie D. 2009. "Managing Age Discrimination: An Examination of the Techniques Used When Seeking Employment." *Gerontologist* 49(3): 317–22.

Berkman, Lisa F., Axel Boersch-Supan, and Mauricio Avendano. 2015. "Labor-Force Participation, Policies, and Practices in an Aging America: Adaptation Essential for a Healthy and Resilient Population." *Daedalus* 144(2): 41–54.

Berkman, Lisa F., Thomas Glass, Ian Brissette, and Teresa E. Seeman. 2000. "From Social Integration to Health: Durkheim in the New Millennium." *Social Science and Medicine* 51(6): 843–57.

Bian, John, Charles Bennett, Gregory Cooper, Alessandra D'Alfonso, Deborah Fisher, Joseph Lipscomb, and Chao-Nan Qian. 2016. "Assessing Colorectal Cancer Screening Adherence of Medicare Fee-for-Service Beneficiaries Age 76 to 95 Years." *Journal of Oncology Practice* 12(6): e670–80.

Bianchi, Suzanne M., Liana C. Sayer, Melissa A. Milkie, and John P. Robinson. 2012. "Housework: Who Did, Does, or Will Do It, and How Much Does It Matter?" *Social Forces* 91(1): 55–63.

Bishop, Tara F., Matthew J. Press, Salomeh Keyhani, and Harold Alan Pincus. 2014. "Acceptance of Insurance by Psychiatrists and the Implications for Access to Mental Health Care." *Journal of the American Medical Association: Psychiatry* 71(2): 176–81.

Blackburn, Justin, Julie L. Locher, Michael Morrisey, David J. Becker, and Meredith L. Kilgore. 2016. "The Effects of State-Level Expenditures for Home- and Community-Based Services on the Risk of Becoming a Long-Stay Nursing Home Resident After Hip Fracture." *Osteoporosis International* 27(3): 953–61.

Blanchflower, David G., and Andrew J. Oswald. 2008. "Is Well-being U-Shaped over the Life Cycle?" *Social Science and Medicine* 66(8): 1733–49.

———. 2017. "Do Humans Suffer a Psychological Low in Midlife? Two Approaches (with and Without Controls) in Seven Data Sets." Working paper 23724. Cambridge, Mass.: National Bureau of Economic Research.

Blau, Melinda, and Karen L. Fingerman. 2010. *Consequential Strangers: The Power of People Who Don't Seem to Matter ... but Really Do.* New York: W. W. Norton & Co.

Blazer, Dan G., Celia F. Hybels, Eleanor M. Simonsick, and Joseph T. Hanlon. 2000. "Marked Differences in Antidepressant Use by Race in an Elderly Community Sample: 1986–1996." *American Journal of Psychiatry* 157(7): 1089–94.

Blue Cross Blue Shield. 2017. "The Health of America Report: America's Opioid Epidemic and Its Effect on the Nation's Commercially-Insured Population." Chicago: Blue Cross Blue Shield Association (June 29). https://www.bcbs.com/sites/default/files/file-attachments/health-of-america-report/BCBS-HealthOfAmericaReport-Opioids.pdf (accessed October 2, 2017).

Bookwala, Jamila. 2012. "Marriage and Other Partnered Relationships in Middle and Late Adulthood." In *Handbook of Families and Aging,* edited by Rosemary Blieszner and Victoria Hilkevitch Bedford. Santa Barbara, Calif.: ABC-CLIO.

Bostock, Clare V., Roy L. Soiza, and Lawrence J. Whalley. 2009. "Genetic Determinants of Ageing Processes and Diseases in Later Life." *Maturitas* 62(3): 225–29.

Bound, John, and Sarah Turner. 2002. "Going to War and Going to College: Did World War II and the GI Bill Increase Educational Attainment for Returning Veterans?" *Journal of Labor Economics* 20(4): 784–815.

Brandl, Bonnie, and Jane Raymond. 2012. "Policy Implications of Recognizing That Caregiver Stress Is *Not* the Primary Cause of Elder Abuse." *Generations* 36(3): 32–39.

Brazil, Kevin, Doris Howell, Michel Bedard, Paul Krueger, and Christine Heidebrecht. 2005. "Preferences for Place of Care and Place of Death Among Informal Caregivers of the Terminally Ill." *Palliative Medicine* 19(6): 492–99.

Bridges, Benjamin, and Robert V. Gesumaria. 2015. "The Supplemental Poverty Measure (SPM) and Children: How and Why the SPM and Official Poverty Estimates Differ." *Social Security Bulletin* 75(3): 55.

Brodie, Mollyann, Elizabeth C. Hamel, and Mira Norton. 2015. "Medicare as Reflected in Public Opinion." *Generations* 39(2): 134–41.

Brody, Jane E. 2016 "Aging in Place." *New York Times*, May 2. https://well.blogs.nytimes.com/2016/05/02/aging-in-place/ (accessed February 22, 2017).

Brokaw, Tom. 2001. *The Greatest Generation*. New York: Random House.

Brown, Jeffrey R., and Amy Finkelstein. 2011. "Insuring Long-Term Care in the United States." *Journal of Economic Perspectives* 25(4): 119–41.

Brown, Susan L., and I-Fen Lin. 2012. "The Gray Divorce Revolution: Rising Divorce Among Middle-Aged and Older Adults, 1990–2010." *Journals of Gerontology Series B: Psychological Sciences and Social Sciences* 67(6): 731–41.

Brown, Susan L., and Matthew R. Wright. 2017. "Marriage, Cohabitation, and Divorce in Later Life." *Innovation in Aging* 1(2). doi.org/10.1093/geroni/igx015.

Brunkard, Joan, Gonza Namulanda, and Raoult Ratard. 2008. "Hurricane Katrina Deaths, Louisiana, 2005." *Disaster Medicine and Public Health Preparedness* 2(4): 215–23.

Bucsko, Mike. 2003. "Elderly McKeesport Couple Die After Using Oven for Heat." *Pittsburgh Post-Gazette*, October 8. http://allnurses.com/general-nursing-discussion/elderly-couple-die-46367.html (accessed February 20, 2017).

Burkle, Christopher M., Paul S. Mueller, Keith M. Swetz, C. Christopher Hook, and Mark T. Keegan. 2012. "Physician Perspectives and Compliance with Patient Advance Directives: The Role External Factors Play on Physician Decision Making." *BMC: Medical Ethics* 13: 31. doi:10.1186/1472-6939-13-31.

Burroughs, Augusten. 2013. *Dry: A Memoir*. New York: Picador.

Burton, John R., Andrew G. Lee, and Jane F. Potter, eds. 2017. *Geriatrics for Specialists*. New York: Springer International.

Butler, Robert N. 1969. "Age-Ism: Another Form of Bigotry." *Gerontologist* 9(4): 243–46.

Butler, Stuart M., and Carmen Diaz. 2015. "How 'Villages' Help Seniors Age at Home." Washington, DC: Brookings Institute, October 19. https://www.brookings.edu/blog/usc-brookings-schaeffer-on-health-policy/2015/10/19/how-villages-help-seniors-age-at-home/ (accessed September 18, 2019).

Byers, Amy L., Kristine Yaffe, Kenneth E. Covinsky, Michael B. Friedman, and Martha L. Bruce. 2010. "High Occurrence of Mood and Anxiety Disorders Among Older Adults: The National Comorbidity Survey Replication." *Archives of General Psychiatry* 67: 489–96.

Cahill, Kevin E., Michael D. Giandrea, and Joseph F. Quinn. 2015. "Evolving Patterns of Work and Retirement." In *Handbook of Aging and the Social Sciences*, edited by Linda K. George and Kenneth Ferraro. New York: Academic Press.

Campbell, John Creighton, Naoki Ikegami, and Mary Jo Gibson. 2010. "Lessons from Public Long-Term Care Insurance in Germany and Japan." *Health Affairs* 29(1): 87–95.

Carlson, Melissa D. Aldridge, Colleen L. Barry, Emily J. Cherlin, Ruth McCorkle, and Elizabeth H. Bradley. 2012. "Hospices' Enrollment Policies May Contribute to Underuse of Hospice Care in the United States." *Health Affairs* 31(12): 2690–98.

Carleton, R. Nicholas, Michel A. Thibodeau, Michelle J. N. Teale, Patrick G. Welch, Murray P. Abrams, Thomas Robinson, and Gordon J. G. Asmundson. 2013. "The Center for Epidemiologic Studies Depression Scale: A Review with a Theoretical and Empirical Examination of Item Content and Factor Structure." *PLoS ONE* 8(3): e58067.

Carney, Maria T., Janice Fujiwara, Brian E. Emmert Jr., Tara A. Liberman, and Barbara Paris. 2016. "Elder Orphans: Hiding in Plain Sight." *Current Gerontology and Geriatrics Research*. doi:10.1155/2016/4723250.

Carr, Deborah. 2003. "A 'Good Death' for Whom? Quality of Spouse's Death and Psychological Distress Among Older Widowed Persons." *Journal of Health and Social Behavior* 44(2): 215–32.

———. 2004. "Black/White Differences in Psychological Adjustment to Spousal Loss Among Older Adults." *Research on Aging* 26(6): 591–622.

———. 2009. "Who's to Blame? Perceived Responsibility for Spouse's Death and Psychological Distress Among Older Widowed Persons." *Journal of Health and Social Behavior* 50(3): 359–75.

———. 2011. "Racial Differences in End-of-Life Planning: Why Don't Blacks and Latinos Prepare for the Inevitable?" *Omega: The Journal of Death and Dying* 63(1): 1–20.

———. 2012. "The Social Stratification of Older Adults' Preparations for End of Life Health Care." *Journal of Health and Social Behavior* 53(3): 297–312.

———. 2014. *Worried Sick: How Stress Hurts Us and How to Bounce Back*. New Brunswick, N.J.: Rutgers University Press.

———. 2016a. "Is Death 'the Great Equalizer'? The Social Stratification of Death Quality in the Contemporary United States." *ANNALS: American Academy of Political and Social Research* 663(1): 331–54.

———. 2016b. "We Don't Die Alone: The Role of Family in End-of-Life Planning and Bereavement." Presentation at RAND Summer Institute on the Demography, Epidemiology, and Economics of Aging, Santa Monica (July 14).

———. 2016c. "Grieving for My Abusive Parent? Childhood Maltreatment and Depressive Symptoms Among Bereaved Older Adult Children." Paper presented to the annual meeting of the American Sociological Association. Seattle (August 22).

Carr, Deborah, and Kathrin Boerner. 2013. "Dating After Late-Life Spousal Loss: Does It Compromise Relationships with Adult Children?" *Journal of Aging Studies* 27(4): 487–98.

Carr, Deborah, Vicki A. Freedman, and Jennifer C. Cornman. 2018. "Beyond Gray Divorce: Remarriage and Emotional Well-being of Older Adults." Paper presented to the annual meeting of the Population Association of America. Denver (April 26).

Carr, Deborah, and Michael Friedman. 2005. "Is Obesity Stigmatizing? Body Weight, Perceived Discrimination, and Psychological Well-being in the United States." *Journal of Health and Social Behavior* 46(3): 244–59.

———. 2006. "Body Weight and Interpersonal Relationships." *Social Psychology Quarterly* 69(2): 127–49.

Carr, Deborah, James S. House, Camille Wortman, Randolph Nesse, and Ronald C. Kessler. 2001. "Psychological Adjustment to Sudden and Anticipated Spousal Loss Among Older Widowed Persons." *Journals of Gerontology Series B: Psychological Sciences and Social Sciences* 56(4): S237–48.

Carr, Deborah, Yoko Ibuka, and Louise Russell. 2010. "How Much Time Do Americans Spend Seeking Health Care? Racial and Ethnic Differences in Patient Experiences." *Research in the Sociology of Health Care* 28: 71–98.

Carr, Deborah, and Dmitry Khodyakov. 2007. "Health Care Proxies in Later Life: Whom Do We Choose and Why?" *Journal of Health and Social Behavior* 48(2): 180–94.

Carr, Deborah, and Elizabeth Luth. 2015. "End-of-Life Planning and Health Care." In *Handbook of Aging and the Social Sciences*, edited by Linda K. George and Kenneth Ferraro. New York: Academic Press.

Carr, Deborah, and Sara Moorman. 2009. "End-of-Life Treatment Preferences Among Older Adults: An Assessment of Psychosocial Influences." *Sociological Forum* 24(4): 754–78.

———. 2011. "Social Relations and Aging." In *Handbook of Sociology of Aging*, edited by Richard A. Settersten and Jacqueline L. Angel. New York: Springer.

Carr, Deborah, Sara Moorman, and Kathrin Boerner. 2013. "End-of-Life Planning in a Family Context: Does Relationship Quality Affect Whether (and with Whom) Older Adults Plan?" *Journals of Gerontology Series B: Psychological Sciences and Social Sciences* 68(4): 586–92.

Carr, Deborah, Kristen W. Springer, and Kristi Williams. 2014. "Health and Families." In *The Wiley Blackwell Companion to the Sociology of Families*, edited by Judith Treas, Jacqueline Scott, and Martin Richards. Hoboken, N.J.: John Wiley and Sons.

Carr, Deborah, and Vera Tsenkova. 2018. "Psychosocial Consequences of Body Weight and Obesity." In *Oxford Handbook of Integrative Health Science*, edited by Carol Ryff and Robert Krueger. New York: Oxford University Press.

Carson, E. Ann, and William J. Sabol. 2016. "Aging of the State Prison Population, 1993–2013." NCJ 248766. Washington: U.S. Department of Justice, Bureau of Justice Statistics. https://www.bjs.gov/content/pub/pdf/aspp9313.pdf (accessed February 20, 2017).

Carstensen, Laura L. 1992. "Social and Emotional Patterns in Adulthood: Support for Socioemotional Selectivity Theory." *Psychology and Aging* 7(3): 331–38.

Carstensen, Laura L., Helene H. Fung, and Susan T. Charles. 2003. "Socioemotional Selectivity Theory and the Regulation of Emotion in the Second Half of Life." *Motivation and Emotion* 27(2): 103–23.

Carstensen, Laura L., Monisha Pasupathi, Ulrich Mayr, and John R. Nesselroade. 2000. "Emotional Experience in Everyday Life Across the Adult Life Span." *Journal of Personality and Social Psychology* 79(4): 644–55.

Case, Anne, and Angus Deaton. 2015. "Rising Morbidity and Mortality in Midlife Among White Non-Hispanic Americans in the 21st Century." *Proceedings of the National Academy of Sciences* 112(49): 15078–83.

Caska, Catherine M., Bethany E. Hendrickson, Michelle H. Wong, Sadia Ali, Thomas Neylan, and Mary A. Whooley. 2009. "Anger Expression and Sleep Quality in Patients with Coronary Heart Disease: Findings from the Heart and Soul Study." *Psychosomatic Medicine* 71: 280–85.

Cavan, Ruth Shone. 1983. "The Chicago School of Sociology, 1918–1933." *Urban Life* 11(4): 407–20.

Center for Medicare and Medicaid Services (CMS). 2013. "Hospice Toolkit." Washington: CMS. https://www.cms.gov/Medicare-Medicaid-Coordination/Fraud-Prevention/Medicaid-Integrity-Education/Downloads/hospice-provideroverview-booklet.pdf (accessed September 18, 2018).

———. 2015. "Estimated Financial Effects of the Medicare Access and CHIP Reauthorization Act of 2015 (H.R. 2)." Baltimore: CMS, Office of the Actuary (April 9). https://www.cms.gov/research-statistics-data-and-systems/research/actuarialstudies/downloads/2015hr2a.pdf (accessed August 24, 2017).

Center on Budget and Policy Priorities. 2016. "Policy Basics: State Earned Income Tax Credits." Washington, D.C.: Center on Budget and Policy Priorities. http://www.cbpp.org/sites/default/files/atoms/files/policybasics-seitc.pdf (accessed June 30, 2017).

———. 2017. "SNAP Helps Millions of Low-Income Seniors." April 26. https://www.cbpp.org/research/food-assistance/snap-helps-millions-of-low-income-seniors (accessed September 24, 2018).

Centers for Disease Control and Prevention (CDC). 1999. "Ten Great Public Health Achievements—United States, 1900–1999." *Morbidity and Mortality Weekly Report* 48(12): 241–43.

———. 2013. "Deaths Associated with Hurricane Sandy—October-November 2012." *Morbidity and Mortality Weekly Report* 62(20): 393–97.

———. 2015. "Suicide: Facts at a Glance." Washington, D.C.: CDC, National Center for Injury Prevention and Control. http://www.cdc.gov/Violence Prevention/pdf/Suicide-DataSheet-a.pdf (accessed September 4, 2016).

———. 2017. "Important Facts About Falls." Atlanta: CDC (updated February 10, 2017). https://www.cdc.gov/homeandrecreationalsafety/falls/adultfalls.html (accessed March 10, 2017).

———. 2018a. "Current Cigarette Smoking Among Adults in the United States." Atlanta: CDC (updated February 15, 2018). https://www.cdc.gov/tobacco/data_statistics/fact_sheets/adult_data/cig_smoking/ (accessed May 1, 2017).

———. 2018b. "National Statistics: Arthritis-Attributable Limitations." Atlanta: CDC (updated July 28, 2018). https://www.cdc.gov/arthritis/data_statistics/national-statistics.html (accessed September 24, 2018).

———. 2018c. "Quarterly Provisional Estimates for Selected Indicators of Mortality, 2016–Quarter 1, 2018." Atlanta: CDC (updated September 4, 2018). https://www.cdc.gov/nchs/nvss/vsrr/mortality.htm (accessed September 24, 2018).

Charles, Susan Turk, and Laura L. Carstensen. 2007. "Emotion Regulation and Aging." In *Handbook of Emotion Regulation*, edited by James J. Gross. New York: Guildford.

Charney, Dennis S., Charles F. Reynolds, Lydia Lewis, Barry D. Lebowitz, Trey Sunderland, George S. Alexopoulos, et al. 2003. "Depression and Bipolar Support Alliance Consensus Statement on the Unmet Needs in Diagnosis and Treatment of Mood Disorders in Late Life." *Archives of General Psychology* 60(7): 664–72.

Chatterji, Pinka, Heesoo Joo, and Kajal Lahiri. 2017. "Diabetes and Labor Market Exits: Evidence from the Health and Retirement Study (HRS)." *Journal of the Economics of Ageing* 9(June): 100–110.

Chen, Edith, and Gregory E. Miller. 2013. "Socioeconomic Status and Health: Mediating and Moderating Factors." *Annual Review of Clinical Psychology* 9(March): 723–49.

Chen, Michelle. 2017. "Our Prison Population Is Getting Older and Older." *Nation*, December 11.

Cherlin, Andrew J. 2014. *Labor's Love Lost: The Rise and Fall of the Working-Class Family in America*. New York: Russell Sage Foundation.

Chesney, Edward, Guy M. Goodwin, and Seena Fazel. 2014. "Risks of All-Cause and Suicide Mortality in Mental Disorders: A Meta-Review." *World Psychiatry* 13(2): 153–60.

Chetty, Raj, Michael Stepner, Sarah Abraham, Shelby Lin, Benjamin Scuderi, Nicholas Turner, Augustin Bergeron, and David Cutler. 2016. "The Association Between Income and Life Expectancy in the United States, 2001–2014." *Journal of the American Medical Association* 315(16): 1750–66.

Chi, Nai-Ching, and George Demiris. 2016. "Family Caregivers' Pain Management in End-of-Life Care: A Systematic Review." *American Journal of Hospice and Palliative Medicine* 34(5): 470–85. doi:10.1177/1049909116637359.

Chipperfield, Judith G., Raymond P. Perry, and Bernard Weiner. 2003. "Discrete Emotions in Later Life." *The Journals of Gerontology Series B: Psychological Sciences and Social Sciences* 58(1): P23–P34.

Chiu, Tina. 2010. "It's About Time: Aging Prisoners, Increasing Costs, and Geriatric Release." New York: Vera Institute of Justice (March). http://archive.vera.org/sites/default/files/resources/downloads/Its-about-time-aging-prisoners-increasing-costs-and-geriatric-release.pdf (accessed February 20, 2017).

Choi, Namkee G., Jinseok Kim, Diana M. DiNitto, and C. Nathan Marti. 2015. "Perceived Social Cohesion, Frequency of Going Out, and Depressive Symptoms in Older Adults: Examination of Longitudinal Relationships." *Gerontology and Geriatric Medicine* (November). doi:10.1177/2333721415615478.

Christakis, Nicholas A. 2001. *Death Foretold: Prophecy and Prognosis in Medical Care.* Chicago: University of Chicago Press.

Cintron, Alexie, and R. Sean Morrison. 2006. "Pain and Ethnicity in the United States: A Systematic Review." *Journal of Palliative Medicine* 9(6): 1454–73.

Clark, Noreen M., Marshall H. Becker, Nancy K. Janz, Kate Lorig, William Rakowski, and Lynda Anderson. 1991. "Self-Management of Chronic Disease by Older Adults: A Review and Questions for Research." *Journal of Aging and Health* 3(1): 3–27.

Clarke, Philippa, and Nancy Ambrose Gallagher. 2013. "Optimizing Mobility in Later Life: The Role of the Urban Built Environment for Older Adults Aging in Place." *Journal of Urban Health* 90(6): 997–1009.

Clarke, Philippa, and Linda K. George. 2005. "The Role of the Built Environment in the Disablement Process." *American Journal of Public Health* 95(11): 1933–39.

Cole, Stephen R., Ichiro Kawachi, Susan J. Maller, and Lisa F. Berkman. 2000. "Test of Item-Response Bias in the CES-D Scale: Experience from the New Haven EPESE Study." *Journal of Clinical Epidemiology* 53(3): 285–89.

Colello, Kirsten J., and Angela Napili. 2016. "Older Americans Act: Background and Overview." Washington: Congressional Research Service (July 16). https://fas.org/sgp/crs/misc/R43414.pdf (accessed February 23, 2018).

Coleman, Eric A. 2003. "Falling through the Cracks: Challenges and Opportunities for Improving Transitional Care for Persons with Continuous Complex Care Needs." *Journal of the American Geriatrics Society* 51(4): 549–55.

Collins, Lauren G., and Kristine Swartz. 2011. "Caregiver Care." *American Family Physician* 83(11): 1309–17.

Congressional Budget Office (CBO). 2017. "Congressional Budget Office Cost Estimate: H.R. 1628 Better Care Reconciliation Act of 2017." Washington: CBO (June 26). https://www.cbo.gov/system/files/115th-congress-2017-2018/costestimate/52849-hr1628senate.pdf (accessed July 1, 2017).

———. 2018. "The Distribution of Household Income, 2014." Washington, D.C.: CBO (March). https://www.cbo.gov/system/files/115th-congress-2017-2018/reports/53597-distribution-household-income-2014.pdf (accessed June 15, 2018).

Conner, Kyaien O., Valire Carr Copeland, Nancy K. Grote, Gary Koeske, Daniel Rosen, Charles F. Reynolds, and Charlotte Brown. 2010. "Mental Health Treatment Seeking Among Older Adults with Depression: The Impact of Stigma and Race." *American Journal of Geriatric Psychiatry* 18(6): 531–43.

Connidis, Ingrid Arnet. 2010. *Family Ties and Aging.* Newbury Park, Calif.: Pine Forge Press.

Conwell, Yeates, Kimberly Van Orden, and Eric D. Caine. 2011. "Suicide in Older Adults." *Psychiatric Clinics of North America* 34(2): 451–68.

Cooper, Claudia, Amber Selwood, Martin Blanchard, Zuzana Walker, Robert Blizard, and Gill Livingston. 2009. "Abuse of People with Dementia by Family Carers: Representative Cross-Sectional Survey." *British Medical Journal* 338: 155. doi:10.1136/bmj.b155.

Cooper, Richard, Charles Rotimi, Susan Ataman, Daniel McGee, Babatunde Osotimehin, Solomon Kadiri, Walinjom Muna, Samuel Kingue, Henry Fraser, Terrence Forrester, Franklyn Bennett, and Rainford Wilks. 1997. "The Prevalence of Hypertension in Seven Populations of West African Origin." *American Journal of Public Health* 87(2): 160–68.

Cooper-Patrick, Lisa, Rosa M. Crum, and Daniel E. Ford. 1994. "Characteristics of Patients with Major Depression Who Received Care in General Medical and Specialty Mental Health Settings." *Medical Care* 32(1): 15–24.

Cornwell, Benjamin. 2015. "Social Disadvantage and Network Turnover." *Journals of Gerontology Series B: Psychological Sciences and Social Sciences* 70(1): 132–42.

Cornwell, Benjamin, and Edward O. Laumann. 2015. "The Health Benefits of Network Growth: New Evidence from a National Survey of Older Adults." *Social Science and Medicine* 125(January): 94–106.

Cornwell, Benjamin, Edward O. Laumann, and L. Philip Schumm. 2008. "The Social Connectedness of Older Adults: A National Profile." *American Sociological Review* 73(2): 185–203.

Corporation for National Community and Service (CNCS). 2016. "Value of Senior Volunteers to U.S. Economy Estimated at $77 Billion." Washington, D.C.: CNCS (May 16). https://www.nationalservice.gov/newsroom/press-releases/2016/value-senior-volunteers-us-economy-estimated-77-billion (accessed October 8, 2017).

Cortright, Joe. 2018. "Gerontopoly: Homeownership, Wealth, and Age." *City Observatory,* April 23. https://cityobservatory.org/gerontopoly-homeownership-wealth-and-age/ (accessed September 21, 2018).

Cotten, Shelia R., George Ford, Sherry Ford, and Timothy M. Hale. 2014. "Internet Use and Depression Among Retired Older Adults in the United States: A

Longitudinal Analysis." *Journals of Gerontology Series B: Psychological Sciences and Social Sciences* 69(5): 763–71.

Crimmins, Eileen M., Mark D. Hayward, and Teresa E. Seeman. 2004. "Race/Ethnicity, Socioeconomic Status, and Health." In *Critical Perspectives on Racial and Ethnic Differences in Health in Late Life*, edited by Norman B. Anderson, Rodolfo A. Bulatao, and Barney Cohen. Washington, D.C.: National Academies Press.

Crosby, Alex E., LaVonne Ortega, and Mark R. Stevens. 2013. "Suicides—United States, 2005–2009." *MMWR Morbidity and Mortality Weekly Report* 62(3): 177–81.

Cruz, Lenika. 2015. "'Dinnertimin' and 'No Tipping': How Advertisers Targeted Black Consumers in the 1970s." *Atlantic*, June 7. https://www.theatlantic.com/entertainment/archive/2015/06/casual-racism-and-greater-diversity-in-70s-advertising/394958/ (accessed July 1, 2017).

Crystal, Stephen, and Dennis Shea. 1990. "Cumulative Advantage, Cumulative Disadvantage, and Inequality Among Elderly People." *Gerontologist* 30(4): 437–43.

Cubanski, Juliette, and Tricia Neuman. 2017. "The Facts on Medicare Spending and Financing." Washington, D.C.: Henry J. Kaiser Family Foundation (June 22). http://www.kff.org/medicare/issue-brief/the-facts-on-medicare-spending-and-financing/ (accessed August 24, 2017).

Cubanski, Juliette, Kendal Orgera, Anthony Damico, and Tricia Neuman. 2018. "How Many Seniors Are Living in Poverty? National and State Estimates under the Official and Supplemental Poverty Measures in 2016." Henry J. Kaiser Family Foundation, March 2. https://www.kff.org/medicare/issue-brief/how-many-seniors-are-living-in-poverty-national-and-state-estimates-under-the-official-and-supplemental-poverty-measures-in-2016/ (accessed June 1, 2018).

Cuijpers, Pim, and Filip Smit. 2002. "Excess Mortality in Depression: A Meta-Analysis of Community Studies." *Journal of Affective Disorders* 72(3): 227–36.

Culhane Dennis P., Stephen Metraux, Thomas Byrne, Magdi Stino, and Jay Bainbridge. 2013. "The Age Structure of Contemporary Homelessness: Evidence and Implications for Public Policy." *Analysis of Social Issues and Public Policy* 13(1): 228–44.

Cumming, Elaine, and William Earl Henry. 1961. *Growing Old: The Process of Disengagement*. New York: Basic Books.

Cutler, David M., and Ellen Meara. 2004. "Changes in the Age Distribution of Mortality over the Twentieth Century." In *Perspectives on the Economics of Aging*, edited by David A. Wise. Chicago: University of Chicago Press.

Cwikel, Julie, Helen Gramotnev, and Christina Lee. 2006. "Never-Married Childless Women: Health and Social Circumstances in Older Age." *Social Science and Medicine* 62(8): 1991–2001.

Daniel, Caitlin. 2016. "Economic Constraints on Taste Formation and the True Cost of Healthy Eating." *Social Science and Medicine* 148(January): 34–41.

Dannefer, Dale. 1987. "Aging as Intracohort Differentiation: Accentuation, the Matthew Effect, and the Life Course." *Sociological Forum* 2(2): 211–36.

Darmon, Nicole, and Adam Drewnowski. 2008. "Does Social Class Predict Diet Quality?" *American Journal of Clinical Nutrition* 87(5): 1107–17.

Darrow, Barb. 2017. "Microsoft Expands Paid Leave for Family Caregivers." *Fortune*, June 27. http://fortune.com/2017/06/27/microsoft-paid-family-care-leave/ (accessed October 8, 2017).

Davies, Curt, with Dameka Williams. 2002. "The Grandparent Study 2002 Report." Washington, D.C.: American Association of Retired Persons (May). http://assets.aarp.org/rgcenter/general/gp_2002.pdf (accessed October 9, 2016).

De Jong Gierveld, Jenny. 2004. "Remarriage, Unmarried Cohabitation, Living Apart Together: Partner Relationships Following Bereavement or Divorce." *Journal of Marriage and Family* 66(1): 236–43.

De Jong Gierveld, Jenny, Marjolein Broese van Groenou, Adriaan W. Hoogendoorn, and Johannes H. Smit. 2009. "Quality of Marriages in Later Life and Emotional and Social Loneliness." *Journals of Gerontology Series B: Psychological Sciences and Social Sciences* 64B(4): 497–506.

De Jong Gierveld, Jenny, and Betty Havens. 2004. "Cross-National Comparisons of Social Isolation and Loneliness: Introduction and Overview." *Canadian Journal on Aging* 23(2): 109–13.

Decker, Sandra L. 2012. "In 2011 Nearly One-Third of Physicians Said They Would Not Accept New Medicaid Patients, but Rising Fees May Help." *Health Affairs* 31(8): 1673–79.

DeNavas-Walt, Carmen, Bernadette D. Proctor, and Jessica Smith. 2004. "Income, Poverty, and Health Insurance Coverage in the United States: 2003." *Current Population Reports*, P60-226. Washington: U.S. Department of Commerce, U.S. Bureau of the Census (August).

DePaulo, Bella. 2013. "Happy Singles." In *The World Book of Love,* edited by Leo Bormans. Tielt, Belgium: Lannoo Publishers.

Desmond, Matthew. 2012. "Disposable Ties and the Urban Poor." *American Journal of Sociology* 117(5): 1295–1335.

Detering, Karen M., Andrew D. Hancock, Michael C. Reade, and William Silvester. 2010. "The Impact of Advance Care Planning on End of Life Care in Elderly Patients: Randomised Controlled Trial." *British Medical Journal* 340: 1345. doi:10.1136/bmj.c1345.

Dick, Danielle M., Arpana Agrawal, Matthew C. Keller, Amy Adkins, Fazil Aliev, Scott Monroe, John K. Hewitt, Kenneth S. Kendler, and Kenneth J. Sher. 2015. "Candidate Gene–Environment Interaction Research: Reflections and Recommendations." *Perspectives on Psychological Science* 10(1): 37–59.

Dickens, Charles. [1861] 1965. *Great Expectations*. Toronto: Macmillan of Canada.
Dilworth-Anderson, Peggye, Beverly H. Brummett, Paula Goodwin, Sharon Wallace Williams, Redford B. Williams, and Ilene C. Siegler. 2005. "Effect of Race on Cultural Justifications for Caregiving." *Journals of Gerontology Series B: Psychological Sciences and Social Sciences* 60(5): S257–62.
Dimah, Keren Patricia, and Agber Dimah. 2004. "Elder Abuse and Neglect Among Rural and Urban Women." *Journal of Elder Abuse and Neglect* 15(1): 75–93.
Ditto, Peter H., Joseph H. Danks, William D. Smucker, Jamila Bookwala, Kristen M. Coppola, Rebecca Dresser, Angela Fagerlin, Mitchell Gready, Renate M. Houts, Lisa K. Lockhart, and Stephen Zyzanski. 2001. "Advance Directives as Acts of Communication." *Annals of Internal Medicine* 161(3): 421–30.
Dowd, Jennifer Beam, and Allison Aiello. 2009. "Socioeconomic Differentials in Immune Response in the U.S." *Epidemiology* 20(6): 902–8.
Dowd, Jennifer B., Jeremy Albright, Trivellore E. Raghunathan, Robert F. Schoeni, Felicia LeClere, and George A. Kaplan. 2011. "Deeper and Wider: Income and Mortality in the USA over Three Decades." *International Journal of Epidemiology* 40: 183–88.
Drewnowski, Adam, and France Bellisle. 2007. "Is Sweetness Addictive?" *Nutrition Bulletin* 32(S1): 52–60.
Drucker, Ernest. 2002. "Population Impact of Mass Incarceration under New York's Rockefeller Drug Laws: An Analysis of Years of Life Lost." *Journal of Urban Health Bulletin of the New York Academy of Medicine* 79(3): 434–35.
Druss, Benjamin G., and Elizabeth R. Walker. 2011. *Mental Disorders and Medical Comorbidity*. Princeton, N.J.: Robert Wood Johnson Foundation, The Synthesis Project. http://www.rwjf.org/content/dam/farm/reports/issue_briefs/2011/rwjf69438/subassets/rwjf69438_1 (accessed September 3, 2016).
Ducharme, Jamie. 2016. "Longevity Tips from the Oldest U.S. Resident." *Boston*, May 17. https://www.bostonmagazine.com/health/2016/05/17/goldie-michelson/ (accessed February 25, 2018).
Duke, Brendan. 2016. "When I Was Your Age: Millennials and the Generational Wage Gap." Washington, D.C.: Center for American Progress (March 3). https://www.americanprogress.org/issues/economy/reports/2016/03/03/131627/when-i-was-your-age/ (accessed October 8, 2017).
Duncan, Greg J., and Jeanne Brooks-Gunn, eds. 1999. *Consequences of Growing up Poor*. New York: Russell Sage Foundation.
Duncan, Greg J., Mary C. Daly, Peggy McDonough, and David R. Williams. 2002. "Optimal Indicators of Socioeconomic Status for Health Research." *American Journal of Public Health* 92(7): 1151–57.
Durkheim, Émile. [1897] 1951. *Suicide: A Study in Sociology*. Translated by John A. Spaulding. New York: Free Press.

Dykstra, Pearl A. 1995. "Loneliness Among the Never and Formerly Married: The Importance of Supportive Friendships and a Desire for Independence." *Journals of Gerontology Series B: Psychological Sciences and Social Sciences* 50B(5): S321–29.

Elder, Glen H., Jr. 1994. "Time, Human Agency, and Social Change: Perspectives on the Life Course." *Social Psychology Quarterly* 57(1): 4–15.

———. 1999. *Children of the Great Depression: Social Change in Life Experience.* Boulder, Colo.: Westview Press.

Elder, Glen H., Jr., Michael J. Shanahan, and Elizabeth Colerick Clipp. 1994. "When War Comes to Men's Lives: Life-Course Patterns in Family, Work, and Health." *Psychology and Aging* 9(1): 5–16.

Ellis, Renee R., and Tavia Simmons. 2014. "Coresident Grandparents and Their Grandchildren: 2012." P20-576. Washington: U.S. Department of Commerce, U.S. Census Bureau, Economics and Statistics Administration (October). https://www.census.gov/content/dam/Census/library/publications/2014/demo/p20-576.pdf (accessed March 25, 2017).

Emanuel, Ezekiel J., and Linda L. Emanuel. 1994. "The Economics of Dying—The Illusion of Cost Savings at the End of Life." *New England Journal of Medicine* 330(8): 540–44.

Emmons, William R., Ana H. Kent and Lowell R. Ricketts. 2018. *The Demographics of Wealth: How Education, Race, and Birth Year Shape Financial Outcomes, An Introduction to the Series.* St. Louis, Mo.: Center for Household Financial Stability/Federal Reserve Board of St. Louis. https://www.stlouisfed.org/~/media/Files/PDFs/HFS/essays/HFS_essay_2_2018.pdf?la=en (accessed September 19, 2018).

Epel, Elissa S., Elizabeth H. Blackburn, Jue Lin, Firdaus S. Dhabhar, Nancy E. Adler, Jason D. Morrow, and Richard M. Cawthon. 2004. "Accelerated Telomere Shortening in Response to Life Stress." *Proceedings of the National Academy* 101(49): 17312–15.

Estes, Carroll. 1979. *The Aging Enterprise.* San Francisco: Jossey-Bass.

Evans, Gary W., and Rochelle C. Cassells. 2014. "Childhood Poverty, Cumulative Risk Exposure, and Mental Health in Emerging Adults." *Clinical Psychological Science* 2(3): 287–96.

Evans, Mavis, and Pat Mottram. 2000. "Diagnosis of Depression in Elderly Patients." *Advances in Psychiatric Treatment* 6(1): 49–56.

Evans, William N., and Craig L. Garthwaite. 2014. "Giving Mom a Break: The Impact of Higher EITC Payments on Maternal Health." *American Economic Journal: Economic Policy* 6(2): 258–90.

Ezop, Paula. 2011. "My Experience with Hospice Care." Open to Hope, May 20. http://www.opentohope.com/my-experience-with-hospice-care/ (accessed September 8, 2016).

Family Caregiving Alliance. 2001. "Selected Long-Term Care Statistics." San Francisco: Family Caregiving Alliance (updated January 13, 2015). https://

www.caregiver.org/selected-long-term-care-statistics (accessed April 22, 2017).

Federal Communications Commission (FCC). 2015. "2015 Broadband Progress Report." Washington: FCC (February 4). https://www.fcc.gov/reports-research/reports/broadband-progress-reports/2015-broadband-progress-report (accessed September 24, 2018).

Federal Interagency Forum on Aging-Related Statistics. 2016. *Older Americans 2016: Key Indicators of Well-being*. Washington: U.S. Government Printing Office.

Federal Reserve. 2015. "Report on the Economic Well-being of U.S. Households in 2014." Washington, D.C.: Board of Governors of the Federal Reserve System (May). https://www.federalreserve.gov/econresdata/2014-report-economic-well-being-us-households-201505.pdf (accessed May 1, 2017).

Feinglass, Joe, Suru Lin, Jason Thompson, Joseph Sudano, Dorothy Dunlop, Jing Song, and David W. Baker. 2007. "Baseline Health, Socioeconomic Status, and 10-Year Mortality Among Older Middle-Aged Americans: Findings from the Health and Retirement Study, 1992–2002." *Journals of Gerontology Series B: Psychological Sciences and Social Sciences* 62(4): S209–17.

Ferraro, Kenneth F., and Melissa M. Farmer. 1999. "Utility of Health Data from Social Surveys: Is There a Gold Standard for Measuring Morbidity?" *American Sociological Review* 64(2): 303–15.

Ferraro, Kenneth F., and Tetyana Pylypiv Shippee. 2009. "Aging and Cumulative Inequality: How Does Inequality Get under the Skin?" *Gerontologist* 49(3): 333–43.

Fiori, Katherine L., and Christy A. Denckla. 2012. "Social Support and Mental Health in Middle-Aged Men and Women: A Multidimensional Approach." *Journal of Aging and Health* 24(3): 407–38.

Fischer, David Hackett. 1978. *Growing Old in America*. New York: Oxford University Press.

Fiske, Amy, Julie Loebach Wetherell, and Margaret Gatz. 2009. "Depression in Older Adults." *Annual Review of Clinical Psychology* 5: 363–89.

Flory, James, Yinong Young-Xu, Ipek Gurol, Norman Levinsky, Arlene Ash, and Ezekiel Emanuel. 2004. "Place of Death: U.S. Trends Since 1980." *Health Affairs* 23: 194–200.

Ford, Earl S., Chaoyang Li, Guixiang Zhao, and J. Tsai. 2011. "Trends in Obesity and Abdominal Obesity Among Adults in the United States from 1999–2008." *International Journal of Obesity* 35(5): 736–43.

Foster, Malcolm. 2018. "How Robots Could Help Care for Japan's Ageing Population." *Independent*, April 9. https://www.independent.co.uk/arts-entertainment/photography/japan-robot-elderly-care-ageing-population-exercises-movement-a8295706.html (accessed June 10, 2018).

Fredriksen-Goldsen, Karen I. 2016. "The Future of LGBT+ Aging: A Blueprint for Action in Services, Policies, and Research." *Generations* 40(2): 6–15.

Freedman, Vicki A., and Brenda C. Spillman. 2014. "The Residential Continuum from Home to Nursing Home: Size, Characteristics, and Unmet Needs of Older Adults." *Journals of Gerontology Series B: Psychological Sciences and Social Sciences* 69(supp. 1): S42–50.

Freeman, Harold P. 1989. "Cancer in the Socioeconomically Disadvantaged." *CA: A Cancer Journal for Clinicians* 39(5): 266–88.

French, Eric B., Jeremy McCauley, Maria Aragon, Pieter Bakx, Martin Chalkley, Stacey H. Chen, Bent J. Christensen, et al. 2017. "End-of-Life Medical Spending in Last Twelve Months of Life Is Lower Than Previously Reported." *Health Affairs* 36(7): 1211–17.

Freudenberg, William R., Robert Gramling, Shirley Laska, and Kai T. Erikson. 2009. *Catastrophe in the Making: The Engineering of Katrina and the Disasters of Tomorrow*. Washington, D.C.: Island Press.

Friedman, Elliot M., and Pamela Herd. 2010. "Income, Education, and Inflammation: Differential Associations in a National Probability Sample (The MIDUS Study)." *Psychosomatic Medicine* 72(3): 290–300.

Friend, Tad. 2017. "Silicon Valley's Quest to Live Forever." *New Yorker*, April 3. http://www.newyorker.com/magazine/2017/04/03/silicon-valleys-quest-to-live-forever (accessed April 15, 2017).

Fuchs, Flávio D. 2011. "Why Do Black Americans Have Higher Prevalence of Hypertension? An Enigma Still Unsolved." *Hypertension* 57(3): 379–80.

Gabler, Ellen, Sheri Fink, and Vivian Yee. 2017. "At Florida Nursing Home, Many Calls for Help, but None That Made a Difference." *New York Times*, September 23. https://www.nytimes.com/2017/09/23/us/nursing-home-deaths.html (accessed August 5, 2018).

Galea, Sandro, Melissa Tracy, Katherine J. Hoggatt, Charles DiMaggio, and Adam Karpati. 2011. "Estimated Deaths Attributable to Social Factors in the United States." *American Journal of Public Health* 101(8): 1456–65.

Garrett, Bowen, and Anuj Gangopadhyaya. 2016. "Who Gained Health Insurance Coverage under the ACA, and Where Do They Live?" Washington, D.C.: Urban Institute (December 21). https://www.urban.org/research/publication/who-gained-health-insurance-coverage-under-aca-and-where-do-they-live (accessed September 22, 2017).

Gaugler, Joseph E. 2016. "Innovations in Long-Term Care." In *Handbook of Aging and the Social Sciences* (8th ed.), edited by Robert H. Binstock. New York: Academic Press.

Gawande, Atul. 2014. *Being Mortal: Medicine and What Matters in the End*. New York: Metropolitan Books.

———. 2017. "If the U.S. Adopts the GOP's Health-Care Bill, It Would Be an Act of Mass Suicide." *New Yorker*, September 22. https://www.newyorker.com/news/news-desk/if-the-us-adopts-the-gops-health-care-bill-it-would-be-an-act-of-mass-suicide (accessed September 23, 2017).

Generations United. 2014. "The State of Grandfamilies in America: 2014." Washington, D.C.: Generations United. https://www.gu.org/app/uploads/2018/05/Grandfamilies-Report-SOGF-2014.pdf (accessed September 24, 2018).

———. 2017. "Generations United's Public Policy Priorities for the 115th Congress." Washington, D.C.: Generations United. https://dl2.pushbulletusercontent.com/aZtUMuvqrfDd1dtMdqqdWKRGVPRXhuas/GU%20115th%20PPA%20-%20Final.pdf (accessed August 22, 2017).

George, Linda K. 1993. "Sociological Perspectives on Life Transitions." *Annual Review of Sociology* 19(August): 353–73.

Geronimus, Arline T., Margaret Hicken, Danya Keene, and John Bound. 2006. "'Weathering' and Age Patterns of Allostatic Load Scores Among Blacks and Whites in the United States." *American Journal of Public Health* 96(5): 826–33.

Gerontological Society of America. 2017. *Oral Health: An Essential Element of Healthy Aging*. Washington, D.C.: Gerontological Society of America (July). https://www.geron.org/images/gsa/documents/gsa2017oralhealthwhitepaper.pdf (accessed July 6, 2017).

Gibbs, K., Sandy J. Slater, N. Nicholson, Diane C. Barker, and Frank J. Chaloupka. 2012. "Income Disparities in Street Features That Encourage Walking—A BTG Research Brief." Chicago, Ill.: Bridging the Gap Program, Health Policy Center, Institute for Health Research and Policy, University of Illinois at Chicago.

Gibson, Mary Jo, and Michele Hayunga. 2006. "We Can Do Better: Lessons Learned for Protecting Older Persons in Disasters." Washington, D.C.: American Association of Retired Persons. https://assets.aarp.org/rgcenter/il/better_1.pdf (accessed September 24, 2018).

Giddan, Jane, and Ellen Cole. 2015. *70 Candles! Women Thriving in Their 8th Decade*. Chagrin Falls, Ohio: Taos Institute Publications.

Gill, Sarah C., Peter Butterworth, Bryan Rodgers, Kaarin J. Anstey, Elena Villamil, and David Melzer. 2006. "Mental Health and the Timing of Men's Retirement." *Social Psychiatry and Psychiatric Epidemiology* 41(7): 515–22.

Glaeser, Edward, and Joseph Gyourko. 2018. "The Economic Implications of Housing Supply." *Journal of Economic Perspectives* 32(1): 3–30.

Glass, Thomas A., and Jennifer L. Balfour. 2003. "Neighborhoods, Aging, and Functional Limitations." In *Neighborhoods and Health*, edited by Ichiro Kawachi and Lisa F. Berkman. New York: Oxford University Press.

Golant, Stephen M. 2015. *Aging in the Right Place*. Baltimore: Health Professions Press.

Goldman, Noreen. 1993. "Marriage Selection and Mortality Patterns: Inferences and Fallacies." *Demography* 30(2): 189–208.

———. 2016. "Will the Latino Mortality Advantage Endure?" *Research on Aging* 38(3): 263–82.

Goldsen, Jayn, Amanda E. B. Bryan, Hyun-Jun Kim, Anna Muraco, Sarah Jen, and Karen I. Fredriksen-Goldsen. 2017. "Who Says I Do: The Changing Context of Marriage and Health and Quality of Life for LGBT Older Adults." *Gerontologist* 57(1): S50–62.

Goldstein, Nathan E., Lewis M. Cohen, Robert M. Arnold, Elizabeth Goy, Stephen Arons, and Linda Ganzini. 2012. "Prevalence of Formal Accusations of Murder and Euthanasia Against Physicians." *Journal of Palliative Medicine* 15(3): 334–39.

Gomes, Barbara, Natalia Calanzani, Jonathan Koffman, and Irene J. Higginson. 2015. "Is Dying in Hospital Better than Home in Incurable Cancer and What Factors Influence This? A Population-Based Study." *BMC Medicine* 13: 235, doi:10.1186/s12916-015-0466-5.

Gomes, Barbara, and Irene J. Higginson. 2006. "Factors Influencing Death at Home in Terminally Ill Patients with Cancer: Systematic Review." *British Medical Journal* 332(7540): 515–21.

Gozalo, Pedro, Michael Plotzke, Vincent Mor, Susan C. Miller, and Joan M. Teno. 2015. "Changes in Medicare Costs with the Growth of Hospice Care in Nursing Homes." *New England Journal of Medicine* 372: 1823–31.

Gozalo, Pedro, Joan M. Teno, Susan L. Mitchell, Jon Skinner, Julie Bynum, Denise Tyler, and Vincent Mor. 2011. "End-of-Life Transitions Among Nursing Home Residents with Cognitive Issues." *New England Journal of Medicine* 365(13): 1212–21.

Grady, Denise. 2000. "Little Access to Pain Drugs in Some Areas." *New York Times*, April 6. http://www.nytimes.com/2000/04/06/us/little-access-to-pain-drugs-in-some-areas.html (accessed August 31, 2016).

Grafova, Irina B., Vicki A. Freedman, Rizie Kumar, and Jeannette Rogowski. 2008. "Neighborhoods and Obesity in Later Life." *American Journal of Public Health* 98(11): 2065–71.

Grafova, Irina B., Vicki A. Freedman, Nicole Lurie, Rizie Kumar, and Jeannette Rogowski. 2014. "The Difference-in-Difference Method: Assessing the Selection Bias in the Effects of Neighborhood Environment on Health." *Economics and Human Biology* 13(1): 20–33.

Graham, Carrie, Andrew E. Scharlach, and Elaine Kurtovich. 2018. "Do Villages Promote Aging in Place? Results of a Longitudinal Study." *Journal of Applied Gerontology* 37(3): 310–31.

Graham, Carrie L., Andrew E. Scharlach, Roscoe Nicholson, and Catherine O'Brien. 2017. "2016 National Survey of U.S. Villages." Research brief. Evanston, Ill.: Mather LifeWays Institute on Aging.

Graham, Judith. 2013. "Medicare to Cover More Mental Health Costs." *New York Times*, December 27, 2013. https://newoldage.blogs.nytimes.com/2013/12/27/medicare-to-cover-more-mental-health-costs/?mcubz=1 (accessed July 1, 2017).

———. 2014. "A Shortage of Caregivers." *New York Times*, February 26. https://newoldage.blogs.nytimes.com/2014/02/26/a-shortage-of-caregivers/ (accessed October 6, 2017).

Granovetter, Mark S. 1973. "The Strength of Weak Ties." *American Journal of Sociology* 78(6): 1360–80.

Grantmakers in Aid. 2017. "Heartache, Pain, and Hope: Rural Communities, Older People, and the Opioid Crisis: An Introduction for Funders." Arlington, Va.: Grantmakers in Aging (August 27). https://www.giaging.org/documents/170823_GIA_Rural_Opioid_Paper_FINAL_for_web.pdf (accessed October 2, 2017).

Gratton, Lynda, and Andrew Scott. 2016. "What Older Workers Can Learn from Younger Workers and Vice-Versa?" *Harvard Business Review*, November 18. https://hbr.org/2016/11/what-younger-workers-can-learn-from-older-workers-and-vice-versa (accessed September 29, 2017).

Gravlee, Clarence C. 2009. "How Race Becomes Biology: Embodiment of Social Inequality." *American Journal of Physical Anthropology* 139(1): 47–57.

Green, Carmen R., Karen O. Anderson, Tamara A. Baker, Lisa C. Campbell, Sheila Decker, Roger B. Fillingim, Donna A. Kalauokalani, Kathyrn E. Lasch, Cynthia Myers, Raymond C. Tait, Knox H. Todd, and April H. Vallerand. 2003. "The Unequal Burden of Pain: Confronting Racial and Ethnic Disparities in Pain." *Pain Medicine* 4(3): 277–94.

Greenfield, Emily A., and Nadine F. Marks. 2006. "Linked Lives: Adult Children's Problems and Their Parents' Psychological and Relational Well-being." *Journal of Marriage and Family* 68(2): 442–54.

Grigoriadis, Sophie, and Gail Erlick Robinson. 2007. "Gender Issues in Depression." *Annals of Clinical Psychiatry* 19(4): 247–55.

Groopman, Jerome E., and Michael Prichard. 2007. *How Doctors Think*. Boston: Houghton Mifflin.

Gruenberg, Ernest M. 1977. "The Failures of Success." *Milbank Memorial Fund Quarterly: Health and Society* 55(1): 3–24.

Gruneir, Andrea, Vincent More, Sherry Weitzen, Rachael Truchil, Joan Teno, and Jason Roy. 2007. "Where People Die: A Multilevel Approach to Understanding Influences on Site of Death in America." *Medical Care Research and Review* 64(4): 351–78.

Gunn, David A., Helle Rexbye, Christopher E. M. Griffiths, Peter G. Murray, Amelia Fereday, Sharon D. Catt, Cyrena C. Tomlin, et al. 2009. "Why Some Women Look Young for Their Age." *PloS One* 4(12): e8021.

Ha, Jung-Hwa. 2008. "Changes in Support from Confidants, Children, and Friends Following Widowhood." *Journal of Marriage and Family* 70(2): 306–18.

Haas Institute. N.d. "Responding to Rising Inequality Policy Interventions to Ensure Opportunity for All." Policy brief. Berkeley: University of California, Haas Institute for a Fair and Inclusive Society. http://haasinstitute.berkeley.edu/sites/default/files/HaasInstitute_InequalityPolicyBrief_FINALforDISTRO_2.pdf (accessed July 15, 2017).

Hagger-Johnson, Gareth, Séverine Sabia, Eric John Brunner, Martin Shipley, Martin Bobak, Michael Marmot, Mika Kivimaki, and Archana Singh-Manoux. 2013. "Combined Impact of Smoking and Heavy Alcohol Use on Cognitive

Decline in Early Old Age: Whitehall II Prospective Cohort Study." *British Journal of Psychiatry* 203(2): 120–25.

Hales, C. Nicholas, David J. Barker, Penelope M. Clark, Lorna J. Cox, Caroline Fall, Clive Osmond, and P. D. Winter. 1991. "Fetal and Infant Growth and Impaired Glucose Tolerance at Age 64." *BMJ* 303(6809): 1019–22.

Halonen, Jaana I., Anna L. Hansell, John Gulliver, David Morley, Marta Blangiardo, Daniela Fecht, Mireille B. Toledano, et al. 2015. "Road Traffic Noise Is Associated with Increased Cardiovascular Morbidity and Mortality and All-Cause Mortality in London." *European Heart Journal* 36(39): 2653–61.

Hammes, Bernard J. 2003. "Updates on Respecting Choices Four Years On." *Innovations in End-of-Life Care Journal* 5(2): 335–40.

Hanchate, Amresh, Andrea C. Kronman, Yinong Young-Xu, Arlene S. Ash, and Ezekiel Emanuel. 2009. "Racial and Ethnic Differences in End-of-Life Costs: Why Do Minorities Cost More than Whites?" *Archives of Internal Medicine* 169(5): 493–501.

Harburg, Ernest, Mara Julius, Niko Kaciroti, Lillian Gleiberman, and Anthony M. Schork. 2003. "Expressive/Suppressive Anger-Coping Responses, Gender, and Types of Mortality: A 17-Year Follow-up (Tecumseh, Michigan, 1971–1988)." *Psychosomatic Medicine* 65(4): 588–97.

Hardy, Melissa, and Lawrence Hazelrigg. 2010. *Pension Puzzles: Social Security and the Great Debate*. New York: Russell Sage Foundation.

Harrington-Meyer, Madonna. 2014. *Grandmothers at Work: Juggling Families and Jobs*. New York: New York University Press.

Harrington-Meyer, Madonna, and Pamela Herd. 2007. *Market Friendly or Family Friendly? The State and Gender Inequality in Old Age*. New York: Russell Sage Foundation.

Harrington-Meyer, Madonna, Douglas A. Wolf, and Christine L. Himes. 2006. "Declining Eligibility for Social Security Spouse and Widow Benefits in the United States?" *Research on Aging* 28(2): 240–60.

Havighurst, Robert J. 1963. "Successful Aging." In *Processes of Aging: Social and Psychological Perspectives*, edited by Richard H. Williams, Clark Tibbits, and Wilma Donohue. New Brunswick, N.J.: Aldine Transaction.

Hawkley, Louise C., and John T. Cacioppo. 2010. "Loneliness Matters: A Theoretical and Empirical Review of Consequences and Mechanisms." *Annals of Behavioral Medicine* 40(2): 218–27.

Hayflick, Leonard. 1994. *How and Why We Age*. New York: Ballantine Books.

Hayslip, Bert, Jr., and Heidemarie Blumenthal. 2016. "Grandparenthood: A Developmental Perspective." In *Gerontology: Changes, Challenges, and Solutions*, edited by Madonna Harrington-Meyer and Elizabeth A. Daniele. Santa Barbara, Calif.: Praeger Publishers.

Hayslip, Bert, Jr., Rebecca J. Glover, Bric E. Harris, Paula B. Miltenberger, Annabel Baird, and Patricia L. Kaminski. 2009. "Perceptions of Custodial Grandparents Among Young Adults." *Journal of Intergenerational Relationships* 7(2/3): 209–24.

Hayslip, Bert, Jr., and Kyle S. Page. 2012. "Grandparenthood: Grandchild and Great-Grandchild Relationships." In *Handbook of Families and Aging*, edited by Rosemary Blieszner and Victoria Hilkevitch Bedford. Santa Barbara, Calif.: ABC-CLIO.

Health Care Cost Institute (HCCI). 2016. "2016 Health Care Cost and Utilization Report." Washington, D.C.: HCCI (November). https://www.healthcostinstitute.org/research/annual-reports/entry/2016-health-care-cost-and-utilization-report/ (accessed September 21, 2018).

Hebert, Liesi E., Jennifer Weuve, Paul A. Scherr, and Denis A. Evans. 2013. "Alzheimer Disease in the United States (2010–2050) Estimated Using the 2010 Census." *Neurology* 80(19): 1778–83.

Hebert, Paul L., Kevin D. Frick, Robert L. Kane, and A. Marshall McBean. 2005. "The Causes of Racial and Ethnic Differences in Influenza Vaccination Rates Among Elderly Medicare Beneficiaries." *Health Services Research* 40(2): 517–38.

Helppie-McFall, Brooke, Amanda Sonnega, Robert J. Willis, and Peter Hudomiet. 2015. "Occupations and Work Characteristics: Effects on Retirement Expectations and Timing." Working Paper 2015-331. Ann Arbor: University of Michigan, Institute for Social Research, Michigan Retirement Research Center (October). http://www.mrrc.isr.umich.edu/publications/papers/pdf/wp331.pdf (accessed September 24, 2018).

Henry, Meghan, Rian Watt, Lily Rosenthal, and Azim Shivji. 2016. *The 2016 Annual Homeless Assessment Report (AHAR) to Congress*. Washington: U.S. Department of Housing and Urban Development (November). https://www.hudexchange.info/resources/documents/2016-AHAR-Part-1.pdf (accessed February 20, 2017).

Henry J. Kaiser Family Foundation. 2015. "State Health Facts." https://www.kff.org/statedata/ (accessed September 21, 2018).

———. 2016. "Medicaid-to-Medicare Fee Index." http://www.kff.org/medicaid/state-indicator/medicaid-to-medicare-fee-index/?currentTimeframe=0&sortModel=%7B%22colId%22:%22Location%22,%22sort%22:%22asc%22%7D (accessed July 6, 2017).

———. 2018. "State Health Facts: Life Expectancy at Birth (in Years)." https://www.kff.org/other/state-indicator/life-expectancy/?currentTimeframe=0&sortModel=%7B%22colId%22:%22Location%22,%22sort%22:%22asc%22%7D (accessed May 20, 2018).

Herd, Pamela. 2005. "Ensuring a Minimum: Social Security Reform and Women." *Gerontologist* 45(1): 12–25.

Herd, Pamela, Melissa Favreault, Madonna Harrington Meyer, and Timothy M. Smeeding. 2018. "A Targeted Minimum Benefit Plan: A New Proposal to Reduce Poverty Among Older Social Security Recipients." *RSF: The Russell Sage Foundation Journal of the Social Sciences* 4(2): 74–90.

Herd, Pamela, Robert F. Schoeni, and James S. House. 2008. "Upstream Solutions: Does the Supplemental Security Income Program Reduce Disability in the Elderly?" *Milbank Quarterly* 86: 5–45.

Hermanson, Bonnie, Gilbert S. Omenn, Richard A. Kronmal, Bernard J. Gersh, and Participants in the Coronary Artery Surgery Study. 1998. "Beneficial Six-Year Outcome of Smoking Cessation in Older Men and Women with Coronary Artery Disease." *New England Journal of Medicine* 319: 1365–69.

Hernandez-Tejada, Melba Alexandra, Ananda B. Amstadter, Wendy Muzzy, and Ron Acierno. 2013. "The National Elder Mistreatment Study: Race and Ethnicity Findings." *Journal of Elder Abuse and Neglect* 25(4): 281–93.

Heron, Melonie. 2016. "Deaths: Leading Causes for 2014." *National Vital Statistics Reports* 65(5, June 30). Hyattsville, Md.: Centers for Disease Control and Prevention, National Center for Health Statistics. https://www.cdc.gov/nchs/data/nvsr/nvsr65/nvsr65_05.pdf (accessed July 7, 2017).

Herring, Stephanie C., Andrew Hoell, Martin P. Hoerling, James P. Kossin, Carl J. Schreck III, and Peter A. Stott. 2016. "Explaining Extreme Events of 2015 from a Climate Perspective." *Bulletin for American Meteorological Society* 97(12). doi: 10.1175/BAMS-ExplainingExtremeEvents2015.1.

Hoffman, Kelly M., Sophie Trawalter, Jordan R. Axt, and M. Norman Oliver. 2016. "Racial Bias in Pain Assessment and Treatment Recommendations, and False Beliefs About Biological Differences Between Blacks and Whites." *Proceedings of the National Academy of Sciences* 113(16): 4296–4301.

Holstein, Martha. 2015. *Women in Late Life: Critical Perspectives on Gender and Age.* Lanham, Md.: Rowman & Littlefield.

Horowitz, Amy, Mark Brennan, Joann P. Reinhardt, and Thalia MacMillan. 2006. "The Impact of Assistive Device Use on Disability and Depression Among Older Adults with Age-Related Vision Impairments." *Journals of Gerontology Series B: Psychological Sciences and Social Sciences* 61(5): S274–80.

House, James S. 2015. *Beyond Obamacare: Life, Death, and Social Policy.* New York: Russell Sage Foundation.

House, James S., Paula M. Lantz, and Pamela Herd. 2005. "Continuity and Change in the Social Stratification of Aging and Health over the Life Course: Evidence from a Nationally Representative Longitudinal Study from 1986 to 2001–2002 (Americans' Changing Lives Study)." *Journals of Gerontology: Series B Psychological Sciences and Social Sciences* 60: S15–26.

Housing Assistance Council. 2014. "Housing an Aging Rural America: Rural Seniors and Their Homes." Washington, D.C.: Housing Assistance Council (October). http://www.ruralhome.org/storage/documents/publications/rrreports/ruralseniors2014.pdf (accessed March 12, 2017).

Hout, Michael, and Erin Cumberworth. 2012. *The Labor Force and the Great Recession.* Stanford, Calif.: Stanford Center on Poverty and Inequality.

Hoynes, Hilary, Doug Miller, and David Simon. 2015. "Income, the Earned Income Tax Credit, and Infant Health." *American Economic Journal: Economic Policy* 7(1): 172–211.

Hoynes, Hilary W., and Diane Whitmore Schanzenbach. 2018. "Safety Net Investments in Children." Working paper 24594. Cambridge, Mass.: National Bureau of Economic Research.

Hoynes, Hilary, Diane Whitmore Schanzenbach, and Douglas Almond. 2016. "Long-Run Impacts of Childhood Access to the Safety Net." *American Economic Review* 106(4): 903–34.

Hughes, Everett Cherrington. 1945. "Dilemmas and Contradictions of Status." *American Journal of Sociology* 50(5): 353–59.

Hughes, Mary Elizabeth, Linda J. Waite, Tracey A. LaPierre, and Ye Luo. 2007. "All in the Family: The Impact of Caring for Grandchildren on Grandparents' Health." *Journals of Gerontology: Series B Psychological Sciences and Social Sciences* 62(2): S108–19.

Human Rights Watch. 2012. "Old Behind Bars: The Aging Prison Population in the United States." New York: Human Rights Watch (January 27). https://www.hrw.org/report/2012/01/27/old-behind-bars/aging-prison-population-united-states (accessed April 22, 2017).

Hummer, Robert A., and Juanita J. Chinn. 2011. "Race/Ethnicity and U.S. Adult Mortality: Progress, Prospects, and New Analyses." *Du Bois Review: Social Science Research on Race* 8(1): 5–24.

Hummer, Robert A., and Elaine M. Hernandez. 2013. "The Effect of Educational Attainment on Adult Mortality in the United States." *Population Bulletin* 68(1): 1–16.

Hunt, Bijou R., Steve Whitman, and Marc S. Hurlbert. 2014. "Increasing Black-White Disparities in Breast Cancer Mortality in the 50 Largest Cities in the United States." *Cancer Epidemiology* 38(2): 118–23.

Hurd, Michael D., and Susann Rohwedder. 2015. "Measuring Economic Preparation for Retirement: Income Versus Consumption." Working paper. Ann Arbor: University of Michigan, Retirement Research Center.

Huynh, Thanh N., Eric C. Kleerup, Joshua F. Wiley, Terrance D. Savitsky, Diana Guse, Bryan J. Garber, and Neil S. Wenger. 2013. "The Frequency and Cost of Treatment Perceived to Be Futile in Critical Care." *Journal of the American Medical Association: Internal Medicine* 173(20): 1887–94.

Iams, Howard, and Christopher R. Tamborini. 2012. "The Implications of Marital History Change on Women's Eligibility for Social Security Wife and Widow Benefits, 1990–2009." *Social Security Bulletin* 72(2): 23–38.

Idler, Ellen L., and Ronald J. Angel. 1990. "Self-Rated Health and Mortality in the NHANES-I Epidemiologic Follow-up Study." *American Journal of Public Health* 80(4): 446–52.

Idler, Ellen L., David A. Boulifard, and Richard J. Contrada. 2012. "Mending

Broken Hearts: Marriage and Survival Following Cardiac Surgery." *Journal of Health and Social Behavior* 53(1): 33–49.

Iezzoni, Lisa I., and Vicki A. Freedman. 2008. "Turning the Disability Tide: The Importance of Definitions." *Journal of the American Medical Association* 299(3): 332–34.

Institute of Medicine. 1997. *Approaching Death: Improving Care at the End of Life.* Washington, D.C.: National Academies Press.

———. 2015. *Dying in America: Improving Quality and Honoring Individual Preferences Near the End of Life.* Washington, D.C.: National Academies Press.

Isaacs, Julia. 2013. "Unemployment from a Child's Perspective." Washington, D.C.: First Focus and Urban Institute (March). https://www.urban.org/research/publication/unemployment-childs-perspective/view/full_report (accessed September 24, 2018).

Jackson, Pamela Braboy, and Quincy Thomas Stewart. 2003. "A Research Agenda for the Black Middle Class: Work Stress, Survival Strategies, and Mental Health." *Journal of Health and Social Behavior* 44(3): 442–55.

Jacobson, Gretchen, Anthony Damico, and Tricia Neuman. 2017. "Medicare Advantage 2018 Data Spotlight: First Look." Issue brief. Menloo Park, Calif.: Henry J. Kaiser Family Foundation (October 13). https://www.kff.org/medicare/issue-brief/medicare-advantage-2018-data-spotlight-first-look/ (accessed September 24, 2018).

Jaffe, In. 2017. "Chicago Neighborhoods Are Trying to Adapt the 'Village Movement' Structure." *National Public Radio*, December 13. https://www.npr.org/2017/12/13/570603485/chicago-neighborhoods-are-trying-to-adapt-the-village-movement-structure (accessed September 21, 2018).

James, Sherman A. 1994. "John Henryism and the Health of African-Americans." *Culture, Medicine, and Psychiatry* 18(2): 163–82.

Janicki-Deverts, Denise, Sheldon Cohen, Karen A. Matthews, Myron D. Gross, and David R. Jacobs Jr. 2009. "Socioeconomic Status, Antioxidant Micronutrients, and Correlates of Oxidative Damage: The Coronary Artery Risk Development in Young Adults (CARDIA) Study." *Psychosomatic Medicine* 71(5): 541–48.

Janssen, Ian, and Amy E. Mark. 2007. "Elevated Body Mass Index and Mortality Risk in the Elderly." *Obesity Reviews* 8(1): 41–59.

Jaquad, Suleika. 2018. "In a California Prison Hospice, Inmates Became Caregivers to Fellow Convicts Who Will Never Make It out Alive." *New York Times*, May 20, 45–56.

Jenkins, J. Lee, Matthew Levy, Lainie Rutkow, and Adam Spira. 2014. "Variables Associated with Effects on Morbidity in Older Adults Following Disasters." *PLoS Currents* (December 5). doi:10.1371/currents.dis.0fe970aa16d51cde6a96 2b7a732e494a.

Jha, Ashish K., Elliott S. Fisher, Zhonghe Li, E. John Orav, and Arnold M. Epstein.

2005. "Racial Trends in the Use of Major Procedures Among the Elderly." *New England Journal of Medicine* 353(7): 683–91.

Jha, Ashish K., E. John Orav, and Arnold M. Epstein. 2011. "Low-Quality, High-Cost Hospitals, Mainly in South, Care for Sharply Higher Shares of Elderly Black, Hispanic, and Medicaid Patients." *Health Affairs* 30(10): 1904–11.

Johnson, Kimberly S. 2013. "Racial and Ethnic Disparities in Palliative Care." *Journal of Palliative Medicine* 16(11): 1329–34.

Johnson, Kimberly S., Maragatha Kuchibhatla, and James A. Tulsky. 2008. "What Explains Racial Differences in the Use of Advance Directives and Attitudes Toward Hospice Care?" *Journal of the American Geriatrics Society* 56(10): 1953–58.

Johnson, Richard W. 2012. "Older Workers, Retirement, and the Great Recession." A Greta Recession Brief. New York and Stanford, Calif.: Russell Sage Foundation and Stanford Center on Poverty and Inequality (October). https://web.stanford.edu/group/recessiontrends-dev/cgi-bin/web/sites/all/themes/barron/pdf/Retirement_fact_sheet.pdf (accessed May 1, 2017).

Johnson, Wendy, Lars Penke, and Frank M. Spinath. 2011. "Heritability in the Era of Molecular Genetics: Some Thoughts for Understanding Genetic Influences on Behavioural Traits." *European Journal of Personality* 25(4): 254–66.

Joint Center for Housing Studies. 2014. "Housing America's Older Adults—Meeting the Needs of an Aging Population." Cambridge, Mass.: Joint Center for Housing Studies of Harvard University. https://www.nado.org/wp-content/uploads/2014/09/Harvard-Housing-Americas-Older-Adults-2014.pdf (accessed April 22, 2017).

Jonas, Daniel E., Yoko Ibuka, and Louise B. Russell. 2011. "How Much Time Do Adults Spend on Health-Related Self-Care? Results from the American Time Use Survey." *Journal of the American Board of Family Medicine* 24(4): 380–90.

Joutsenniemi, Kaisla E., Tuija P. Martelin, Seppo V. Koskinen, Pekka T. Martikainen, Tommi T. Härkänen, Riitta M. Luoto, and Arpo J. Aromaa. 2006. "Official Marital Status, Cohabiting, and Self-Rated Health—Time Trends in Finland, 1978–2001." *European Journal of Public Health* 16(5): 476–83.

Kahneman, Daniel, and Angus Deaton. 2010. "High Income Improves Evaluation of Life but Not Emotional Well-being." *Proceedings of the National Academy of Sciences* 107(38): 16489–93.

Kaiser, Paulina, Ana V. Diez Roux, Mahasin Mujahid, Mercedes Carnethon, Alain Bertoni, Sara D. Adar, Steven Shea, Robyn McClelland, and Lynda Lisabeth. 2016. "Neighborhood Environments and Incident Hypertension in the Multi-Ethnic Study of Atherosclerosis." *American Journal of Epidemiology* 183(11): 988–97.

Kaiser Commission on Medicaid and the Uninsured. 2017. "Key Facts About the Uninsured Population (November 2017)." Menlo Park, Calif.: The Henry J. Kaiser Family Foundation. http://files.kff.org/attachment/Fact-Sheet-Key-Facts-about-the-Uninsured-Population (accessed September 20, 2018).

Karel, Michelle J., Margaret Gatz, and Michael A. Smyer. 2012. "Aging and Mental Health in the Decade Ahead: What Psychologists Need to Know." *American Psychologist* 67(3): 184–98.

Karlamangla, Arun S., Dana Miller-Martinez, Carol S. Aneshensel, Teresa E. Seeman, Richard G. Wight, and Joshua Chodosh. 2009. "Trajectories of Cognitive Function in Late Life in the United States: Demographic and Socioeconomic Predictors." *American Journal of Epidemiology* 170(3): 331–42.

Karlamangla, Arun S., Burton H. Singer, and Teresa E. Seeman. 2006. "Reduction in Allostatic Load in Older Adults Is Associated with Lower All-Cause Mortality Risk: MacArthur Studies of Successful Aging." *Psychosomatic Medicine* 68(3): 500–507.

Katz, Sidney, and C. Amechi Akpom. 1976. "A Measure of Primary Sociobiological Functions." *International Journal of Health Services* 6(3): 493–508.

Kaufman, Gayle, and Glen H. Elder Jr. 2003. "Grandparenting and Age Identity." *Journal of Aging Studies* 17(3): 269–82.

Kaufman, Gayle, and Peter Uhlenberg. 1998. "Effects of Life Course Transitions on the Quality of Relationships Between Adult Children and Their Parents." *Journal of Marriage and the Family* 60(4): 924–38.

Kawachi, Ichiro, Norman Daniels, and Dean E. Robinson. 2005. "Health Disparities by Race and Class: Why Both Matter." *Health Affairs* 24(2): 343–52.

Kelley, Amy S., Partha Deb, Qingling Du, Melissa D. Aldridge Carlson, and R. Sean Morrison. 2013. "Hospice Enrollment Saves Money for Medicare and Improves Care Quality Across a Number of Different Lengths-of-Stay." *Health Affairs* 32(3): 552–61.

Kenen, Joanne. 2017. "Hospice in Crisis: The Most Important End-of-Life Movement in a Generation Struggles in an Era of Changing Families and Prolonged Deaths." *Politico*, September 27. https://www.politico.com/agenda/story/2017/09/27/how-hospice-works-000526 (accessed September 24, 2018).

Kessler, Ronald C., Patricia Berglund, Olga Demler, Robert Jin, Kathleen R. Merikangas, and Ellen E. Walters. 2005. "Lifetime Prevalence and Age-of-Onset Distributions of DSM-IV Disorders in the National Comorbidity Survey Replication." *Archives of General Psychiatry* 62(6): 593–602.

Kessler, Ronald C., Cindy L. Foster, William B. Saunders, and P. E. Stang. 1995. "Social Consequences of Psychiatric Disorders, I: Educational Attainment." *American Journal of Psychiatry* 152(7): 1026–32.

Kessler, Ronald C., Kristen D. Mickelson, and David R. Williams. 1999. "The Prevalence, Distribution, and Mental Health Correlates of Perceived Discrimination in the United States." *Journal of Health and Social Behavior* 40(3): 208–30.

Khera, Amit V., Connor A. Emdin, Isabel Drake, Pradeep Natarajan, Alexander G. Bick, Nancy R. Cook, Daniel I. Chasman, Usman Baber, Roxana Mehran, Daniel J. Rader, Valentin Fuster, Eric Boerwinkle, Olle Melander, Marju Orho-Melander, Paul M Ridker, and Sekar Kathiresan. 2016. "Genetic Risk, Adherence to a Healthy Lifestyle, and Coronary Disease." *New England Journal of Medicine* 375(24): 2349–58.

Kim, Giyeon, David A. Chiriboga, and Yuri Jang. 2009. "Cultural Equivalence in Depressive Symptoms in Older White, Black, and Mexican-American Adults." *Journal of the American Geriatrics Society* 57(5): 790–96.

Kim, Giyeon, Jason M. Parton, Jamie DeCoster, Ami N. Bryant, Katy L. Ford, and Patricia A. Parmelee. 2013. "Regional Variation of Racial Disparities in Mental Health Service Use Among Older Adults." *Gerontologist* 53(4): 618–26.

Kington, Raynard, and James P. Smith. 1997. "Socioeconomic Status and Racial and Ethnic Differences in Functional Status Associated with Chronic Diseases." *American Journal of Public Health* 87(5): 805–10.

Klinenberg, Eric. 2015. *Heat Wave: A Social Autopsy of Disaster in Chicago.* 2nd ed. Chicago: University of Chicago Press.

Kochanek, Kenneth D., Sherry L. Murphy, Jiaquan Xu, and Elizabeth Arias. 2017. "Mortality in the United States, 2016." Data Brief 293. Hyattsville, Md.: Centers for Disease Control and Prevention, National Center for Health Statistics (December). https://www.cdc.gov/nchs/data/databriefs/db293.pdf (accessed September 24, 2018).

Koenig, Harold, Dana King, and Verna B. Carson. 2012. *Handbook of Religion and Health.* New York: Oxford University Press.

Kong, Jooyoung, and Sara M. Moorman. 2015. "Caring for My Abusers: Childhood Maltreatment and Caregiver Depression." *Gerontologist* 55(4): 656–66.

Kontis, Vasilis, James E. Bennett, Colin D. Mathers, Guangquan Li, Kyle Foreman, and Majid Ezzati. 2017. "Future Life Expectancy in 35 Industrialised Countries: Projections with a Bayesian Model Ensemble." *Lancet* 389(10076): 1323–35.

Koropeckyj-Cox, Tanya. 2005. "Singles, Society, and Science: Sociological Perspectives." *Psychological Inquiry* 16(2/3): 91–97.

Kramer, Betty J., and James A. Yonker. 2011. "Perceived Success in Addressing End-of-Life Care Needs of Low-Income Elders and Their Families: What's Family Conflict Got to Do with It?" *Journal of Pain and Symptom Management* 41(1): 35–48.

Krause, Neal. 2006. "Gratitude Toward God, Stress, and Health in Late Life." *Research on Aging* 28(2): 163–83.

Kreider, Rose M., and Renee Ellis. 2011. "Number, Timing, and Duration of Marriages and Divorces: 2009." *Current Population Reports,* P70-125. Washington: U.S. Department of Commerce, U.S. Census Bureau (May). https://www.census.gov/prod/2011pubs/p70-125.pdf (accessed October 3, 2017).

Krieger, Nancy, Jarvis T. Chen, and Pamela D. Waterman. 2010. "Decline in U.S. Breast Cancer Rates After the Women's Health Initiative: Socioeconomic and Racial/Ethnic Differentials." *American Journal of Public Health* 100(April): S132–39.

Kris, Alison E., Emily J. Cherlin, Holly Prigerson, Melissa D. Aldridge Carlson, Rosemary Johnson-Hurzeler, Stanislav V. Kasl, and Elizabeth H. Bradley. 2006. "Length of Hospice Enrollment and Subsequent Depression in Family Caregivers: 13-Month Follow-up Study." *American Journal of Geriatric Psychiatry* 14(3): 264–69.

Kroenke, Kurt, and Robert L. Spitzer. 1998. "Gender Differences in the Reporting of Physical and Somatoform Symptoms." *Psychosomatic Medicine* 60(2): 150–55.

Krugman, Paul. 2015. "Twin Peaks Planet." *New York Times*, January 1. https://www.nytimes.com/2015/01/02/opinion/paul-krugman-twin-peaks-planet.html?_r=0 (accessed October 1, 2017).

Kuh, Diana, and Yoav Ben-Shlomo, eds. 1997. *A Life Course Approach to Chronic Disease Epidemiology*. New York: Oxford University Press.

Kushel, Margot. 2016. "How the Homeless Population Is Changing: It's Older and Sicker." *The Conversation*, January 8. http://theconversation.com/how-the-homeless-population-is-changing-its-older-and-sicker-50632 (accessed February 20, 2017).

Kwan, Elaine, and Chanaka Wijeratne. 2016. "Presentations of Anxiety in Older People." *Medicine Today* 17(12): 34–41.

Lachs, Mark, and Jacquelin Berman. 2011. *Under the Radar: New York State Elder Abuse Prevalence Study*. New York: Lifespan of Greater Rochester, Inc., Weill Cornell Medical Center of Cornell University, and New York City Department for the Aging.

Lachs, Mark S., Jeanne A. Teresi, Mildred Ramirez, Kimberly Van Haitsma, Stephanie Silver, Joseph P. Eimicke, Gabriel Boratgis, et al. 2016. "The Prevalence of Resident-to-Resident Elder Mistreatment in Nursing Homes." *Annals of Internal Medicine* 165(4): 229–36.

Lachs, Mark S., Christianna S. Williams, Shelley O'Brien, Karl A. Pillemer, and Mary E. Charlson. 1998. "The Mortality of Elder Mistreatment." *Journal of the American Medical Association* 280(5): 428–32.

Laditka, James N., and Sarah B. Laditka. 2001. "Adult Children Helping Older Parents: Variations in Likelihood and Hours by Gender, Race, and Family Role." *Research on Aging* 23(4): 429–56.

Langa, Kenneth M., Eric B. Larson, Eileen M. Crimmins, Jessica D. Faul, Deborah A. Levine, Mohammed U. Kabeto, and David R. Weir. 2017. "A Comparison of the Prevalence of Dementia in the United States in 2000 and 2012." *Journal of the American Medical Association: Internal Medicine* 177(1): 51–58.

Langford, Catherine Penny Hinson, Juanita Bowsher, Joseph P. Maloney, and Patricia P. Lillis. 1997. "Social Support: A Conceptual Analysis." *Journal of Advanced Nursing* 25(1): 95–100.

Lantz, Paula M., James S. House, James M. Lepkowski, David R. Williams, Richard P. Mero, and Jieming Chen. 1998. "Socioeconomic Factors, Health Behaviors, and Mortality Results from a Nationally Representative Prospective

Study of U.S. Adults." *Journal of the American Medical Association* 279(21): 1703–8.

La Roche, Julie. 2015. "Warren Buffett: 'Retirement Is Not My Idea of Living.'" *Business Insider,* October 14. http://www.businessinsider.com/why-buffett-says-he-wont-retire-2015-10 (accessed August 22, 2017).

Latham, Kenzie, and Philippa J. Clarke. 2013. "The Role of Neighborhood Safety in Recovery from Mobility Limitations: Findings from a National Sample of Older Americans (1996–2008)." *Research on Aging* 35(4): 481–502.

Latham, Kenzie, and Monica M. Williams. 2015. "Does Neighborhood Disorder Predict Recovery from Mobility Limitation? Findings from the Health and Retirement Study." *Journal of Aging and Health* 27(8): 1415–42.

Leigh, J. Paul, Daniel J. Tancredi, and Richard L. Kravitz. 2009. "Physician Career Satisfaction Within Specialties." *BMC Health Services Research* 9: 166. https://bmchealthservres.biomedcentral.com/articles/10.1186/1472-6963-9-166 (accessed September 9, 2017).

Leland, John. 2008. "In 'Sweetie' and 'Dear,' a Hurt for the Elderly." *New York Times,* October 6. http://www.nytimes.com/2008/10/07/us/07aging.html?_r=0 (accessed September 20, 2016).

Lenzer, Jeanne. 2012. "Unnecessary Care: Are Doctors in Denial and Is Profit Driven Healthcare to Blame?" *British Medical Journal* 345: doi:10.1136/bmj.e6230.

Levenson, Robert W., Laura L. Carstensen, Wallace V. Friesen, and Paul Ekman. 1991. "Emotion, Physiology, and Expression in Old Age." *Psychology and Aging* 6(1): 28–35.

Levy, Becca R., and Mahzarin R. Banaji. 2004. "Implicit Ageism." In *Ageism: Stereotyping and Prejudice Against Older Persons,* edited by Todd D. Nelson. Cambridge, Mass.: MIT Press.

Levy, Daniel, Satish Kenchaiah, Martin G. Larson, Emelia J. Benjamin, Michelle J. Kupka, Kalon K. L. Ho, Joanne M. Murabito, and Ramachandran S. Vasan. 2002. "Long-Term Trends in the Incidence of and Survival with Heart Failure." *New England Journal of Medicine* 347(18): 1397–1402.

Lewis, Joanne M., Michelle DiGiacomo, David C. Currow, and Patricia M. Davidson. 2011. "Dying in the Margins: Understanding Palliative Care and Socioeconomic Deprivation in the Developed World." *Journal of Pain and Symptom Management* 42(1): 105–18.

Li, Yunqing, and Kenneth F. Ferraro. 2005. "Volunteering and Depression in Later Life: Social Benefit or Selection Processes?" *Journal of Health and Social Behavior* 46(1): 68–84.

———. 2006. "Volunteering in Middle and Later Life: Is Health a Benefit, Barrier, or Both?" *Social Forces* 85(1): 497–519.

Lima, Julie C., Susan M. Allen, Frances Goldscheider, and Orna Intrator. 2008. "Spousal Caregiving in Late Midlife Versus Older Ages: Implications of Work and Family Obligations." *Journals of Gerontology Series B: Psychological Sciences and Social Sciences* 63(4): S229–38.

Lin, I-Fen, Susan L. Brown, and Anna M. Hammersmith. 2017. "Marital Biography, Social Security Receipt, and Poverty." *Research on Aging* 39(1): 86–110.

Lin, I-Fen, Holly R. Fee, and Hsueh-Sheng Wu. 2012. "Negative and Positive Caregiving Experiences: A Closer Look at the Intersection of Gender and Relationship." *Family Relations* 61(2): 343–58.

Lines, Lisa M., and Joshua M. Wiener. 2014. "Racial and Ethnic Disparities in Alzheimer's Disease: A Literature Review." Washington: U.S. Department of Health and Human Services, Office of the Assistant Secretary for Planning and Evaluation, Office of Disability, Aging, and Long-Term Care Policy (February).

Link, Bruce G., and Jo Phelan. 1995. "Social Conditions as Fundamental Causes of Disease." *Journal of Health and Social Behavior* 35: 80–94.

Livingston, Gretchen, Kim Parker, and Molly Rohal. 2014. "Four-in-Ten Couples Are Saying 'I Do,' Again: Growing Number of Adults Have Remarried." Washington, D.C.: Pew Research Center.

Lofton, Kara Leigh. 2016. "West Virginia Struggles with Shortage of Geriatric Physicians." *West Virginia Public Radio*, May 5. http://wvpublic.org/post/west-virginia-struggles-shortage-geriatric-physicians#stream/0 (accessed October 2, 2017).

Loggers, Elizabeth Trice, Paul K. Maciejewski, Elizabeth Paulk, Susan DeSanto-Madeva, Matthew Nilsson, Kasisomayajula Viswanath, Alexi Anne Wright, Tracy A. Balboni, Jennifer Temel, Heather Stieglitz, Susan Block, and Holly G. Prigerson. 2009. "Racial Differences in Predictors of Intensive End-of-Life Care in Advanced Cancer Patients." *Journal of Clinical Oncology* 27(33): 5559–64.

Long, Michelle, Matthew Rae, Gary Claxton, and Anthony Damico. 2016. "Trends in Employer-Sponsored Insurance Offer and Coverage Rates, 1999–2014." Issue brief. Menlo Park, Calif.: Henry J. Kaiser Family Foundation (March). http://files.kff.org/attachment/issue-brief-trends-in-employer-sponsored-insurance-offer-and-coverage-rates-1999-2014-2 (accessed October 5, 2017).

Luhmann, Maike, and Louise C. Hawkley. 2016. "Age Differences in Loneliness: From Late Adolescence to Oldest Old Age." *Developmental Psychology* 52(6): 943–59.

Lumsdaine, Robin L., and Stephanie J. C. Vermeer. 2015. "Retirement Timing of Women and the Role of Care Responsibilities for Grandchildren." *Demography* 52(2): 433–54.

Lunney, June R., Joanne Lynn, and Christopher Hogan. 2002. "Profiles of Older Medicare Decedents." *Journal of the American Geriatrics Society* 50(6): 1108–12.

Luth, Elizabeth. 2017. "A Case for Death as Equalizer: Fundamental Causes as

Non-Predictors of Multidimensional End-of-Life Care Quality." Ph.D. diss., Rutgers University, New Brunswick, N.J.

Luthra, Shefali. 2016. "Fueled by Health Law, 'Concierge Medicine' Reaches New Markets." *Kaiser Health News*, January 14. https://khn.org/news/fueled-by-health-law-concierge-medicine-reaches-new-markets/ (accessed September 21, 2018).

Lye, Diane N. 1996. "Adult Child–Parent Relationships." *Annual Review of Sociology* 22(August): 79–102.

MacLean, Alair, and Glen H. Elder Jr. 2007. "Military Service in the Life Course." *Annual Review of Sociology* 33: 175–96.

Magee, William, and Patricia Louie. 2016. "Did the Difference Between Black and White Americans in Anger-Out Decrease During the First Decade of the Twenty-First Century?" *Race and Social Problems* 8(3): 256–70.

Malloy-Weir, Leslie J., Cathy Charles, Amiram Gafni, and Vikki A. Entwistle. 2015. "Empirical Relationships Between Health Literacy and Treatment Decision Making: A Scoping Review of the Literature." *Patient Education and Counseling* 98(3): 296–309.

Mandelblatt, Jeanne S., Vanessa B. Sheppard, and Alfred I. Neugut. 2013. "Black-White Differences in Breast Cancer Outcomes Among Older Medicare Beneficiaries Does Systemic Treatment Matter?" *Journal of the American Medical Association* 310: 376–77.

Maniam, Shiva, and Samantha Smith. 2017. "A Wider Partisan and Ideological Gap Between Younger, Older Generations." Washington, D.C.: Pew Research Center (March 20). http://www.pewresearch.org/fact-tank/2017/03/20/a-wider-partisan-and-ideological-gap-between-younger-older-generations/ (accessed October 3, 2017).

Manning, Wendy D., and Susan L. Brown. 2011. "The Demography of Unions Among Older Americans, 1980–Present: A Family Change Approach." In *Handbook of Sociology of Aging*, edited by Richard A. Settersten Jr. and Jacqueline L. Angel. New York: Springer.

Manton, Kenneth G., XiLiang Gu, and Gene R. Lowrimore. 2008. "Cohort Changes in Active Life Expectancy in the U.S. Elderly Population: Experience from the 1982–2004 National Long-Term Care Survey." *Journals of Gerontology Series B: Psychological Sciences and Social Sciences* 63(5): S269–81.

Marans, David. 2017. "Senate Democrats Introduce Bill Allowing Medicare Buy-In at 55." *Huffington Post*, August 4. http://www.huffingtonpost.com/entry/democrats-medicare-expansion_us_598491c6e4b041356ebf7569 (accessed September 24, 2017).

Marmot, Michael. 2005. "Social Determinants of Health Inequalities." *Lancet* 365: 1099–1104.

———. 2006. "Status Syndrome: A Challenge to Medicine." *Journal of the American Medical Association* 295(11): 1304–7.

Marshall Project. 2018. "Old, Sick, and Dying in Shackles." New York: Marshall

Project (March 7). https://www.themarshallproject.org/2018/03/07/old-sick-and-dying-in-shackles (accessed June 1, 2018).

Martikainen, Pekka T., and Tapani Valkonen. 1996. "Mortality After the Death of a Spouse: Rates and Causes of Death in a Large Finnish Cohort." *American Journal of Public Health* 86(8): 1087–93.

Martin, Erika, and Mary Beth McDade. 2017. "Long Beach Police Search for Leads in Series of Robberies, Sexual Assault at Senior Housing Complex." *KTLA5*, February 8. http://ktla.com/2017/02/08/long-beach-police-search-for-leads-in-series-of-robberies-sexual-assault-at-senior-housing-complex/ (accessed March 13, 2017).

Mather, Mara. 2012. "The Emotion Paradox in the Aging Brain." *Annals of the New York Academy of Sciences* 1251(1): 33–49.

Mather, Mark, Linda A. Jacobsen, and Kelvin M. Pollard. 2015. "Aging in the United States." *Population Bulletin* 70(2): 1–21.

Mathews, T. J., and Marian F. MacDorman. 2013. "Infant Mortality Statistics from the 2010 Period Linked Birth/Infant Death Data Set." *National Vital Statistics Reports* 62(8). Hyattsville, Md.: Centers for Disease Control and Prevention, National Center for Health Statistics (December 18). https://www.cdc.gov/nchs/data/nvsr/nvsr62/nvsr62_08.pdf (accessed September 24, 2018).

McCurry, Justin. 2018. "'Dementia Towns': How Japan Is Evolving for Its Ageing Population." *Guardian*, January 14. https://www.theguardian.com/world/2018/jan/15/dementia-towns-japan-ageing-population (accessed August 7, 2018).

McPherson, Christine J., and Julia M. Addington-Hall. 2003. "Judging the Quality of Care at the End of Life: Can Proxies Provide Reliable Information?" *Social Science and Medicine* 56(1): 95–109.

McPherson, Christine J., Keith G. Wilson, Michelle M. Lobchuk, and Susan Brajtman. 2007. "Self-Perceived Burden to Others: Patient and Family Caregiver Correlates." *Journal of Palliative Care* 23(3): 135–42.

Meals on Wheels Association of America (MOWAA). 2016. "Meals on Wheels Annual Report." Washington, D.C.: MOWAA. https://www.mowp.org/wp-content/uploads/MOWP_2016-annual-report-final-rev4.pdf (accessed September 24, 2018).

Mechanic, David, and Donna D. McAlpine. 2011. "Mental Health and Aging: A Life-Course Perspective." In *Handbook of Sociology of Aging*, edited by Richard A. Settersten Jr. and Jacqueline L. Angel. New York: Springer.

Medicare Payment Advisory Commission (MedPAC). 2017. "Hospice Services." Chapter 12 in *Report to the Congress: Medicare Payment Policy*. Washington, D.C.: MedPAC (March). http://www.medpac.gov/docs/default-source/reports/mar18_medpac_entirereport_sec.pdf (accessed September 24, 2018).

Meghani, Salimah H., Eeeseung Byun, and Rollin M. Gallagher. 2012. "Time to Take Stock: A Meta-analysis and Systematic Review of Analgesic Treatment Disparities for Pain in the United States." *Pain Medicine* 13(2): 150–74.

Meier, Diane E. 2010. "The Development, Status, and Future of Palliative Care." In *Palliative Care: Transforming the Care of Serious Illness*, edited by Diane E. Meier, Stephen L. Isaacs, and Robert Hughes. San Francisco: Jossey-Bass.

Mendes de Leon, Carlos F., Thomas A. Glass, and Lisa F. Berkman. 2003. "Social Engagement and Disability in a Community Population of Older Adults: The New Haven EPESE." *American Journal of Epidemiology* 157(7): 633–42.

Mendez-Luck, Carolyn A., and Katherine P. Anthony. 2016. "*Marianismo* and Caregiving Role Beliefs Among U.S.-Born and Immigrant Mexican Women." *Journals of Gerontology Series B: Psychological Sciences and Social Sciences* 71(5): 926–35.

Merrick, Elizabeth L., Constance M. Horgan, Dominic Hodgkin, Deborah W. Garnick, Susan F. Houghton, Lee Panas, Richard Saitz, and Frederic C. Blow. 2008. "Unhealthy Drinking Patterns in Older Adults: Prevalence and Associated Characteristics." *Journal of the American Geriatrics Society* 56(2): 214–23.

Merton, Robert K. 1968. "The Matthew Effect in Science." *Science* 159(3810): 56–63.

MetLife Mature Market Institute. 2011. "The MetLife Study of Elder Financial Abuse: Crimes of Occasion, Desperation, and Predation Against America's Elders." New York: MetLife (June). https://ltcombudsman.org/uploads/files/issues/mmi-elder-financial-abuse.pdf (accessed September 24, 2018).

Meyer, Ilan H. 1995. "Minority Stress and Mental Health in Gay Men." *Journal of Health and Social Behavior* 36(1): 38–56.

Miller, Baila, and Lynda Cafasso. 1992. "Gender Differences in Caregiving: Fact or Artifact?" *Gerontologist* 32(4): 498–507.

Miller, Nancy A. 2011. "Relations Among Home- and Community-Based Services Investment and Nursing Home Rates of Use for Working-Age and Older Adults: A State-Level Analysis." *American Journal of Public Health* 101(9): 1735–41.

Mills, C. Wright. 1959. *The Sociological Imagination*. New York: Oxford University Press.

Mitchell, Susan L., Vincent Mor, Pedro L. Gozalo, Joseph L. Servadio, and Joan M. Teno. 2016. "Tube Feeding in U.S. Nursing Home Residents with Advanced Dementia, 2000–2014." *Journal of the American Medical Association* 316(7): 769–70.

Moen, Phyllis. 2016. *Encore Adulthood: Boomers on the Edge of Risk, Renewal, and Purpose*. New York: Oxford University Press

Mojtabai, Ramin. 2009. "Unmet Need for Treatment of Major Depression in the United States." *Psychiatric Services* 60(3): 297–305.

Molinari, Victor A., Lisa M. Brown, Kathryn A. Frahm, John A. Schinka, and Roger Casey. 2013. "Perceptions of Homelessness in Older Homeless Veterans, VA Homeless Program Staff Liaisons, and Housing Intervention Providers." *Journal of Health Care for the Poor and Underserved* 24(2): 487–98.

Montez, Jennifer Karas, Mark D. Hayward, and Douglas A. Wolf. 2017. "Do U.S.

States' Socioeconomic and Policy Contexts Shape Adult Disability?" *Social Science and Medicine* 178: 115–26.

Montez, Jennifer Karas, Anna Zajacova, and Mark D. Hayward. 2016. "Explaining Inequalities in Women's Mortality Between U.S. States." *SSM: Population Health* 2(December): 561–71.

Moodie, Susanna. [1853] 2010. *Life in the Clearings Versus the Bush*. Toronto: New Canadian Library.

Moorman, Sara M. 2011. "Older Adults' Preferences for Independent or Delegated End-of-Life Medical Decision-Making." *Journal of Aging and Health* 23(1): 135–57.

Moorman, Sara M., and Deborah Carr. 2008. "Spouses' Effectiveness as End-of-Life Health Care Surrogates: Accuracy, Uncertainty, and Errors of Overtreatment or Undertreatment." *Gerontologist* 48(6): 811–19.

Moorman, Sara M., and Megumi Inoue. 2013. "Predicting a Partner's End-of-Life Preferences, or Substituting One's Own?" *Journal of Marriage and Family* 75(3): 734–45.

Moorman, Sara M., and Cameron Macdonald. 2012. "Medically Complex Home Care and Caregiver Strain." *Gerontologist* 53(3): 407–17.

Moorman, Sara M., Jeffrey E. Stokes, and Jeremiah C. Morelock. 2016. "Mechanisms Linking Neighborhood Age Composition to Health." *Gerontologist* 57(4): 667–78.

Mora, Pablo A., Gabriela Orsak, Marco D. DiBonaventura, and Elaine A. Leventhal. 2013. "Why Do Comparative Assessments Predict Health? The Role of Self-Assessed Health in the Formation of Comparative Health Judgments." *Health Psychology* 32(11): 1175–78.

Morgan, Rachel E., and Britney J. Mason. 2014. "Crimes Against the Elderly, 2003–2013." NCJ 248339. Washington: U.S. Department of Justice, Bureau of Justice Statistics (November). https://www.bjs.gov/content/pub/pdf/cae0313.pdf (accessed March 13, 2017).

Morrison, R. Sean, Sylvan Wallenstein, Dana K. Natale, Richard S. Senzel, and Lo-Li Huang. 2000. "'We Don't Carry That'—Failure of Pharmacies in Predominantly Nonwhite Neighborhoods to Stock Opioid Analgesics." *New England Journal of Medicine* 342(14): 1023–26.

Mouzon, Dawne M. 2013. "Can Family Relationships Explain the Race Paradox in Mental Health?" *Journal of Marriage and Family* 75(2): 470–85.

Musich, Shirley, Shaohung S. Wang, Kevin Hawkins, and Charlotte S. Yeh. 2015. "Homebound Older Adults: Prevalence, Characteristics, Health Care Utilization and Quality of Care." *Geriatric Nursing* 36(6): 445–50.

Mutchler, Jan E., and Ceara R. Somerville. 2016. "Gender, Race, and Ethnicity and the Life Course." In *Gerontology: Changes, Challenges, and Solutions*, edited by Madonna Harrington Meyer and Elizabeth A. Daniele. Santa Barbara, Calif.: Praeger Publishers.

Nápoles, Anna M., Letha Chadiha, Rani Eversley, and Gina Moreno-John. 2010.

"Developing Culturally Sensitive Dementia Caregiver Interventions: Are We There Yet?" *American Journal of Alzheimer's Disease and Other Dementias* 25(5): 398–406.

National Academy of Science. 2016. *Relieving Pain in America: A Blueprint for Transforming Prevention, Care, Education, and Research.* Washington, D.C.: National Academies Press.

National Academies of Sciences, Engineering, and Medicine. 2015. *The Growing Gap in Life Expectancy by Income: Implications for Federal Programs and Policy Responses.* Washington, D.C.: National Academies Press.

———. 2016. *Families Caring for an Aging America.* Washington, D.C.: National Academies Press.

———. 2017. *Pain Management and the Opioid Epidemic: Balancing Societal and Individual Benefits and Risks of Prescription Opioid Use.* Washington, D.C.: National Academies Press.

National Alliance for Caregiving and American Association of Retired Persons (AARP). 2015. "Caregiving in the U.S. 2015." Washington, D.C.: National Alliance for Caregiving in collaboration with AARP (November). https://www.caregiving.org/caregiving2015/ (accessed October 22, 2016).

National Center for Health Statistics (NCHS). 2011. *Health, United States, 2010: With Special Feature on Death and Dying.* Hyattsville, Md.: Centers for Disease Control and Prevention, NCHS.

———. 2016. *Health, United States, 2015: With Special Feature on Racial and Ethnic Health Disparities.* Hyattsville, Md.: Centers for Disease Control and Prevention, NCHS.

———. 2017. "LCWK1. Deaths, Percent of Total Deaths, and Death Rates for the 15 Leading Causes of Death in 5-Year Age Groups, by Race and Sex: United States, 2015." In *National Vital Statistics System: Mortality 2015* (September 29). https://www.cdc.gov/nchs/data/dvs/LCWK1_2015.pdf (accessed September 24, 2018).

National Council on Aging. 2015. "2015 Results: The United States of Aging Survey." https://www.ncoa.org/news/resources-for-reporters/usoa-survey/2015-results/ (accessed September 27, 2016).

National Hospice and Palliative Care Organization (NHPCO). 2010. *Standards of Practice for Hospice Programs.* Alexandria, Va.: NHPCO.

———. 2012. "NHPCO Facts and Figures: Hospice Care in America." Washington, D.C.: NHPCO.

———. 2015. "NHPCO Facts and Figures: Hospice Care in America." Washington, D.C.: NHPCO.

———. 2016. "NHPCO Facts and Figures: Hospice Care in America." Washington, D.C.: NHPCO.

National Institute on Alcohol Abuse and Addiction. 2010. "Older Adults." https://www.niaaa.nih.gov/alcohol-health/special-populations-co-occurring-disorders/older-adults (accessed September 20, 2018).

National Institute on Drug Abuse (NIDA). 2018. "Overdose Death Rates." Washington, D.C.: NIDA (updated 2018). https://www.drugabuse.gov/related-topics/trends-statistics/overdose-death-rates (accessed July 1, 2017).

National Institutes of Health (NIH). 2016. "Rates of Nonmedical Prescription Opioid Use and Opioid Use Disorder Double in 10 Years." Washington, D.C.: NIH (June 22). https://www.nih.gov/news-events/rates-nonmedical-prescription-opioid-use-opioid-use-disorder-double-10-years (accessed June 22, 2016).

National Opinion Research Center (NORC) and the Associated Press. 2015. "Long-Term Care in America: Americans' Outlook and Planning for Future Care." Chicago: Associated Press and NORC at the University of Chicago (July). https://www.longtermcarepoll.org/wp-content/uploads/2017/11/AP-NORC-Long-term-Care-2015_Trend_Report.pdf (accessed September 24, 2018).

National Research Council. 2004. Measuring Racial Discrimination. Washington, D.C.: The National Academies Press.

———. 2011a. Explaining Divergent Levels of Longevity in High-Income Countries. Washington, D.C.: National Academies Press.

———. 2011b. *Health Care Comes Home: The Human Factors.* Washington, D.C.: National Academies Press.

———. 2013. *New Directions in the Sociology of Aging.* Washington, D.C.: National Research Council of the National Academies.

National Resident Matching Program (NRMP). 2018. "Results and Data: Specialties Matching Service: 2018 Appointment Year." Washington, D.C.: NRMP. http://www.nrmp.org/wp-content/uploads/2018/02/Results-and-Data-SMS-2018.pdf (accessed September 24, 2018).

Needham, Belinda L., Nancy Adler, Steven Gregorich, David Rehkopf, Jue Lin, Elizabeth H. Blackburn, and Elissa S. Epel. 2013. "Socioeconomic Status, Health Behavior, and Leukocyte Telomere Length in the National Health and Nutrition Examination Survey, 1999–2002." *Social Science and Medicine* 85(May): 1–8.

Needham, Belinda L., Jose R. Fernandez, Jue Lin, Elissa S. Epel, and Elizabeth H. Blackburn. 2012. "Socioeconomic Status and Cell Aging in Children." *Social Science and Medicine* 74(12): 1948–51.

Neikrug, Ariel B., and Sonia Ancoli-Israel. 2009. "Sleep Disorders in the Older Adult: A Mini-Review." *Gerontology* 56(2): 181–89.

Nelson, Lorene M., W. T. Longstreth, Thomas D. Koepsell, and Gerald Van Belle. 1990. "Proxy Respondents in Epidemiologic Research." *Epidemiologic Reviews* 12(1): 71–86.

Nelson, Todd D. 2005. "Ageism: Prejudice Against Our Feared Future Self." *Journal of Social Issues* 61(2): 207–21.

Neumark, David, Ian Burn, and Patrick Button. 2017. "Age Discrimination and

Hiring of Older Workers." Working Paper 21669. Cambridge, Mass.: National Bureau of Economic Research.

Newport, Frank, and Joy Wilke. 2013. "Most in U.S. Want Marriage, but Its Importance Has Dropped." *Gallup*, August 2. http://www.gallup.com/poll/163802/marriage-importance-dropped.aspx (accessed March 25, 2017).

Newsweek. 1946. "Books vs. Babies." *Newsweek*, January 14, p. 79.

New York Times. 2012. "Mapping Hurricane Sandy's Deadly Toll." *New York Times*, November 17. http://www.nytimes.com/interactive/2012/11/17/nyregion/hurricane-sandy-map.html?_r=0 (accessed February 10, 2017).

Nicholas, Lauren Hersch, Kenneth M. Langa, Theodore J. Iwashyna, and David R. Weir. 2011. "Regional Variation in the Association Between Advance Directives and End-of-Life Medicare Expenditures." *Journal of the American Medical Association* 306(13): 1447–53.

Noah, Timothy. 2012. *The Great Divergence: America's Growing Inequality Crisis and What We Can Do About It*. New York: Bloomsbury Publishing USA.

Noël-Miller, Claire M. 2011. "Partner Caregiving in Older Cohabiting Couples." *Journals of Gerontology Series B: Psychological Sciences and Social Sciences* 66B(3): 341–53.

———. 2013. "Repartnering Following Divorce: Implications for Older Fathers' Relations with Their Adult Children." *Journal of Marriage and Family* 75(3): 697–712.

North, Michael S., and Susan T. Fiske. 2013. "Act Your (Old) Age: Prescriptive, Ageist Biases over Succession, Consumption, and Identity." *Personality and Social Psychology Bulletin* 39(6): 720–34.

Northcutt, Wendy. 2008. *The Darwin Awards Next Evolution: Chlorinating the Gene Pool*. New York: Penguin.

Noymer, Andrew, Andrew M. Penner, and Aliya Saperstein. 2011. "Cause of Death Affects Racial Classification on Death Certificates." *PLoS One* (January 26). doi:10.1371/journal.pone.0015812.

Nusselder, Wilma J., Marcel T. Slockers, Luuk Krol, Colette T. Slockers, Caspar W. N. Looman, and Ed F. van Beeck. 2013. "Mortality and Life Expectancy in Homeless Men and Women in Rotterdam: 2001–2010." *PLoS One* 8(1): e73979.

Nyce, Steven A., and Sylvester J. Schieber. 2005. *The Economic Implications of Aging Societies: The Costs of Living Happily Ever After*. New York: Cambridge University Press.

O'Rand, Angela M. 1996. "The Precious and the Precocious: Understanding Cumulative Disadvantage and Cumulative Advantage over the Life Course." *Gerontologist* 36(2): 230–38.

Olivero, Magaly. 2015. "Doctor Shortage: Who Will Take Care of the Elderly?" *U.S. News & World Report*, April 21. https://health.usnews.com/health-news/patient-advice/articles/2015/04/21/doctor-shortage-who-will-take-care-of-the-elderly (accessed October 8, 2017).

Olshansky, S. Jay, and A. Brian Ault. 1986. "The Fourth Stage of the Epidemiologic Transition: The Age of Delayed Degenerative Diseases." *Milbank Quarterly* 64(3): 355–91.

Omran, Abdel R. 1971. "The Epidemiologic Transition: A Theory of the Epidemiology of Population Change." *Milbank Memorial Fund Quarterly* 49(4): 509–38.

Organization for Economic Cooperation and Development (OECD). 2011. "Compendium of OECD Well-being Indicators." http://www.oecd.org/sdd/47917288.pdf (accessed May 24, 2018).

Ornstein, Charles, and Jessica Huseman. 2016. "Federal Officials Seek to Stop Social Media Abuse of Nursing Home Residents." *Shots: Health News from NPR*, August 8. http://www.npr.org/sections/health-shots/2016/08/08/489195484/federal-officials-seek-to-stop-social-media-abuse-of-nursing-home-residents (accessed March 25, 2017).

Ornstein, Katherine A., Bruce Leff, Kenneth E. Covinsky, Christine S. Ritchie, Alex D. Federman, Laken Roberts, Amy S. Kelley, Albert L. Siu, and Sarah L. Szanton. 2015. "Epidemiology of the Homebound Population in the United States." *JAMA Internal Medicine* 175(7): 1180–86.

Osterman, Paul. 2017. *Who Will Care for Us? Long-Term Care and the Long-Term Workforce.* New York: Russell Sage Foundation.

Palmore, Erdman. 2005. "Three Decades of Research on Ageism." *Generations* 29(3): 87–90.

Pampel, Fred C., Patrick M. Krueger, and Justin T. Denney. 2010. "Socioeconomic Disparities in Health Behaviors." *Annual Review of Sociology* 36: 349–70.

Pan, Liping, Heidi M. Blanck, Bettylou Sherry, Karen Dalenius, and Laurence M. Grummer-Strawn. 2012. "Trends in the Prevalence of Extreme Obesity Among U.S. Preschool-Aged Children Living in Low-Income Families, 1998–2010." *Journal of the American Medical Association* 308(24): 2563–65.

Papanicolas Irene, Liana R. Woskie, and Ashish K. Jha. 2018. "Health Care Spending in the United States and Other High-Income Countries." *Journal of the American Medical Association* 319(10): 1024–39. doi:10.1001/jama.2018.1150.

Pasupathi, Monisha, and Corinna E. Löckenhoff. 2002. "Ageist Behavior." In *Ageism: Stereotyping and Prejudice Against Older Persons*, edited by Todd D. Nelson. Cambridge, Mass.: MIT Press.

Patel, Kushang V., Jack M. Guralnik, Elizabeth J. Dansie, and Dennis C. Turk. 2013. "Prevalence and Impact of Pain Among Older Adults in the United States: Findings from the 2011 National Health and Aging Trends Study." *Pain* 154(12): 2649–57.

Pavalko, Eliza K., and Glen H. Elder Jr. 1990. "World War II and Divorce: A Life-Course Perspective." *American Journal of Sociology* 95(5): 1213–34.

Pearlin, Leonard I., Scott Schieman, Elena M. Fazio, and Stephen C. Meersman. 2005. "Stress, Health, and the Life Course: Some Conceptual Perspectives." *Journal of Health and Social Behavior* 46(2): 205–19.

Pearlin, Leonard I., and Carmi Schooler. 1978. "The Structure of Coping." *Journal of Health and Social Behavior* 19(1): 2–21.
Perelli-Harris, Brienna, and Nora Sánchez Gassen. 2012. "How Similar Are Cohabitation and Marriage? Legal Approaches to Cohabitation Across Western Europe." *Population and Development Review* 38(3): 435–67.
Perkins, Martinique, Virginia J. Howard, Virginia G. Wadley, Michael Crowe, Monika M. Safford, William E. Haley, George Howard, and David L. Roth. 2013. "Caregiving Strain and All-Cause Mortality: Evidence from the REGARDS Study." *Journals of Gerontology Series B: Psychological Sciences and Social Sciences* 68(4): 504–12.
Petrolia, Daniel R., and Sanjoy Bhattacharjee. 2010. "Why Don't Coastal Residents Choose to Evacuate for Hurricanes?" *Coastal Management* 38(2): 97–112.
Pew Research Center. 2010. "A Balance Sheet at 30 Months: How the Great Recession Has Changed Life in America." Washington, D.C.: Pew Research Center (June 30). http://www.pewsocialtrends.org/2010/06/30/how-the-great-recession-has-changed-life-in-america/ (accessed October 1, 2017).
———. 2011. "Fighting Poverty in a Tough Economy, Americans Move in with Their Relatives." Social & Demographic Trends. Washington, D.C.: Pew Research Center (October 3). http://assets.pewresearch.org/wp-content/uploads/sites/3/2011/10/Multigenerational-Households-Final1.pdf (accessed September 24, 2018).
———. 2013. "Views on End-of-Life Medical Treatments." Washington, D.C.: Pew Research Center (November 21). http://www.pewforum.org/files/2013/11/end-of-life-survey-report-full-pdf.pdf (accessed November 25, 2014).
———. 2015. "Family Support in Graying Societies: How Americans, Germans, and Italians Are Coping with an Aging Population." Social & Demographic Trends Project. Washington, D.C.: Pew Research Center (May 21). http://www.pewsocialtrends.org/2015/05/21/family-support-in-graying-societies/ (accessed May 31, 2017).
Pham, Sheriesse. 2011. "Government Report Finds Elder Abuse on the Rise." *New York Times,* March 3. http://newoldage.blogs.nytimes.com/2011/03/03/government-report-finds-elder-abuse-on-the-rise/ (accessed September 18, 2016).
Phelan, Jo C., Bruce G. Link, and Parisa Tehranifar. 2010. "Social Conditions as Fundamental Causes of Health Inequalities Theory, Evidence, and Policy Implications." *Journal of Health and Social Behavior* 51: S28–40.
Piketty, Thomas. 2014. *Capital in the Twenty-First Century.* Cambridge, Mass.: Harvard University Press.
Pillemer, Karl, Marie-Therese Connolly, Risa Breckman, Nathan Spreng, and Mark S. Lachs. 2015. "Elder Mistreatment: Priorities for Consideration by the White House Conference on Aging." *Gerontologist* 55(2): 320–27.
Pinquart, Martin, and Silvia Sörensen. 2005. "Ethnic Differences in Stressors,

Resources, and Psychological Outcomes of Family Caregiving: A Meta-analysis." *Gerontologist* 45(1): 90–106.

Poon, Leonard W., Gloria M. Clayton, Peter Martin, Mary Ann Johnson, Bradley C. Courtenay, Anne L. Sweaney, Sharan B. Merriam, Betsy S. Pless, and Samuel B. Thielman. 1992. "The Georgia Centenarian Study." *International Journal of Aging and Human Development* 34(1): 1–17.

Preston, Samuel H., Yana C. Vierboom, and Andrew Stokes. 2018. "The Role of Obesity in Exceptionally Slow U.S. Mortality Improvement." *Proceedings of the National Academy of Sciences of the United States of America* 115(5): 957–61.

Price, Rebecca Anhang, Layla Parast, Ann Haas, Joan M. Teno, and Marc N. Elliott. 2017. "Black and Hispanic Patients Receive Hospice Care Similar to That of White Patients When in the Same Hospices." *Health Affairs* 36(7): 1283–90.

Proulx, Jeffrey, and Carolyn M. Aldwin. 2016. "Effects of Coping on Psychological and Physical Health." In *The Encyclopedia of Adulthood and Aging*, edited by Susan Krauss Whitbourne. West Sussex, U.K.: John Wiley & Sons.

Pudrovska, Tetyana, Scott Schieman, and Deborah Carr. 2006. "Strains of Singlehood in Later Life: Do Race and Gender Matter?" *Journals of Gerontology Series B: Psychological Sciences and Social Sciences* 61(6): S315–22.

Quadagno, Jill, and Jennifer Reid. 1999. "The Political Economy Perspective in Aging." In *Handbook of Theories of Aging*, edited by Vern L. Bengtson and K. Warner Schaie. New York: Springer Publishing Co.

Quinn, Brian C. 2011. "State-Level Health Policy Research: Looking Back, Looking Ahead." *Health Services Research* 46(1p2): 243–45.

Radloff, Lenore Sawyer. 1977. "The CES-D Scale: A Self-Report Depression Scale for Research in the General Population." *Applied Psychological Measurement* 1(3): 385–401.

Rainie, Lee, and Barry Wellman. 2012. *Networked: The New Social Operating System*. Cambridge, Mass.: MIT Press.

Raley, R. Kelly, Megan M. Sweeney, and Danielle Wondra. 2015. "The Growing Racial and Ethnic Divide in U.S. Marriage Patterns." *The Future of Children* 25(2): 89–109.

Rau, Jordan. 2017. "Medicaid Cuts May Force Retirees Out of Nursing Homes." *New York Times*, June 24.

Ray, Kristen N., Amalavoyal V. Chari, John Barker Engberg, Marianne Bertolet, and Ateev Mehrotra. 2015. "Disparities in Time Spent Seeking Medical Care in the United States." *Journal of the American Medical Association: Internal Medicine* 175(12):1983–86.

Read, Jen'nan Ghazal, and Bridget K. Gorman. 2010. "Gender and Health Inequality." *Annual Review of Sociology* 36: 371–86.

Reaves, Erica L., and MaryBeth Musumeci. 2015. "Medicaid and Long-Term Services and Supports: A Primer." Menlo Park, Calif.: Henry J. Kaiser Family Foundation (December). http://files.kff.org/attachment/report-medicaid-and-long-term-services-and-supports-a-primer (accessed August 5, 2018).

Redfoot, Donald, Lynn Feinberg, and Ari Houser. 2013. "The Aging of the Baby Boom and the Growing Care Gap: A Look at Future Declines in the Availability of Family Caregiver." Washington, D.C.: AARP Public Policy Institute.

Rehnberg, Johan, and Johan Fritzell. 2016. "The Shape of the Association Between Income and Mortality in Old Age: A Longitudinal Swedish National Register Study." *Social Science and Medicine: Population Health* 2: 750–56.

Renwick, Trudi, and Liana Fox. 2016. "The Supplemental Poverty Measure: 2015." *Current Population Reports*, P60-258. Washington: U.S. Department of Commerce, U.S. Census Bureau (September). https://www.census.gov/content/dam/Census/library/publications/2016/demo/p60-258.pdf (accessed September 21, 2018).

Rexbye, Helle, Inge Petersen, Mette Johansens, Louise Klitkou, Bernard Jeune, and Kaare Christensen. 2006. "Influence of Environmental Factors on Facial Ageing." *Age and Ageing* 35(2): 110–15.

Reynolds, Kristin, Robert H. Pietrzak, Renée El-Gabalawy, Corey S. Mackenzie, and Jitender Sareen. 2015. "Prevalence of Psychiatric Disorders in U.S. Older Adults: Findings from a Nationally Representative Survey." *World Psychiatry* 14(1): 74–81.

Rhee, Nari. 2013. *Race and Retirement Insecurity in the United States*. Washington, D.C.: National Institute on Retirement Security.

Rhodes, Ramona, and Joan M. Teno. 2009. "What's Race Got to Do with It?" *Journal of Clinical Oncology* 27(33): 5496–98.

Rhodes, Ramona L., Joan M. Teno, and Lisa C. Welch. 2006. "Access to Hospice for African Americans: Are They Informed About the Option of Hospice?" *Journal of Palliative Medicine* 9(2): 268–72.

Richardson, Todd J., Soo J. Lee, Marla Berg-Weger, and George T. Grossberg. 2013. "Caregiver Health: Health of Caregivers of Alzheimer's and Other Dementia Patients." *Current Psychiatry Reports* 15(7): 1–7.

Riley, Gerald F., and James D. Lubitz. 2010. "Long-Term Trends in Medicare Payments in the Last Year of Life." *Health Services Research* 45(2): 565–76.

Ripple, Gregory P. 2014. "Federal Court: Mandatory Retirement Age for Pilots Is Not Age Discrimination." National Business Aviation Association, May 2. https://www.nbaa.org/admin/personnel/age-65/20140502-federal-court-mandatory-retirement-age-for-pilots-is-not-age-discrimination.php (accessed May 20, 2018).

Roberto, Karen A. 2016. "Abusive Relationships in Late Life." In *Handbook of Aging and the Social Sciences*, edited by Linda K. George and Kenneth F. Ferraro. New York: Academic Press.

Roberts, William Clifford. 2001. "High Salt Intake, Its Origins, Its Economic Impact, and Its Effect on Blood Pressure." *American Journal of Cardiology* 88(11): 1338–46.

Roepke-Buehler, Susan K., Melissa Simon, and XinQi Dong. 2015. "Association Between Depressive Symptoms, Multiple Dimensions of Depression, and

Elder Abuse: A Cross-Sectional, Population-Based Analysis of Older Adults in Urban Chicago." *Journal of Aging and Health* 27(6): 1003–25.

Rogers, Richard G., Robert A. Hummer, and Charles B. Nam. 1999. *Living and Dying in the USA: Behavioral, Health, and Social Differentials of Adult Mortality.* New York: Elsevier.

Rogers, Tanya. 2009. "Hospice Myths: What Is Hospice Really About?" *Pennsylvania Nurse* 64(4): 4–7.

Rogers, Wendy A., and Tracy L. Mitzner. 2017. "Envisioning the Future for Older Adults: Autonomy, Health, Well-being, and Social Connectedness with Technology Support." *Futures* 87: 133–39.

Rohe, William M., and Leslie S. Stewart. 1996. "Homeownership and Neighborhood Stability." *Housing Policy Debate* 7(1): 37–81.

Romano, Antonino D., Gaetano Serviddio, Angela de Matthaeis, Francesco Bellanti, and Gianluigi Vendemiale. 2010. "Oxidative Stress and Aging." *Journal of Nephrology* 23(15): S29–36.

Romig, Kathleen, and Arloc Sherman. 2016. "Social Security Keeps 22 Million Americans Out of Poverty: A State-by-State Analysis." Center for Budget and Policy Priorities, October 25. http://www.cbpp.org/research/social-security-keeps-22-million-americans-out-of-poverty-a-state-by-state-analysis (accessed May 1, 2017).

Roschelle, Anne R. 1997. *No More Kin: Exploring Race, Class, and Gender in Family Networks.* New York: Sage Publications.

Rose, Miriam S., Linda S. Noelker, and Jill Kagan. 2015. "Improving Policies for Caregiver Respite Services." *Gerontologist* 55(2): 302–8.

Rosenfield, Sarah, and Dawne Mouzon. 2013. "Gender and Mental Health." In *Handbook of the Sociology of Mental Health*, edited by Carol S. Aneshensel, Jo C. Phelan, and Alex Bierman. New York: Springer.

Rossin-Slater, Maya, Christopher Ruhm, and Jane Waldfogel. 2013. "The Effects of California's Paid Family Leave Program on Mothers' Leave-Taking and Subsequent Labor Market Outcomes." *Journal of Public Policy Analysis and Management* 32(2): 224–45.

Rothstein, Richard. 2017. *The Color of Law: A Forgotten History of How Our Government Segregated America.* New York: W. W. Norton.

Rowe, John W., and Robert L. Kahn. 1998. "Successful Aging." *Gerontologist* 37(4): 433–40.

———. 2015. "Successful Aging 2.0: Conceptual Expansions for the 21st Century." *Journal of Gerontology: Social Sciences* 70(4): 593–96.

Roy, Abhik, and Jake Harwood. 1997. "Underrepresented, Positively Portrayed: Older Adults in Television Commercials." *Journal of Applied Communications Research* 25(1): 39–56.

Russell, Dan, Letitia A. Peplau, and Carolyn E. Cutrona. 1980. "The Revised UCLA Loneliness Scale: Concurrent and Discriminant Validity Evidence." *Journal of Personality and Social Psychology* 39(3): 472–80.

Salive, Marcel E. 2013. "Multimorbidity in Older Adults." *Epidemiologic Reviews* 35(1): 75–83.

Sampson, Deborah, and Katherine Hertlein. 2015. "The Experience of Grandparents Raising Grandchildren." *Grandfamilies: The Contemporary Journal of Research, Practice, and Policy* 2(1): 75–96.

Sanko, John. 2014. "Thermoregulation: Considerations for Aging People." In *A Comprehensive Guide to Geriatric Rehabilitation*, edited by Timothy L. Kauffman, Ronald W. Scott, John O. Barr, and Michael L. Moran. Previously titled *Geriatric Rehabilitation Manual*. London: Elsevier.

Sapolsky, Robert M. 2005. "The Influence of Social Hierarchy on Primate Health." *Science* 308(5722): 648–52.

Saraceno, Benedetto, Itzhak Levav, and Robert Kohn. 2005. "The Public Mental Health Significance of Research on Socio-Economic Factors in Schizophrenia and Major Depression." *World Psychiatry* 4(3): 181–85.

Sarkisian, Natalia, and Naomi Gerstel. 2008. "Till Marriage Do Us Part: Adult Children's Relationships with Their Parents." *Journal of Marriage and Family* 70(2): 360–76.

Sarkisian, Catherine A., Mary H. Lee-Henderson, and Carol M. Mangione. 2003. "Do Depressed Older Adults Who Attribute Depression to 'Old Age' Believe It Is Important to Seek Care?" *Journal of General Internal Medicine* 18(12): 1001–05.

Savage, Mark. 2016. "Colonel Abrams: U.S. House Singer Dies Aged 67." *BBC*, November 28. http://www.bbc.com/news/entertainment-arts-38129229 (accessed April 22, 2017).

Sawyer, Patricia, Eric V. Bodner, Christine S. Ritchie, and Richard M. Allman. 2006. "Pain and Pain Medication Use in Community-Dwelling Older Adults." *American Journal of Geriatric Pharmacotherapy* 4(4): 316–24.

Sayer, Liana C. 2005. "Gender, Time, and Inequality: Trends in Women's and Men's Paid Work, Unpaid Work, and Free Time." *Social Forces* 84(1): 285–303.

Schade, William J., and G. Marie Swanson. 1988. "Comparison of Death Certificate Occupation and Industry Data with Lifetime Occupational Histories Obtained by Interview: Variations in the Accuracy of Death Certificate Entries." *American Journal of Industrial Medicine* 14(2): 121–36.

Schafer, Markus H., and Jonathan Koltai. 2014. "Does Embeddedness Protect? Personal Network Density and Vulnerability to Mistreatment Among Older American Adults." *Journals of Gerontology Series B: Psychological Sciences and Social Sciences* 70(4): 597–606.

Scharlach, Andrew. 2012. "Creating Aging-Friendly Communities in the United States." *Ageing International* 37(1): 25–38.

Schanzenbach, Diane Whitmore, and Lauren Bauer. 2016. "The Long-Term Impact of the Head Start Program." Washington, D.C.: Brookings Institution

(August 19). https://www.brookings.edu/research/the-long-term-impact-of-the-head-start-program/ (accessed September 20, 2017).

Schlessinger, Joel, Daniel Schlessinger, and Bernard Schlessinger. 2010. "Prospective Demographic Study of Cosmetic Surgery Patients." *Journal of Clinical and Aesthetic Dermatology* 3(11): 30–35.

Schmitt, John. 2008. "The Decline of Good Jobs: How Have Jobs with Adequate Pay and Benefits Done?" *Challenge* 51(1): 5–25.

Schnittker, Jason. 2015. "Natural Symptoms? The Intersection of Social, Biological, and Genetic Determinants of Depression in Later Life." In *Genetics, Health, and Society*, edited by Brea L. Perry. Bingley, U.K.: Emerald Group Publishing.

Schoen, Cathy, Karen Davis, and Amber Willink. 2017. "Medicare Beneficiaries' High Out-of-Pocket Costs: Cost Burdens by Income and Health Status." Commonwealth Fund, May. https://www.commonwealthfund.org/publications/issue-briefs/2017/may/medicare-beneficiaries-high-out-pocket-costs-cost-burdens-income (accessed September 24, 2018).

Schoeni, Robert F., Linda G. Martin, Patricia M. Andreski, and Vicki A. Freedman. 2005. "Persistent and Growing Socioeconomic Disparities in Disability Among the Elderly: 1982–2002." *American Journal of Public Health* 95(11): 2065–70.

Schroeder, Steven A. 2007. "We Can Do Better—Improving the Health of the American People." *New England Journal of Medicine* 357(12): 1221–28.

Schulz, Richard, and Paula R. Sherwood. 2008. "Physical and Mental Health Effects of Family Caregiving." *American Journal of Nursing* 108(9): 23–27.

Schwartz, Christine R. 2013. "Trends and Variation in Assortative Mating: Causes and Consequences." *Annual Review of Sociology* 39(July): 23.1–20.

Scommegna, Paola. 2012. "More U.S. Children Raised by Grandparents." Washington, D.C.: Population Reference Bureau.

Seelye, Katharine Q. 2016. "Children of Heroin Crisis Find Refuge in Grandparents' Arms." *New York Times*, May 5. http://www.nytimes.com/interactive/2016/05/05/us/grandparents-heroin-impact-kids.html (accessed May 21, 2016).

Seery, Mark D. 2011. "Resilience: A Silver Lining to Experiencing Adverse Life Events?" *Current Directions in Psychological Science* 20(6): 390–94.

Seltzer, Judith A., and Suzanne M. Bianchi. 2013. "Demographic Change and Parent-Child Relationships in Adulthood." *Annual Review of Sociology* 39(July): 275–90.

Semega, Jessica L., Kayla R. Fontenot, and Melissa A. Kollar. 2017. "Income and Poverty in the United States: 2016." *Current Population Reports*, P60-259. Washington: U.S. Department of Commerce, U.S. Census Bureau (September). https://www.census.gov/content/dam/Census/library/publications/2017/demo/P60-259.pdf (accessed September 21, 2018).

Severson, Kim. 2014. "Grandma's Meat Loaf? Hardly. Her Retirement Home

Now Has a 3-Star Chef." *New York Times*, September 7. https://www.nytimes.com/2014/09/08/dining/grandmas-meat-loaf-hardly-her-retirement-home-now-has-a-3-star-chef.html (accessed September 21, 2018).

Sewell, William H., and Robert M. Hauser. 1975. *Education, Occupation, and Earnings. Achievement in the Early Career*. New York: Academic Press.

Shadel, Doug, and Karla Pak. 2017. *AARP Investment Fraud Vulnerability Study*. Washington, D.C.: AARP Research (February).

Shanahan, Michael J., and Scott M. Hofer. 2005. "Social Context in Gene-Environment Interactions: Retrospect and Prospect." *Journals of Gerontology Series B: Psychological Sciences and Social Sciences* 60(special issue 1): 65–76.

Shapiro, Thomas, Tatjana Meschede, and Sam Osoro. 2013. *The Roots of the Widening Racial Wealth Gap: Explaining the Black-White Economic Divide*. Waltham, Mass.: Institute on Assets and Social Policy.

Sharp, Emily Schoenhofen, and Margaret Gatz. 2011. "The Relationship Between Education and Dementia: An Updated Systematic Review." *Alzheimer Disease and Associated Disorders* 25(4): 289–304.

Shaw, Benjamin A., and Neda Agahi. 2012. "A Prospective Cohort Study of Health Behavior Profiles After Age 50 and Mortality Risk." *BMC Public Health* 12: 803.

Shellman, Juliette, Camella Granara, and Gabrielle Rosengarten. 2011. "Barriers to Depression Care for Black Older Adults: Practice and Policy Implications." *Journal of Gerontological Nursing* 37(6): 13–17.

Sherman, Carey Wexler, Noah J. Webster, and Toni C. Antonucci. 2013. "Dementia Caregiving in the Context of Late-Life Remarriage: Support Networks, Relationship Quality, and Well-being." *Journal of Marriage and Family* 75: 1149–63.

Shierholz, Heidi. 2014. "Six Years from Its Beginning, the Great Recession's Shadow Looms over the Labor Market." Issue brief 374. Washington, D.C.: Economic Policy Institute (January 9). http://www.epi.org/files/2014/six-years-after-start-of-great-recession.pdf (accessed October 1, 2017).

Shirley, James. [1659] 1919. *The Oxford Book of English Verse, 1250–1900*, edited by Arthur Quiller-Couch. Oxford: Oxford University Press.

Siegel, Michael, and Emily F. Rothman. 2016. "Firearm Ownership and Suicide Rates Among US Men and Women, 1981–2013." *American Journal of Public Health* 106(7): 1316–22.

Silber, Jeffrey H., Paul R. Rosenbaum, Amy S. Clark, Bruce J. Giantonio, Richard N. Ross, Yun Teng, Min Wang, et al. 2013. "Characteristics Associated with Differences in Survival Among Black and White Women with Breast Cancer." *Journal of American Medical Association* 310: 389–97.

Skolnick, Andrew A. 1998. "MediCaring Project to Demonstrate, Evaluate Innovative End-of-Life Program for Chronically Ill." *Journal of the American Medical Association* 279(19): 1511–12.

Skopek, Jan, and Thomas Leopold. 2017. "Who Becomes a Grandparent and

When? Educational Differences in the Chances and Timing of Grandparenthood." *Demographic Research* 37(article 29): 917–28.

Smith, Aaron, and Monica Anderson. 2017. "Automation in Everyday Life." Washington, D.C.: Pew Research Center (October 4). http://assets.pewresearch.org/wp-content/uploads/sites/14/2017/10/03151500/PI_2017.10.04_Automation_FINAL.pdf (accessed June 10, 2018).

Smith, Alexander K., Craig C. Earle, and Ellen P. McCarthy. 2009. "Racial and Ethnic Differences in End-of-Life Care in Fee-for-Service Medicare Beneficiaries with Advanced Cancer." *Journal of the American Geriatrics Society* 57(1): 153–58.

Smith, Dylan M., Kenneth M. Langa, Mohammed U. Kabeto, and Peter A. Ubel. 2005. "Health, Wealth, and Happiness: Financial Resources Buffer Subjective Well-being After the Onset of a Disability." *Psychological Science* 16(9): 663–66.

Smoldt, Robert, Denis Cortese, Natalie Landman, and David Gans. 2017. "Medicare Physician Payment: Why It's Still a Problem, and What to Do Now." *Health Affairs Blog,* January 27. http://healthaffairs.org/blog/2017/01/27/medicare-physician-payment-why-its-still-a-problem-and-what-to-do-now/ (accessed August 23, 2017).

Social Security Administration (SSA). 2013. "Chart Description—Women's Eligibility Basis for Social Security Retirement Benefits Is Changing." Washington: SSA, Office of Retirement Policy (September). https://www.ssa.gov/retirementpolicy/research/womens-eligibility-alt.html (accessed September 24, 2018).

———. 2018. "Retirement Estimator." https://www.ssa.gov/benefits/retirement/estimator.html (accessed September 21, 2018).

Solt, Frederick. 2008. "Economic Inequality and Democratic Political Engagement." *American Journal of Political Science* 52(1): 48–60.

Span, Paula. 2011a. "In Sickness and in Health." *New York Times,* January 7. https://newoldage.blogs.nytimes.com/2011/01/07/in-sickness-and-in-health/?mcubz=1&_r=0 (accessed July 1, 2017).

———. 2011b. "The Undeserving Parent." *New York Times,* October 20. http://newoldage.blogs.nytimes.com/2011/10/20/the-undeserving-parent/ (accessed October 8, 2016).

———. 2013a. "The Reluctant Caregiver." *New York Times,* February 20. http://newoldage.blogs.nytimes.com/2013/02/20/the-reluctant-caregiver/ (accessed September 25, 2016).

———. 2013b. "When Aggression Follows Dementia." *New York Times,* July 12. http://newoldage.blogs.nytimes.com/2013/07/12/when-aggression-follows-dementia/ (accessed September 18, 2016).

———. 2016a. "Alone on the Range, Seniors Often Lack Access to Health Care." *New York Times,* April 8. http://www.nytimes.com/2016/04/12/health/alone

-on-the-range-seniors-often-lack-access-to-health-care.html?_r=0 (accessed August 31, 2016).

———. 2016b. "New Opioid Limits Challenge the Most Pain-Prone." *New York Times*, June 6.

Spevick, Jeremy. 2003. "The Case for Racial Concordance Between Patients and Physicians." *Virtual Mentor* 5(6): 163–65.

Spillman, Brenda C., Jennifer Wolff, Vicki A. Freedman, and Judith D. Kasper. 2014. "Informal Caregiving for Older Americans: An Analysis of the 2011 National Study of Caregiving." Washington: U.S. Department of Health and Human Services, Assistant Secretary for Planning and Evaluation, Office of Disability, Aging, and Long-Term Care Policy.

Springer, Kristen W., and Dawne M. Mouzon. 2011. "'Macho Men' and Preventive Health Care: Implications for Older Men in Different Social Classes." *Journal of Health and Social Behavior* 52(2): 212–27.

Starr, Paul. 1982. *The Social Transformation of American Medicine.* New York: Basic Books.

Steenland, Kyle, and James Beaumont. 1984. "The Accuracy of Occupation and Industry Data on Death Certificates." *Journal of Occupational and Environmental Medicine* 26(4): 288–96.

Steiger, Douglas. 2017. "Trump Budget Abuses the Elderly." *Democracy*, May 24. http://democracyjournal.org/briefing-book/trump-budget-abuses-the-elderly/ (accessed July 4, 2017).

Steinhauser, Karen E., Nicholas A. Christakis, Elizabeth Clipp, Maya McNeilly, Lauren M. McIntyre, and James A. Tulsky. 2000. "Factors Considered Important at the End of Life by Patients, Family, Physicians, and Other Care Providers." *Journal of the American Medical Association* 284(19): 2476–82.

Steinhorn, Leonard. 2006. *The Greater Generation: In Defense of the Baby Boom Legacy.* New York: Thomas Dunne Books.

Stevenson, David G., Jesse B. Dalton, David C. Grabowski, and Haiden A Huskamp. 2015. "Nearly Half of All Medicare Hospice Enrollees Received Care from Agencies Owned by Regional or National Chains." *Health Affairs* 34(1): 30–38.

Stoltzfus, Eli R. 2016. "Defined Contribution Retirement Plans: Who Has Them and What Do They Cost?" *Beyond the Numbers* (U.S. Bureau of Labor Statistics) 5(17, December). https://www.bls.gov/opub/btn/volume-5/pdf/defined-contribution-retirement-plans-who-has-them-and-what-do-they-cost.pdf (accessed May 31, 2017).

Strully, Kate W., David H. Rehkopf, and Ziming Xuan. 2010. "Effects of Prenatal Poverty on Infant Health: State Earned Income Tax Credits and Birth Weight." *American Sociological Review* 75(4): 534–62.

Stuber, Jennifer, Kathleen Maloy, Sara Rosenbaum, and Karen C. Jones. 2000. "Beyond Stigma: What Barriers Actually Affect the Decisions of Low-Income

Families to Enroll in Medicaid?" Paper 53. Health Policy and Management Issue Briefs. Washington, D.C.: George Washington University.

Studenski, Stephanie, Subashan Perera, Kushang Patel, Caterina Rosano, Kimberly Faulkner, Marco Inzitari, Jennifer Brach, et al. 2011. "Gait Speed and Survival in Older Adults." *Journal of the American Medical Association* 305(1): 50–58.

Subramanian, S. V., Feliz Elwert, and Nicholas Christakis. 2008. "Widowhood and Mortality Among the Elderly: The Modifying Role of Neighborhood Concentration of Widowed Individuals." *Social Science and Medicine* 66(4): 873–84.

Suitor, J. Jill, Megan Gilligan, and Karl Pillemer. 2016. "Stability, Change, and Complexity in Later Life Families." In *Handbook of Aging and the Social Sciences*, edited by Linda K. George and Kenneth F. Ferraro. New York: Academic Press.

Sullivan, Patrick F., Michael C. Neale, and Kenneth S. Kendler. 2000. "Genetic Epidemiology of Major Depression: Review and Meta-analysis." *American Journal of Psychiatry* 157(10): 1552–62.

Sykes, Kathy. 2017. "Trends in Social Research, Policy, and Practice: A Time for Commitment: Economic and Health Equity for Older Americans." Washington, D.C.: Gerontological Society of America. https://www.geron.org/images/membership/SRPPTrends2017.pdf (accessed September 15, 2017).

Tach, Laura M., and Alicia Eads. 2015. "Trends in the Economic Consequences of Marital and Cohabitation Dissolution in the United States." *Demography* 52(2): 401–32.

Tait, Raymond C., and John T. Chibnall. 2014. "Racial/Ethnic Disparities in the Assessment and Treatment of Pain: Psychosocial Perspectives." *American Psychologist* 69(2): 131–41.

Tamborini, Christopher R. 2007. "The Never-Married in Old Age: Projections and Concerns for the Near Future." *Social Security Bulletin* 67(2): 25–40.

Taylor, Shelley E., and Teresa E. Seeman. 1999. "Psychosocial Resources and the SES-Health Relationship." *Annals of the New York Academy of Sciences* 896(1): 210–25.

Taylor, Tiffany, and Barbara J. Risman. 2006. "Doing Deference or Speaking Up: Deconstructing the Experience and Expression of Anger." *Race, Gender, and Class* 13: 60–80.

Teaster, Pamela B., Karen A. Roberto, and Tyler A. Dugar. 2006. "Intimate Partner Violence of Rural Aging Women." *Family Relations* 55(5): 636–48.

Temel, Jennifer S., Joseph A. Greer, Alona Muzikansky, Emily R. Gallagher, Sonal Admane, Vicki A. Jackson, Constance M. Dahlin, et al. 2010. "Early Palliative Care for Patients with Metastatic Non–small-cell Lung Cancer." *New England Journal of Medicine* 363(8): 733–42.

Teno, Joan M., Vicki A. Freedman, Judith D. Kasper, Pedro Gozalo, and Vincent Mor. 2015. "Is Care for the Dying Improving in the United States?" *Journal of Palliative Medicine* 18(8): 662–66.

Teno, Joan M., Pedro L. Gozalo, Julie P. W. Bynum, Natalie E. Leland, Susan C. Miller, Nancy E. Morden, Thomas Scupp, David C. Goodman, and Vincent Mor. 2013. "Change in End-of-Life Care for Medicare Beneficiaries: Site of Death, Place of Care, and Health Care Transitions in 2000, 2005, and 2009." *Journal of the American Medical Association* 309(5): 470–77.

Teno, Joan M., Susan L. Mitchell, Pedro L. Gozalo, David Dosa, Amy Hsu, Orna Intrator, and Vincent Mor. 2010. "Hospital Characteristics Associated with Feeding Tube Placement in Nursing Home Residents with Advanced Cognitive Impairment." *Journal of the American Medical Association* 303(6): 544–50.

Thomas, John, D. Johniene Thomas, Thomas Pearson, Michael Klag, and Lucy Mead. 1997. "Cardiovascular Disease in African American and White Physicians: The Meharry Cohort and Meharry-Hopkins Cohort Studies." *Journal of Health Care for the Poor and Underserved* 8(3): 270–83.

Thompson, Christie. 2014. "What Happens to the Homeless When They Die." *ThinkProgress,* June 26. https://thinkprogress.org/what-happens-to-the-homeless-when-they-die-3fe40560edc5/ (accessed May 20, 2018).

Thorne, Deborah, Pamela Foohey, Robert M. Lawless, and Katherine M. Porter. 2018. "Graying of U.S. Bankruptcy: Fallout from Life in a Risk Society." Consumer Bankruptcy Project (August 5). SSRN: https://ssrn.com/abstract=3226574 (accessed August 6, 2018).

Tilly, Jane. 2016. "Promoting Community Living for Older Adults Who Need Long-Term Services and Support." Washington: Administration for Community Living. https://www.acl.gov/sites/default/files/triage/Issue-Brief-Promoting-Community-Living.pdf (accessed September 21, 2018).

Traub, Amy, Laura Sullivan, Tatjana Meschede, and Tom Shapiro. 2017. *The Asset Value of Whiteness: Understanding the Racial Wealth Gap.* Demos, February 6. https://www.demos.org/publication/asset-value-whiteness-understanding-racial-wealth-gap (accessed August 3, 2018).

Travis, Shirley S. 1995. "Families and Formal Networks." In *Aging and the Family: Theory and Research,* edited by Rosemary H. Blieszner and Victoria Hilkevitch Bedford. Westport, Conn.: Greenwood Press.

Turner, R. Jay, and William R. Avison. 2003. "Status Variations in Stress Exposure: Implications for the Interpretation of Research on Race, Socioeconomic Status, and Gender." *Journal of Health and Social Behavior* 44(4): 488–505.

Turney, Kristin. 2014. "The Intergenerational Consequences of Mass Incarceration: Implications for Children's Co-residence and Contact with Grandparents." *Social Forces* 93(1): 299–327.

Tweedy, Damon. 2015. "The Case for Black Doctors." *New York Times,* May 15. https://www.nytimes.com/2015/05/17/opinion/sunday/the-case-for-black-doctors.html?mcubz=0 (accessed July 1, 2017).

Umberson, Debra. 1992. "Gender, Marital Status, and the Social Control of Health Behavior." *Social Science and Medicine* 34(8): 907–17.

Umberson, Debra, Julie Skalamera Olson, Robert Crosnoe, Hui Liu, Tetyana

Pudrovska, and Rachel Donnelly. 2017. "Death of Family Members as an Overlooked Source of Racial Disadvantage in the United States." *Proceedings of the National Academy of Sciences of the United States of America* 114(5): 915–20.

Umberson, Debra, Tetyana Pudrovska, and Corinne Reczek. 2010. "Parenthood, Childlessness, and Well-being: A Life Course Perspective." *Journal of Marriage and Family* 72(3): 612–29.

Urban Institute. 2015. "Nine Charts About Wealth Inequality in America." Washington, D.C.: Urban Institute (updated October 5, 2017). http://apps.urban.org/features/wealth-inequality-charts/ (accessed September 24, 2018).

———. 2017. "Mapping America's Futures." Washington, D.C.: Urban Institute (updated December 1, 2017). https://apps.urban.org/features/mapping-americas-futures/ (accessed September 24, 2018).

U.S. Bureau of Labor Statistics (BLS). 2014. "Employee Benefits Survey: Table 32: Leave Benefits: Access, Civilian Workers, National Compensation Survey, March 2014." Washington: U.S. Department of Labor, BLS. https://www.bls.gov/ncs/ebs/benefits/2014/ownership/civilian/table32a.htm (accessed September 24, 2018).

——— 2015. "Table 5. Fastest Growing Occupations, 2014–24 (Numbers in Thousands)." Washington: U.S. Department of Labor, BLS. https://www.bls.gov/news.release/ecopro.t05.htm (accessed October 4, 2017).

U.S. Census Bureau. 2010. *Census Atlas of the United States*. Chapter 1, "Education." Washington: U.S. Department of Commerce. https://www.census.gov/population/www/cen2000/censusatlas/ (accessed September 20, 2018).

———. 2014. *Current Population Survey: Annual Social and Economic Supplement*. Washington: U.S. Department of Commerce. https://www2.census.gov/programs-surveys/cps/techdocs/cpsmar14R.pdf (accessed September 24, 2018).

———. 2015. *Current Population Survey: 2015 Annual Social and Economic Supplement*. Washington: U.S. Department of Commerce. ftp://ftp2.census.gov/programs-surveys/cps/techdocs/cpsmar15.pdf (accessed May 1, 2017).

———. 2017. "Historical Income Tables: Income Inequality." Washington: U.S. Department of Commerce (updated August 10). https://www.census.gov/data/tables/time-series/demo/income-poverty/historical-income-inequality.html (accessed September 24, 2018).

U.S. Department of Health and Human Services (HHS). 2008. "Advance Directives and Advance Care Planning: Report to Congress." Washington: HHS, Office of the Assistant Secretary for Planning and Evaluation (August). http://aspe.hhs.gov/daltcp/reports/2008/adcongrpt.htm (accessed November 25, 2014).

U.S. Department of Labor. 2015. "The Cost of Doing Nothing: The Price We All Pay Without Paid Leave Policies to Support America's 21st Century Working Families." Washington: U.S. Department of Labor (September 4).

https://ia801900.us.archive.org/11/items/TheCostOfDoingNothing/The_Cost_of_Doing_Nothing.pdf (accessed September 24, 2018).

Van den Beuken–van Everdingen, M. H. J., J. M. de Rijke, A. G. Kessels, H. C. Schouten, M. Van Kleef, and J. Patijn. 2007. "Prevalence of Pain in Patients with Cancer: A Systematic Review of the Past 40 Years." *Annals of Oncology* 18(9): 1437–49.

Van den Hoonaard, Deborah Kestin. 2012. *By Himself: The Older Man's Experience of Widowhood.* Toronto: University of Toronto Press.

Van Hasselt, Martijn, Judy Kruger, Beth Han, Ralph S. Caraballo, Michael A. Penne, Brett Loomis, and Joseph C. Gfroerer. 2015. "The Relation Between Tobacco Taxes and Youth and Young Adult Smoking: What Happened Following the 2009 U.S. Federal Tax Increase on Cigarettes?" *Addictive Behaviors* 45(June): 104–9.

Van Rijn, Rogier M., Suzan J. W. Robroek, Sandra Brouwer, and Alex Burdorf. 2013. "Influence of Poor Health on Exit from Paid Employment: A Systematic Review." *Occupational and Environmental Medicine* 71(4): 295–301.

Varney, Sarah. 2015. "A Racial Gap in Attitudes Toward Hospice Care." *New York Times,* August 21. http://www.nytimes.com/2015/08/25/health/a-racial-gap-in-attitudes-toward-hospice-care.html (accessed August 31, 2016).

Vickers, Margaret H. 2000. "Stigma, Work, and 'Unseen' Illness: A Case and Notes to Enhance Understanding." *Illness, Crisis, and Loss* 8(2): 131–51.

Vig, Elizabeth K., Janelle S. Taylor, Helene Starks, Elizabeth K. Hopley, and Kelly Fryer-Edwards. 2006. "Beyond Substituted Judgment: How Surrogates Navigate End-of-Life Decision-Making." *Journal of the American Geriatrics Society* 54(11): 1688–93.

Wachterman, Melissa W., E. R. Marcantonio, R. B. Davis, and E. P. McCarthy. 2011. "Association of Hospice Agency Profit Status with Patient Diagnosis, Location of Care, and Length of Stay." *Journal of American Medical Association* 305(5): 472–79.

Waite, Katherine R., Alex D. Federman, Danielle M. McCarthy, Rebecca Sudore, Laura M. Curtis, David W. Baker, Elizabeth A. Wilson, Romana Hasnain-Wynia, Michael S. Wolf, and Michael K. Paasche-Orlow. 2013. "Literacy and Race as Risk Factors for Low Rates of Advance Directives in Older Adults." *Journal of the American Geriatrics Society* 61(3): 403–6.

Wang, Wendy, and Kim Parker. 2011. "Women See Value and Benefits of College; Men Lag on Both Fronts, Survey Finds." Washington, D.C.: Pew Research Center (August 17).

Wang, XiaoRong, Karen M. Robinson, and Heather K. Hardin. 2015. "The Impact of Caregiving on Caregivers' Medication Adherence and Appointment Keeping." *Western Journal of Nursing Research* 37(12): 1548–62.

Warren, John Robert. 2009. "Socioeconomic Status and Health Across the Life Course: A Test of the Social Causation and Health Selection Hypotheses." *Social Forces* 87(4): 2125–53.

Waxman, Elaine, and Linda Giannarelli. 2017. "The Impact of Proposed 2018 Changes to Key Safety Net Programs on Family Resources." Washington, D.C.: Urban Institute.

Weil, David. 2014. *The Fissured Workplace: Why Work Became So Bad for So Many and What Can Be Done to Improve It.* Cambridge, Mass.: Harvard University Press.

Weintraub, Arlene. 2010. *Selling the Fountain of Youth: How the Anti-Aging Industry Made a Disease Out of Getting Old—And Made Billions.* New York: Basic Books.

Weiss, Robert S. 1973. *Loneliness: The Experience of Emotional and Social Isolation.* Cambridge, Mass.: MIT Press.

West, Loraine A., Samantha Cole, Daniel Goodkind, and Wan He. 2014. "65+ in the United States: 2010." *Current Population Reports,* P23-212. Washington: U.S. Department of Commerce, U.S. Census Bureau (June). https://www.census.gov/content/dam/Census/library/publications/2014/demo/p23-212.pdf (accessed May 5, 2018).

Weuve, Jennifer. 2014. "Invited Commentary: How Exposure to Air Pollution May Shape Dementia Risk, and What Epidemiology Can Say About It." *American Journal of Epidemiology* 180(4): 367–71.

Whalen, Jeanne. 2018. "After Addiction Comes Families' Second Blow: The Crushing Cost of Rehab." *Wall Street Journal,* March 8. https://www.wsj.com/articles/after-addiction-comes-families-second-blow-crushing-cost-of-rehab-1520528850 (accessed June 10, 2018).

Whedon, James M., Todd A. Mackenzie, Reed B. Phillips, and Jon D. Lurie. 2015. "Risk of Traumatic Injury Associated with Chiropractic Spinal Manipulation in Medicare Part B Beneficiaries Aged 66–99." *Spine* 40(4): 264–70.

White, Helene R., Erich W. Labouvie, and Vasiliki Papadaratsakis. 2005. "Changes in Substance Use During the Transition to Adulthood: A Comparison of College Students and Their Noncollege Age Peers." *Journal of Drug Issues* 35(2): 281–306.

Whitehead, Margaret. 1992. *Inequalities in Health: The Black Report/The Health Divide.* New York: Penguin.

Wiglesworth, Aileen, Laura Mosqueda, Ruth Mulnard, Solomon Liao, Lisa Gibbs, and William Fitzgerald. 2010. "Screening for Abuse and Neglect of People with Dementia." *Journal of the American Geriatrics Society* 58(3): 493–500.

Wilcox, W. Bradford, and Wendy Wang. 2017. "The Marriage Divide: How and Why Working-Class Families Are More Fragile Today." Washington, D.C.: AEI/Brookings Institute (September). http://www.aei.org/wp-content/uploads/2017/09/The-Marriage-Divide.pdf (accessed October 5, 2017).

Wilkinson, Richard G., and Kate Pickett. 2009. *The Spirit Level: Why More Equal Societies Almost Always Do Better.* London: Allen Lane.

Williams, Brie, Rebecca L. Sudore, Robert Greifinger, and R. Sean Morrison. 2011.

"Balancing Punishment and Compassion for Seriously Ill Prisoners." *Annals of Internal Medicine* 155(2):122–26.

Williams, David R., Yan Yu, James S. Jackson, and Norman B. Anderson. 1997. "Racial Differences in Physical and Mental Health: Socio-economic Status, Stress, and Discrimination." *Journal of Health Psychology* 2(3): 335–51.

Williams, Joah L., Melba Hernandez-Tejada, Emily S. Fanguy, and Ron Acierno. 2016. "Elder Abuse." In *Gerontology: Changes, Challenges, and Solutions,* edited by Madonna Harrington-Meyer and Elizabeth A. Daniele. Santa Barbara, Calif.: Praeger Publishers.

Williams, Sally. 2016. "Sixty, Female, and All Living under One Roof (Just Don't Call It a Commune)." *Telegraph,* August 19. http://www.telegraph.co.uk/women/life/sixty-female-middle-class---and-all-living-under-one-roof-just-d/ (accessed October 7, 2017).

Wilson, C., and B. Moulton. 2010. "Loneliness Among Older Adults: A National Survey of Adults 45+." Prepared by Knowledge Networks and Insight Policy Research. Washington, D.C.: American Association of Retired Persons (September).

Wilson, William Julius. 1987. *The Truly Disadvantaged: The Inner City, the Underclass, and Public Policy.* Chicago: University of Chicago Press.

Winter, Laraine, and Susan M. Parks. 2012. "Acceptors and Rejecters of Life-Sustaining Treatment: Differences in Advance Care Planning Characteristics." *Journal of Applied Gerontology* 31(6): 734–42.

Wolf, Douglas. 2016. "Late-Life Disability Trends and Trajectories." In *Handbook of Aging and the Social Sciences,* edited by Linda K. George and Kenneth Ferraro. New York: Academic Press.

Wolitzky-Taylor, Kate B., Natalie Castriotta, Eric J. Lenze, Melinda A. Stanley, and Michelle G. Craske. 2010. "Anxiety Disorders in Older Adults: A Comprehensive Review." *Depression and Anxiety* 27(2): 190–211.

World Health Organization. 2016. "Health Topics: Mental Health." http://www.who.int/about/mission/en/ (accessed September 20, 2016).

Wray, Linda A., A. Regula Herzog, Robert J. Willis, and Robert B. Wallace. 1998. "The Impact of Education and Heart Attack on Smoking Cessation Among Middle-Aged Adults." *Journal of Health and Social Behavior* 39(4): 271–94.

Wright, Alexi A., Nancy L. Keating, Tracy A. Balboni, Ursula A. Matulonis, Susan D. Block, and Holly G. Prigerson. 2010. "Place of Death: Correlations with Quality of Life of Patients with Cancer and Predictors of Bereaved Caregivers' Mental Health." *Journal of Clinical Oncology* 28(29): 4457–64.

Xu, Jiaquan, Sherry L. Murphy Kenneth D. Kochanek, and Brigham A. Bastian. 2016. "Deaths: Final Data for 2013." *National Vital Statistics Reports* 64(2, February 16). Hyattsville, Md.: Centers for Disease Control and Prevention, NCHS. https://www.cdc.gov/nchs/data/nvsr/nvsr64/nvsr64_02.pdf (accessed September 24, 2018).

Yaffe, Kristine, Alexandra J. Fiocco, Karla Lindquist, Eric Vittinghoff, Eleanor M. Simonsick, Anne B. Newman, Suzanne Satterfield, Caterina Rosano, Susan M. Rubin, Hilsa N. Ayonayon, and Tamara B. Harris. 2009. "Predictors of Maintaining Cognitive Function in Older Adults: The Health ABC Study." *Neurology* 72(23): 2029–35.

Yilmazer, Tansel, Patryk Babiarz, and Fen Liu. 2015. "The Impact of Diminished Housing Wealth on Health in the United States: Evidence from the Great Recession." *Social Science and Medicine* 130(April): 234–41.

Yuan, Anastasia S. Vogt. 2007. "Perceived Age Discrimination and Mental Health." *Social Forces* 86(1): 291–311.

Zarit, Steven H., and Judy M. Zarit. 2011. *Mental Disorders in Older Adults: Fundamentals of Assessment and Treatment.* New York: Guilford Press.

Zeng Chenjie, Wanqing Wen, Alicia K. Morgans, William Pao, Xiao-Ou Shu, and Wei Zheng. 2015. "Disparities by Race, Age, and Sex in the Improvement of Survival for Major Cancers: Results from the National Cancer Institute Surveillance, Epidemiology, and End Results (SEER) Program in the United States, 1990 to 2010." *Journal of the American Medical Association: Oncology* 1(1): 88–96.

Zhang, Baohui, Alexi A. Wright, Haiden A. Huskamp, Matthew E. Nilsson, Matthew L. Maciejewski, Craig C. Earle, Susan D. Block, Paul K. Maciejewski, and Holly G. Prigerson. 2009. "Health Care Costs in the Last Week of Life: Associations with End-of-Life Conversations." *Archives of Internal Medicine* 169(5): 480–88.

Ziettlow, Amy, and Naomi Cahn. 2017. *Homeward Bound: Modern Families, Elder Care, and Loss.* New York: Oxford University Press.

Zilberberg, Marya D., and Andrew F. Shorr. 2012. "Economics at the End of Life: Hospital and ICU Perspectives." *Seminars in Respiratory and Critical Care Medicine* 33(4): 362–69.

Zimmer, Zachary, and Sara Rubin. 2016. "Life Expectancy with and Without Pain in the U.S. Elderly Population." *Journals of Gerontology Series A: Biological Sciences and Medical Sciences* 71(9): 1171–76.

Zoeckler, Jeanette M., and Michael Silverstein. 2016. "Work and Retirement." In *Gerontology: Changes, Challenges, and Solutions,* edited by Madonna Harrington Meyer and Elizabeth A. Daniele. Santa Barbara, Calif.: Praeger Publishers.

Index

Boldface numbers refer to figures and tables.

AARP (American Association of Retired Persons), 124, 132, 226–227
ACA. *See* Affordable Care Act
access to health care: expanding, 230–233; in hospice settings, 196–197; insurance and, 81–85, 173, 234–235; mental health and, 91–92, **92,** 109–111, 230, 263n25; mortality rates and, 52, **53**; racial disparities in, 15, 58, 84, 103, 190–192, 206, 256n31; socioeconomic status (SES) and, 81–85, 103
activities of daily living (ADL), 61–62, 64–65, 141, 175, 271n137
activity theory, 38–39
advance care planning, 200–209, **208,** 240, 282n118
Affordable Care Act (ACA, 2010), 81–82, 110, 139, 204, 234–235
African-Americans. *See* Blacks
Agahi, Neda, 78
Age Discrimination in Employment Act (ADEA, 1967), 17, 28
ageism, 8, 96, 99–101, 111, 127, 249n21, 265n63
age segregation, 4–5, 157, 158, 164–165
aging alone, 18, 120, 134
aging in place, 25, 153–158, 273–274n17
Ailshire, Jennifer, 168
alcohol use, 2, 18, 55, 62, 78, 94–95, 109, 261n6
Aldridge, Melissa, 281n94
allostatic load (AL), 63, 163
Alzheimer's disease, **64,** 68, 83, 146, 224–226, **225**

American Association of Retired Persons (AARP), 124, 132, 226–227
American Community Survey (ACS), 221
American Geriatrics Society (AGS), 230, 231
American Psychological Association, 259n91
Americans' Changing Lives (ACL), 168, 264n33
American Time Use Study (ATUS), 103
AmeriCorps, 243
anger, 94, 264n33
anxiety, 73, 93–94, 101, 106, 143
Arpino, Bruno, 268n49
Asian Americans: demographics of older adults, **19,** 19–20; education and, 21, **21;** living arrangements and, **152;** marriage and divorce rates of, **116;** mental health disparities and, **92;** multigenerational families and, 268–269n58; retirement plans and, 251–252n51
Assets and Health Dynamics among the Oldest Old (AHEAD), 188–189
assisted living facilities (ALFs), 24, 152, 155, 158–160
Azar, Alex, 272n171

baby boom cohort: aging of, 5, 14, 211; caregivers for, 148, 159, 226–227, **227;** childlessness and, 220–221; compared to earlier cohort, 211; as consumer market, 5–6; economic downturns and, 212; incarceration rates and, 176; marriage and divorce rates, 24, 115; social networks and, 134

345

Index

Barker, David, 44, 57, 254*n*22
Barrett, Anne, 17
biological models of aging, 36–38, 54–57, 72
biomarker data, 62–63, 257*n*45
birth rates, 13–14, 20
Black Report, 81, 236
Blacks: access to health care and, 15, 58, 84, 103, 190–192, 206; advance care planning and, 205–206; caregiving role and, 141–142, 288*n*105; death rates of, 2, 18, 20, 188–189; demographics of older adults, **19**, 19–20; disease rates and, 58, 65, 68–70, 76, 256*n*31; education and, 21, **21**, 46; employment and, 29, 49; grandparenting and, 123, 125–126, **127**, 268–269*n*58; hospice care and, 197–199, 281*n*92; incarceration of, 126, 176; income of, 7, 30, 33–34, 212, 251*n*49; life expectancy rates and, 66, **68**; living arrangements and, **152**; marriage and divorce of, 115, **116**, 122, 189, 267*n*6; mental health disparities and, 90–92, **92**, 110, 230, 263*n*25, 264*n*33; physical health disparities and, 52, 79, 218, 255*n*9; retirement and, 251–252*n*51; social networks and, 131, 133; stress exposure and, 73–76, 98, 107; suicide rates of, **95**, 95–96. *See also* racism
Blanchflower, David, 261*n*1
body mass index (BMI), 260*n*100, 285*n*27
Bonilla, Jacinto, 5, 78
Bordone, Valeria, 268*n*49
Bound, John, 254*n*31
Brody, Jane E., 153
Brown, Karen, 196–197
Brown v. Board of Education of Topeka (1954), 42
built environment, 12, 150, 164, 166–169, **167**
Bureau of Prisons, 177
Burn, Ian, 265*n*63
Burroughs, Augusten, 51
Butler, Robert, 99
Button, Patrick, 265*n*63

cancer: advance care planning and, 282*n*118; hospice care and, 196; increases in, 15; as leading causes of death, 66; mortality rates from, 64, **64**; place of death and, 186, 187; public health campaigns and, 15; racial disparities in, 58, 65, 256*n*31; screenings for, 58, 65, 84, 256*n*31; socioeconomic disparities in, 58, 65
Cantwell, Laura, 17
Caregiver Corps Act, 239
caregiving and caregivers: abusive elders and, 145–147; for cancer patients, 186, 187; decision-making and, 237–240; elder abuse and mistreatment, 8, 134–140; gender and, 18–19, 117, 124–125, 140–142, 268*n*49; grandparenting and, 124–127, **127**; health and well-being and, 143–144; hospice requirements for, 197–198, 226; lack of, 226–227, **227**; paid caregivers, 135, 156, 227–228; pain management and, 190; racial disparities in, 141, 188–189; resources for, 147–148, 237–240, 272*n*171; risks of, 144–145; stress and, 118–119, 140–148, 238. *See also* hospice care
Carstensen, Laura, 128, 262*n*9
Case, Anne, 219
CBO. *See* Congressional Budget Office
cellular aging models, 54–55
Census Bureau data, 42, 162, 248*n*11, 283*n*3
centenarians, 2, 224. *See also* oldest-old
Center for Epidemiologic Studies Depression Scale (CES-D), 88, 262–263*n*17
Centers for Disease Control and Prevention (CDC), 78, 218, 273*n*11, 284–285*n*23
Centers for Medicare and Medicaid Services (CMS), 135, 232
Changing Lives of Older Couples (CLOC), 184, 200
Chen, Edith, 46
Cherlin, Andrew, 115
Chesney, Edward, 262*n*11
Chicago: heat wave (1995), 132, 149, 170–171; residential areas in, 166; Villages programs in, 157
Chicago Health and Aging Project (CHAP), 262*n*11
Chicago School, 161
childhood adversity: abuse and, 145–146; cumulative inequality resulting from, 47–50; life-course perspectives and, 36; maternal nutrition and, 44, 57, 254*n*22; overcoming, 46; parent experiences and traits, 44–45, 55; poverty and, 7,

Index   347

45, 248*n*17; public policy to mitigate, 236
childlessness, 207, **208,** 220–221
Children's Health Insurance Program (CHIP), 82, 234
Chinn, Juanita, 255*n*9
chronic illness, 102–104, 180–182, 226. *See also specific illnesses*
cigarettes. *See* smoking
Clarke, Philippa, 166
CMS (Centers for Medicare and Medicaid Services), 135, 232
cognitive functioning: coping style and, 104–106; disengagement theory and, 38; education level and, 69, 105; elder abuse and, 138; emotional regulation and, 262*n*9; grandparenting and, 124, 268*n*49; heart disease and, 102; neighborhood characteristics and, 163; pollution and, 168; smoking and alcohol use, 78; stress and, 105
cohorts, 42, 51, 89, 120
co-housing, 119, 221, 223
Collaborative Psychiatric Epidemiology Surveys (CPES), 92, 263*n*25
community centers and services, 39, 110, 151, 156–158, 239, 252*n*8
community development block grant (CDBG), 239–240
comorbidity, 61, 93, 102
Composite International Diagnostic Interview (CIDI), 88
Congressional Budget Office (CBO), 82, 213, 233, 283–284*n*4, 284*n*7
Consumer Assessment of Healthcare Providers and Systems (CAHPS), 281*n*92
continuing care retirement communities (CCRCs), 152, 159
continuity theory, 39–40
coping, 46, 74–77, 90, 104–106, 111, 131
Cornwell, Benjamin, 129
Coronary Artery Surgery Study (CASS), 77
Corporation for National and Community Service (CNCS), 243–244
Cotton, Cassandra, 199
Credit for Caring Act (2017), 148
Crimmins, Eileen, 255*n*9
Cronkite, Walter, 5
culture: advance care planning and, 205; caregiver role and, 141–142; life extension and, 181; marriage and, 115, 267*n*6; media images of aging, 5, 17, 112, 241–242, 244
Cumming, Elaine, 38
cumulative inequality perspectives: early-origin theories and, 57; economic downturns and, 212, 217; elder abuse and, 139; employment and, 49; explanation of, 8, 37, 47–50; imprisonment and, 175, 178; mental health and, 87, 89, 94; physical health and, 63; preventing late-life inequality and, 233; social isolation and, 133; Social Security and, 35; stress exposure and, 49–50, 105
Current Population Survey (CPS), 248*n*11, 251–252*n*51

Daniel, Caitlin, 79–80
Dartmouth Atlas, 184–185
Darwin Awards, 70
death. *See* end-of-life care; good death; mortality
Deaton, Angus, 108, 219
defined benefit (DB) and defined contribution (DC) plans, 27–28, 237, 251*n*37
dementia, 69, 138, 144, 146–147, 159, 168, 176–177, 228. *See also* Alzheimer's disease
demographic and economic characteristics of older adults, 9–10, 13–35; diversity of, 17–18; economic resources and income sources, 29–30, **31, 33**; education rates, 20–22, **21**; employment and work history, 25–29, **27**; gender, 18–19; increase in older adult population, 13; life expectancy and, 13–16; marital status, **22–23,** 23–25; master status and, 16–17; race and ethnicity, **19,** 19–20. *See also* income inequality
Department of Housing and Urban Development, 174, 247*n*10, 272*n*171
depression: of caregivers, 142, 143, 147; components and symptoms of, 89–90, 102, 262–263*n*17; genetics and, 109; health care access and, 110; hospice care and, 194; measures for, 88, 261*n*7; negative beliefs about old age and, 100; rates of, 88–89, 230, 261*n*6; stress exposure and, 55, 73, 106, 107; suicide and, 96; trends and disparities in, 88–93, **91–92**
Desmond, Matthew, 130

Developmental Origins of Health and Disease (DOHaD) model, 57
developmental theories of late-life well-being, 37–40
diabetes, 57, 64, **64,** 76
Diagnostic Interview Schedule (DIS), 88
diet and nutrition, 2, 79–80, 83
dignity, 8, 135, 169, 175, 183–184, 199–200, 236. *See also* ageism
disability and functional limitations, 103–104, 152, 161, 189–190, 224–225
discrimination, 78, 98, 117–118, 197–198, 218, 260*n*100, 264*n*32. *See also* ageism; racism
disease: health behaviors and, 77; life-expectancy and, 14–15; low-birth-weight infants and, 57, 254*n*22; mortality rates and, 64, **64,** 66; parental effects on, 44; policy to reduce, 234; racial disparities in, 58, 65, 68–70, 76, 256*n*31, 257*n*55; socioeconomic status and, 52, 58, 65, 68–69; stress exposure and, 72–73. *See also specific diseases*
disengagement theory, 38
divorce: advance care planning and, 240; among older adults, 24, 119, 221; employment and, 26; racial and gender disparities in, **22–23,** 23–24, 115, **116;** Social Security benefits and, 31–32, 118, 221; stress and, 119
doctor-patient interactions, 182–183, 190, 193, 202, 232, 240
Dowd, Jennifer, 258*n*62
dual-earner households, 7, 221
dual eligibles, 82, 274*n*17
Dunlap, Adele, 2
durable power of attorney for health care (DPAHC), 201–204, 207–208, 240
Durkheim, Émile, *Suicide,* 114

early origins models, 44, 57
Earned Income Tax Credit (EITC), 76, 236–237, 259*n*94
Educational attainment: activities of daily life and, 64–65; advance care planning and, 206–207; childhood adversity and, 45–46; cognitive functioning and, 69, 105; coping mechanisms for stress and, 75; cumulative inequality resulting from lack of, 48–49; demographics of older adults, 20–22, **21;** employment and, 21, 29, 213; gender and, 21, 42; grandparenting and, 125; Great Recession and, 216–218; health insurance and, 235; knowledge-based economy and, 213; longevity and, 2; marriage and, 115, 121; mental health and, 92, 93, 261*n*6; physical health and, 3, 21–22, 55, 56, 69, 79, 218, 236; public policy on, 49; racial disparities in, 20–21, **21,** 34, 42, 46, 254*n*31; social networks and, 130, 133; socioeconomic status and, 123
EITC (Earned Income Tax Credit), 76, 236–237, 259*n*94
Elder, Glen, 41; *Children of the Great Depression,* 43–44, 253*n*19
elder abuse and mistreatment, 8, 134–140
Elder Justice Act (2010), 139
elder orphans, 134, 226–227
employment: ageism and, 8, 101, 127, 249*n*21, 265*n*63; caregivers and, 142–143, 238; childhood adversity and, 45; cumulative inequality and, 49; demographics of older adults, 25–29, **27;** education level and, 21, 29, 213; gender and, 26–27, **27,** 49, 117–118; globalization and, 213–214; Great Recession and, 216; health insurance and, 81, 118; home health aides, 135, 156, 227; income inequality and, 32, 34–35, 213; mortality rates and, 59–60; non-standard (gig), 28, 217; paid family leave programs and, 238–239; public policy on, 42; racism in, 49; retirement and, 242–243, 251–252*n*51; safety and, 15, 18, 21. *See also* retirement
end-of-life care, 183, 277*n*20. *See also* good death; hospice care
environmental hazards, 53, **53,** 55, 58, 161–162
epidemiologic transition, 66, 257*n*54
estate planning, 206
Estes, Carroll, 165
exercise, 69, 105–106

Fair Treatment for Experienced Pilots Act (Public Law 110-135), 249*n*12
families of choice, 120, 223
Family and Medical Leave Act (FMLA, 1993), 238–239, 288*n*105
family structure, 189, 220–224
Fazel, Seena, 262*n*11

FCT (fundamental cause theory), 65, 81, 82, 200
Federal Bureau of Prisons, 247n10
Federal Communications Commission (FCC), 271n131
Federal Housing Administration (FHA), 46
federal policies: for caregiver needs, 147–148, 272n171; on elder abuse, 136, 139–140; on immigration, 227; incarceration rates and, 176–178; on long-term care insurance, 160; for utility bill assistance, 173. *See also specific acts*
Federal Reserve Board, 217
Feinglass, Joe, 59
Fetal Origins of Adult Disease (FOAD), 57
financial exploitation, 8, 136
Fingerman, Karen, 128
food stamps. *See* Supplemental Nutrition Assistance Program
friendships. *See* social relationships and networks
frustration, 51, 76, 94
fundamental cause theory (FCT), 65, 81, 82, 200
future trends and policy considerations, 12, 210–246, 283n3; access to and quality of health care, 230–233; decision-making and caregivers, 237–240; disparities in well-being, 212–213; economic inequality and, 214–216, **215**; Great Recession and, 216–218; health behaviors and, 218–220, **219**; inequalities, roots of, 233–237; longevity and, 224–229, **225, 227**; nontraditional families and, 220–224

Galea, Sandro, 3
Gawande, Atul, 235
gender: ageism and, 101; aging outlook and, 6–7; alcohol use and, 94; caregiver role and, 18–19, 117, 124–125, 140–142, 268n49; demographics of older adults, 18–19; division of work and family roles based on, 49, 71, 211; education and, 21, 42; employment and, 26–27, **27,** 49, 117–118; income and, 33–34, 119, 212, 251n49; intergenerational relationships and, 123; life expectancy rates, 2, 6, 14, 66, **67–68,** 70–71, 249n23; living arrangements and, 24–25, **24–25,** 151, **152,** 153;

marriage and divorce, **22–23,** 23–25, 115, **116,** 119, 121–122, 221; mental health disparities, 90, **91,** 93, 110, 230, 261n6, 262–263nn16–17; mortality rates, 18, 70–71, 247n4; physical health disparities, 52; poverty and, 3, 7, 18, 30–31, **31,** 249n22; Social Security and, 31–32, 222, 251n49; social support and, 121–122, 130–131, 133; stress and, 98; successful aging theories and, 40, 253n13; suicide rates and, 86, 90, **95,** 95–96
Generation X cohort, 115, 120, 134, 211, 217–218, 242–243
genetics, 2, 53, **53,** 56, 63, 69–70, 108–109, 261n4
George, Linda, 166
Georgia Centenarian Study, 2
geriatrics, 99, 134, 141–142, 153, 230–232, 286–287n75
Geronimus, Arline, 74, 75
GI Bill (1944), 37, 43–44, 46, 212, 254n31
globalization, 213–214
good death: advance care planning for, 200–209, **208**; criteria for, 179–180; defined, 183–184; dignity and, 183–184, 199–200; hospice care and, 193, 197; place of death and, 185–189, **187**; research on attainability of, 184–185, 278n28
Goodwin, Guy, 262n11
grandparenthood, 123–128, **127,** 268–269n58, 268n49, 268n53
Great Depression, 212
Greatest Generation cohort, 51, 212
Great Recession (2007–2009), 26, 27, 126, 174, 212, 216–218

happiness, 107–108, 131–132, 261n1. *See also* quality of life
Harrington-Meyer, Madonna, 125
Hauser, Robert, 45
Hayward, Mark, 255n9
health. *See* mental health; physical health
Health and Retirement Study (HRS): on caregiving, 271n137; on cognitive function and pollution, 168; on crime and safety fears, 169; on dementia and education level, 69; on elder orphans, 134; on health behaviors, 22, 78; on intergenerational relationships, 125, 267–268n34, 268n53; on mental health, 108; mortality

Health and Retirement Study (HRS) (cont.)
data and, 59; on neighborhood characteristics and health, 163; on Social Security benefits for unmarried people, 121; sociological perspectives on aging and, 253n14; on working after retirement, 26, 252n6
health behaviors: cognitive ability and, 105–106; high-risk, increase in, 218–220, **219**; marriage and, 117; multiplicative effects of, 78; oxidative stress and, 55; physical health and, 77–81, 101, 265n65; premature mortality and, 53, **53**; self-reported data on, 62; socioeconomic disparities in, 58. *See also specific behaviors*
health care, 7, 15, 62, 230–233. *See also* access to health care
health disparities, 69–84; access to care and, 81–84; health behaviors and, 77–81; stress exposure and, 72–77. *See also* mental health; physical health
health insurance, 3, 81–85, 118, 173, 234–235. *See also* Medicaid; Medicare
Healthy Longevity Grand Challenge of National Academy of Medicine, 6
heart disease: cognitive functioning and, 102; education levels and, 3; gender and, 18; genetics and, 56; health behaviors and, 77–78, 94, 105–106, 264n33; increases in, 15; as leading cause of death, 66; mortality rates from, 64, **64**; racial disparities in, 68
Henry, William, 38
Herd, Pamela, 77, 221, 237
Hertlein, Katherine, 128
Higher Education Act (1965), 48
Hispanics. *See* Latinos
historical context for aging, 63–65, **64**
Hoffman, Kelly, 191
Holstein, Martha, *Women in Late Life*, 100
home- and community-based services (HCBS), 155–156, 273–274n17, 286n60
homebound older adults, 4–5, 155, 169, 171–172, 247n10. *See also* social isolation
home health aides, 135, 156, 227–228
homelessness, 3, 4, 8, 173–175, 178, 247n10
homeownership, 34, 163, 206
hospice care: disenrollment from, 197, 281n94; disparities in use of, 197–199, 226; expansion of, 209, 226; for-profit providers of, 194–197, **195**, 277n8, 280n88, 280n90; Medicare coverage for, 192–194, 196, 199, 226, 279–280n75, 280n90; misconceptions of, 193–194, 198–199, 280n83; PAS vs., 193
House, James S., 53, 77, 84, 230
housing. *See* living arrangements and housing
Hoynes, Hilary, 248n17
HRS. *See* Health and Retirement Study
Hughes, Everett, 16
Human Rights Watch, 177
Hummer, Robert, 255n9
Hurricane Katrina (2005), 170–172
hypertension, 70, 76

immigration, 13–14, 98, 136, 227, 257n55
immune system perspectives, 18, 55–56
Implicit Attitude Tests (IATs), 100
incarceration, 4, 8, 126, 175–178, 247n10
income inequality: activities of daily life and, 64–65; cumulative inequalities and, 48; demographics of older adults, 29–30, **31**; gender and, 33–34, 119, 212, 251n49; lifelong singlehood and, 120–121; mental health and, 92, 215; minimum benefit plan for, 237; physical health and, 2, 55, 56, 69, 258n62; racial disparities in, 33–34; rates of, 214–216, **215**, 284n7, 284n10; sources of income and, 32–35, **33**, 251n50. *See also* socioeconomic status; *specific sources*
infant mortality rates, 20, 70
Institute of Medicine (IOM), 182, 209
instrumental activities of daily living (IADL), 61–62, 64–65, 141
intergenerational relationships, 123–128, **127**, 267–268n34, 268n49, 268n53, 268–269n58
Internet use, 139, 271n131

James, Sherman, 75
Johnson, Lyndon B., 5
Jones, Susannah Mushatt, 1–3, 224

Kahn, Robert, 40, 253n13
Kahneman, Daniel, 108
Kennedy, John F., 48
Kington, Raynard, 255n9
Klinenberg, Eric, 170; *Heat Wave*, 132
Kong, Jooyoung, 145

Krugman, Paul, 214
Kuhn, Maggie, 158

Latinos: access to health care and, 103, 190–192, 206; advance care planning and, 205–206; caregiving role and, 141–142, 288*n*105; cumulative lifetime earnings of, 251*n*49; demographics of older adults, **19**, 19–20; education and, 21, **21**; hospice care and, 197–198, 281*n*92; income sources for, 33–34; life expectancy rates and, 66, 257*n*55; living arrangements and, **152**; marriage and divorce rates of, **116**, 189; mental health disparities and, 90–92, **92**; mortality disparities and, 188–189; multigenerational families and, **127**, 268–269*n*58; obesity and, 218; poverty rates of, 7, 30; retirement plans and, 251–252*n*51; social isolation and, 133; stress and, 98
Leslie, Michael, 3
Levy, Becca, 100
Lewis, Joanne, 278*n*28
LGBTQ adults, 136, 221, 223
life-course perspectives, 10, 41–50; agency with constraints, 46–47; childhood adversity and, 36; cumulative inequality perspectives, 47–50; economic impact of Great Recession and, 217; foundational assumptions of, 41; historical context and, 41–42, 212; linked lives and, 44–46; suicide and, 96; timing of life events, 43–44, 97
life events and transitions, 42, 43, 96–97
life expectancy: active life expectancy, 62; at birth, 14, 63–64, **68**, 249*n*23, 257*n*48; challenges of extended, 224–229, **225**, **227**; decreases in, 218, 284–285*n*23; depression and, 89, 262*n*11; disparities in, 13–16; gender and, 2, 6, 14, 66, **67–68**, 70–71, 249*n*23; global comparison of, 65; homelessness and, 175, 276*n*83; income inequality and, 215; increases in, 14–15, 42, 181; predicting, 62; race and ethnicity and, 2, 6, 66, **68**; socioeconomic status and, 2, 6, 66, 71
life-extending technologies, 181–183
lifelong singlehood, **22–23**, 23, 32, **116**, 118, 120, 221
Lifespan Respite Care Act (2006), 147–148
Lima, Julie, 271*n*137

Link, Bruce, 52, 65
living apart together (LAT), 119, 221, 223
living arrangements and housing, 11–12, 149–178; accommodations and adaptations for, 154–155; assisted living facilities (ALFs), 24, 152, 155, 158–160; crime victimization and, 169–170; gender and, 24–25, **24–25**, 151, **152**, 153; Great Recession and, 216–217; hazards of, 8; homelessness and, 173–175; homeownership and, 216, 284*n*18; importance of, 160–162; incarceration and, 175–178; independent in the community, 153–158; in institutions, 158–160; natural disasters and, 170–173; neighborhood characteristics and, 163–169, **167**; neighborhood composition and, 162–163; race and ethnicity, 24–25, **24–25**, 46, 151, **152**, 216, 254*n*31. *See also* nursing homes
living will, 201, 205
loneliness, 107, 132–134. *See also* social isolation
Longitudinal Study of Aging Danish Twins, 265*n*65
long-term care facilities, 152, 158–160. *See also* nursing homes
long-term care insurance, 83, 159, 235, 286*n*60
long-term services and supports (LTSS), 40, 273–274*n*17
Low-Income Energy Assistance Program (LIHEAP), 172–173
Luth, Elizabeth, 200

Mandelblatt, Jeanne, 256*n*31
Marmot, Michael, 69
marriage: advance care planning and, 207, **208**; benefits of, 114; caregiving and, 140, 145, 188–189, 240, 271*n*137; delaying or avoiding, 220–221; demographics of older adults, **22–23**, 23–25; health behaviors and, 79; isolation and, 133; for LGBTQ adults, 221, 223; pensions and, 34; poverty and, 30; race and ethnicity, 25, 115, **116**, 122, 189, 267*n*6; remarriage, 23–24, 115, 119, 221–223; social relationships and, 114–120, **116**; Social Security benefits and, 7, 31–32, 210, 221–222; socioeconomic status and, 115, 117–118, 221, 267*n*6. *See also* divorce; widowhood
McEwen, Bruce, 63

Meals on Wheels Association of America (MOWAA), 239–240
media images of aging, 5, 17, 112, 241–242, 244
Medicaid: caregivers, resources for, 148, 228; cumulative inequalities, correcting, 210; dementia care and, 226; eligibility for, 81–82, 156; expansion of, 234–235; expenditures on, 248n17; home- and community-based services and, 156, 273–274n17; low reimbursement rates from, 82–83; nursing home coverage and, 159–160, 188, 274n18; purpose of, 3; to supplement Medicare, 7
Medical Expenditure Panel Survey (MEPS), 102
medical expenditures: advance care planning and, 282n118; of caregivers, 147; dementia care and, 225–226; end-of-life care, 183, 277n20; gaps in Medicare coverage and, 7, 84, 210, 248n19; global comparison of, 257n51; homelessness and, 173–174; hospice care and, 194, 280n83; Medicaid expansion and, 235; for pain medication, 190–191; premature onset of disease and, 234; public policy to reduce, 236; racial disparities in, 206; socioeconomic status and, 7, 29–30, 248n18
medical innovations, 15, 65, 211, 228–229
medicalization of dying, 181–183, 200
Medicare: advance care planning and, 204, 240, 282n118; caregivers, resources for, 228; cumulative inequalities, correcting, 48, 52, 210; dementia care and, 226; for end-of-life care, 186, 188, 226, 277n20; expansion of, 236; expenditures on, 248n17; gaps in coverage, 7, 83–85, 210, 248n19; hospice care coverage, 192–194, 196, 199, 226, 279–280n75, 280n90; long-term care coverage, 83–84; low reimbursement rates from, 110, 230, 232–233; mental health care coverage, 110; pain medication prescriptions, 190; purpose of, 3
Medicare Access and CHIP Reauthorization Act (MACRA, 2015), 232
Medicare Current Beneficiary Survey (MCBS), 84
Medicare Improvements for Patients and Providers Act (MIPPA, 2008), 110

medications, 102–103, 109–110, 190–192, 219–220, 279n60
Meier, Diane, 182
mental health, 10–11, 86–111; access to health care and, 91–92, **92,** 109–111, 230, 263n25; ageism and, 99–101; alcohol use and, 94–95; anger and frustration, 94; anxiety and, 73, 93–94, 101, 106, 143; coping style and cognitive ability, 104–106; defined, 88; depression trends and disparities, 88–93, **91–92** (*see also* depression); economic stability and, 35, 215, 217; education level and, 92, 93, 261n6; elder abuse and, 139; gender and, 90, **91,** 93, 110, 230, 261n6, 262–263nn16–17; genetic factors and, 108–109; homelessness and, 174; lifelong singlehood and, 121; marriage and, 114–115; neighborhood characteristics and, 92, 161–163; physical health and, 102–104; policies and practices for, 109–111; race and ethnicity, 90–92, **92,** 110, 230, 262–263n17, 264n33; social support and, 106–107; socioeconomic status and, 92–93, 106, 107–108, 111; stress and, 49, 73, 96–104 (*see also* stress); suicide ideation and, **95,** 95–96
mental health paradox, 90, 263n21
Mental Health Parity Act (1996), 109
Mental Health Parity and Addiction Equity Act (MHPAEA, 2010), 110
Meredith, James, 48
Merton, Robert, 47
Michelson, Goldie Korash, 1–3, 224
Midlife in the United States (MIDUS) study, 63, 260n100
migration, 13–14, 20
millennial cohort, 120, 211, 217–218, 242–243
Miller, Greg, 46
Miller, Nancy A., 273–274n17
Mills, C. Wright, *The Sociological Imagination,* 42
minimum benefit plan (MBP), 77, 237, 287n103
minorities. *See* gender; race and ethnicity; *specific minority groups*
Moen, Phyllis, 26
Moorman, Sara, 145
morbidity, 62, 74, 231
Morrison, R. Sean, 192

mortality, 13–15, 179–209; advance care planning and, 200–209, **208**; anger suppression and, 94, 264*n*33; biomarkers and, 63; caregivers and, 143; causes of, 180; data sources for, 58–60, 184–185; disengagement theory and, 38; gender differences in, 18, 70–71, 247*n*4; good death, attaining, 183–184; health behaviors contributing to, 77–78; history of dying, 180–181; hospice and, 192–200, **195**; income levels and, 258*n*62; inequities in, study of, 184–185; later-life statistics on, 66–67; leading causes of, 66; medicalization of dying, 181–183, 200; natural disasters and heat waves, 132, 149, 170–173; obesity and, 285*n*27; pain and pain management, 189–192; place of death and, 185–189, **187**; premature, 52–53, **53,** 77, 81, 230, 234; racial disparities in, 19–20; selective, 48, 66; socioeconomic status and, 52, 185, 278*n*28; widowhood and, 119. *See also* good death; life expectancy
multigenerational families, 125–127, **127,** 268–269*n*58

National Academy of Medicine, 6, 181
National Academy of Sciences, 215, 251*n*40
National Comorbidity Survey (NCS), 261*n*6, 263*n*30
National Death Index (NDI), 59
National Elder Mistreatment Study (NEMS), 137
National Family Caregiver Support Program and Lifespan Respite Care Act (2006), 147
National Health and Aging Trends Study (NHATS), 155, 184, 190, 200, 247*n*10
National Health and Nutrition Examination Survey (NHANES), 55, 56, 285*n*27
National Health Interview Survey (NHIS), 64
National Home and Hospice Care Survey, 281*n*94
National Hospice and Palliative Care Organization (NHPCO), 197, 199
National Institute of Mental Health (NIMH), 92
National Longitudinal Mortality Study, 247*n*4

National Longitudinal Study (NLS), 267–268*n*34
National Social Life, Health and Aging Project (NSHAP), 129–130, 137
National Survey of American Life (NSAL), 262–263*n*17
National Survey of Caregivers (NSOC), 144
natural disasters, 8, 132, 149, 170–173
neighborhood characteristics: age segregation and, 164–166; built environment and, 12, 150, 164, 166–169, **167**; crime victimization and, 169–170; mental health and, 92, 161–163; physical health and, 161–164, 167–168; socioeconomic status and, 79, 163–164, 166–168, **167**
Neugut, Alfred, 256*n*31
Neumark, David, 265*n*63
New England Centenarian Study, 2, 247*n*2
New Jersey End of Life Study, 200, 205–206
Nicholas, Lauren, 282*n*118
noise, 161–162, 168–169
Noymer, Andrew, 60
nursing homes: ageism and, 101; criminal records of residents, 178; death in, 186; dementia patients in, 146–147; gender and, 24; Latinos and, 142; Medicaid for, 159–160, 188, 274*n*18; mistreatment of elders in, 135; rates of use, 150–152, 156, 273–274*n*17

Obama, Barack, 110, 139, 204, 234
obesity, 77–79, 218, 260*n*100, 285*n*27
Old Age Social Insurance (OASDI), 31
Older Americans' Act (OAA, 1965), 252*n*8
oldest-old, 13, 137, 144, 150–151, **151,** 210–211, 224
Open to Hope Foundation, 193–194
opioids, 190–192, 218–220, **219,** 279*n*60, 285*n*23
Oswald, Andrew, 261*n*1
Overton, Richard, 2

paid caregivers, 135, 156, 227–228
paid family leave programs, 238–239
pain and pain management, 183, 189–192, 200, 220
Panel Study of Income Dynamics (PSID), 258*n*62

parent-child relationships, 44, 98, 123–124, 222, 267–268n34
Parks, Susan, 204
Patient Self-Determination Act (PSDA, 1990), 200–201, 205
Pearlin, Leonard, 49, 97
Penner, Andrew, 60
pensions, 28, 32–34, **33**, 118, 215, 237
performance measures, 63, 257n45
Pew Research Center, 183, 216, 229
Phelan, Jo, 52, 65
physical health, 10, 51–85; access to health care and, 81–85; ageism and, 8; biological perspectives on aging and, 54–57; of caregivers, 143–144; childhood adversity and, 45; crime and safety fears, 169; cumulative inequalities and, 48; disparities in, 69–72; economic stability and, 35; education level and, 3, 21–22, 55, 56, 69, 79, 218, 236; employment options and, 29, 35; health behaviors and, 77–81, 101, 265n65; homebound older adults and, 4–5; housing hazards and, 154, 273n11; life expectancy and, 2, 15; lifelong singlehood and, 121; living arrangements and, 151–152; marriage and, 114–115, 117; measuring, 57–63; mental health and, 102–104; natural disasters and, 170–173; neighborhood characteristics and, 161–164, 167–168; obesity and, 218; patterns in, 63–69, **64, 67–68**; premature death and, 51–54, **53**; race and ethnicity, 52, 79, 218, 255n9; retirement based on, 38, 252nn5–6; scientific research on, 6; social networks and, 129, 133; socioeconomic status and, 16, 52, 65, 71, 108, 218, 236–237, 255n6, 258n74; stress exposure and, 49, 72–77, 102–104, 108
physician-assisted suicide, 193
place of death, 185–189, **187**
pollution, 168, 170
population growth, 13–14
Porchon-Lynch, Tāo, 5, 78, 224
poverty: childhood adversity and, 7, 45, 248n17; of children, 7; custodial grandparents and, 127; gender and, 3, 7, 18, 30–31, **31**, 249n22; health behaviors and, 79–80; lifelong singlehood and, 121; longevity and, 3; measurement of, 248n18; minimum benefit plan for, 237; of older

adults, 4–5, 7, 9, 29–30, 248n11, 249n22, 251n40; public health campaigns and, 15; public policy to correct, 76–77, 259n94; race and ethnicity, 7, 30–31, **31**; sociological perspectives on aging and, 253n14; stress and, 108
problem-focused coping, 104–105
public health initiatives, 15–16, 65, 78, 81, 218–220
public policy: for caregivers, 148, 238–240; to combat racism, 76; cumulative inequalities, correcting, 48–49; dietary choices and, 80; on health insurance, 234–236; Medicare reimbursements and, 232; mental health and, 109–111; racial disparities and, 34; retirement age and, 28; shortcomings of, 7–8. *See also* future trends and policy considerations
public spending, 248n17, 283–284n4

quality of death. *See* good death
quality of life: for cancer patients, 186; education and, 20; health care availability and, 233; hospice care and, 192–193; life satisfaction, 261n1; living arrangements and, 158; pain reduction and, 190; social inequality and, 3; social networks and, 128, 131–132, 157

race and ethnicity: access to health care and, 15, 58, 84, 103, 190–192, 206, 256n31; advance care planning and, 205–206; affirmative action programs and, 236; aging outlook and, 6–7; bias in health care and, 7, 15; caregiving role and, 141–142, 288n105; cumulative lifetime earnings and, 251n49; demographics of older adults, **19**, 19–20; disease rates and, 58, 65, 68–70, 76, 256n31, 257n55; education rates and, 20–21, **21**, 34, 42, 46, 254n31; grandparenting and, 125–127, **127**; health insurance access and, 81–82; hospice care and, 197–199, 281n92; housing issues and living arrangements, 24–25, **24–25**, 46, 151, **152**, 216, 254n31; incarceration and, 175; income sources and, 33–34; labor force participation and, 26; life expectancy and, 2, 6, 66, **68**; marriage and divorce rates, 25, 115, **116**, 122, 189, 267n6; mental health disparities and, 90–92, **92**, 110,

230, 262–263*n*17, 264*n*33; mortality disparities and, 60, 185, 188–189, 278*n*28; physical health disparities and, 52, 79, 218, 255*n*9; poverty rates and, 7, 30–31, **31**, 249*n*22; segregation and, 3, 42; social networks and, 131; Social Security, disparities in benefits, 7, 18, 31–32, 251*n*49; sociological perspectives on aging and, 253*n*14; stress and, 73–75, 98; successful aging theories and, 40, 253*n*13; suicide rates and, **95**, 95–96; wealth and assets, 34. *See also specific races and ethnicities*
racism: in employment, 49; in healthcare, 189; in medication access, 190–192; mortgage approval and, 46, 216, 254*n*31; public policy to correct, 76; stress exposure and, 73–74, 76, 96; wealth accumulation and, 34
Recognize, Assist, Include, Support, and Engage (RAISE) Family Caregivers Act (2018), 272*n*171
religion, 107, 199, 205
remarriage, 23–24, 115, 119, 221–223
resilience, 109, 263*n*21
retirement: average age for, 26; communities for, 149, 158–160, 164–166; delaying, 27, 127, 242–243; financing, 28–29; forced, 17, 28, 249–250*n*12; physical health requiring, 38, 252*nn*5–6; plans for, 26–29; social roles and, 38–39
Robert Wood Johnson Foundation, 167, 235
Robinson, Maisha, 198–199
robots, 228–229
Rothblatt, Martine, 6
Rowe, Jack, 40, 253*n*13
rural areas: community services in, 156; elder abuse and neglect, 139; hospice availability and, 198; Internet access in, 139, 271*n*131; Medicare coverage and, 84; naturally occurring retirement communities in, 164–165; opioid crisis in, 126, 220; place of death and, 188

Sampson, Deborah, 128
Sanders, Bernie, 236
Saperstein, Aliya, 60
savings and investments, 32–34, **33**, 237
Schanzenbach, Diane, 248*n*17
Schoeni, Robert, 64, 77
Schultz, Richard, 144

Seeman, Teresa, 255*n*9
selection-causation debates, 93, 120, 163
selective migration, 13–14, 257*n*55
selective mortality, 48, 66, 263*n*21
senescence, 51–52, 102
Senior Corps, 243
senior support centers, 39, 110, 252*n*8
Serve America Act (2009), 243
Servicemen's Readjustment Act (1944), 43
Sewell, William, 45
sex ratio. *See* gender
sexual abuse. *See* elder abuse and mistreatment
Shaw, Benjamin, 78
Sheppard, Vanessa, 256*n*31
shift and persist model, 46
Silber, Jeffrey, 256*n*31
single-for-life. *See* lifelong singlehood
slavery hypertension hypothesis, 70
sleep, 102, 145, 169, 264*n*33
Smith, James, 255*n*9
smoking: education level and, 22; gender and, 18; heart disease and, 77–78; longevity and, 2; oxidative stress and, 55; poverty and, 79; public health campaigns and, 15; public policy and, 80–81; quitting, 78; rates, state policies and, 80; self-reported data on, 62; socioeconomic status and, 16
social inequality, 10, 36–50; biomarkers and, 63; cumulative inequality perspectives, 47–50; developmental theories of late-life well-being, 37–40; gender and, 18; quality of life and, 3; sociological perspectives on aging, 41–47
social isolation: advance care planning and, 207–209; aging in place and, 25, 155, 156; dangers of, 11, 132–134; elder abuse and, 8, 138–139; health problems and, 83; loneliness and, 107, 132–133; natural disasters and, 171; place of death and, 187–188
social relationships and networks, 11, 112–148; advance care planning and, 200–202, 207; caregiving strains and, 140–148; changes in later life, 128–129; elder abuse and mistreatment, 134–140; employment and, 26; families of choice, 120, 223; importance of, 114, 128–131; intergenerational relationships, 122–128, **127**; Latinos and, 257*n*55; lifelong

social relationships and networks (*cont.*)
singlehood and, 120–122; longevity and, 2; marriage and, 114–120, **116**; mental health and, 106–107; neighborhood characteristics and, 163; place of death and, 187; of released prisoners, 178; residential churning and, 75; sociological perspectives on aging, 44–45

Social Security: calculating benefits from, 28, 250*n*36; cost-of-living adjustments for, 30; cumulative inequalities, correcting, 48, 210; eligibility requirements for, 7, 28, 31–32, 113, 118, 221–222; expansion of (1960s), 5; expenditures on, 248*n*17; gender disparities in benefits, 31–32, 251*n*49; as income source, 32–33, **33**, 35; lifelong singlehood and, 121; purpose of, 3; racial disparities in benefits, 7, 18, 31–32, 118, 251*n*49

Social Security Act (1935), 30

Social Security Caregiver Credit Act (2017), 239

socioeconomic status (SES): access to health care and, 81–85, 103; activities of daily life and, 64–65; advance care planning and, 206–207; ageism and, 101, 265*n*65; aging outlook and, 6–7; caregiver role and, 125, 142–143, 268*n*53; childhood adversity and, 44–45; dietary choices and, 80; dimensions of, 6; disease rates and, 58, 62, 65, 68–69; incarceration and, 175; intergenerational relationships and, 123–124; life expectancy rates and, 2, 6, 66, 71; living arrangements and, 155–156; marriage and, 115, 117–118, 221, 267*n*6; mental health and, 92–93, 106, 107–108, 111, 215; mortality disparities and, 52, 185, 278*n*28; neighborhood characteristics and, 79, 163–164, 166–168, **167**; opioid addiction and, 219–220; oxidative stress and, 55; physical health and, 16, 52, 65, 71, 108, 218, 236–237, 255*n*6, 258*n*74; public health campaigns, effectiveness of, 81; retirement plans and, 26, 28–29; stress and, 107–108, 259*n*91; successful aging theories and, 40, 253*n*13; utilities, public assistance for, 172–173. *See also* income inequality; poverty

socioemotional selectivity theory (SST), 129

sociological perspectives on aging, 40, 41–47, 253*n*14. *See also* life-course perspectives

state policies: on advance care planning, 204; on crime, 176; on elder abuse, 140; family caregivers, resources for, 148; gun ownership and suicide rates, 96; health outcomes and availability of welfare, 70, 72; longevity and, 3; long-term care insurance, 160; to mitigate poverty, 76–77, 259*n*94; paid family leave programs, 238; smoking rates and, 80

Steinhauser, Karen, 183

stigma: of lifelong singlehood, 120; of mental health issues, 78, 89, 91, 110, 230; race and, 74

stress: ageism and, 96, 99–101, 111; aging and, 7, 86; alcohol use and, 94, 95; of caregiving, 118–119, 140–148, 238; chronic, 96–98, 132, 146; crime and safety fears, 169; cumulative inequality and, 49–50; dangers of, 72–73; differential exposure to, 73–74; divorce and widowhood, 118–119; DNA, effect on, 55; longevity and, 2; mental health and, 93, 96–104; noise and, 169; physical health and, 49, 72–77, 102–104, 108; reducing, 111; social networks and, 131; socioeconomic status and, 107–108, 259*n*91. *See also* coping strategies

Stress in America survey, 259*n*91

structural inequalities, 42, 46–47, 79

Studenski, Stephanie, 257*n*45

successful aging, 8–9, 21, 40–41, 175, 253*n*13

suicide and suicidal ideation, 86, 90, **95**, 95–96, 114, 285*n*23

Supplemental Nutrition Assistance Program (SNAP), 80, 248*nn*17–18

Supplemental Poverty Measure (SPM), 7, 248*n*11, 248*n*18, 249*n*22, 251*n*40

Supplemental Security Income (SSI), 3, 76–77, 175

Survey of Consumer Finance (SCF), 34

Survey of Health, Ageing, and Retirement in Europe (SHARE), 268*n*49

taxes: on cigarettes, 80–81; income inequality and, 214, 284*n*7, 284*n*10; tax credits, 76, 148, 236–237

Teaster, Pamela, 139

technology, 139, 213, 228–229, 271*n*131
Trump, Donald J., 160, 235, 239
Turner, Sarah, 254*n*31

UCLA Loneliness Scale, 133
United States Aging Survey, 131

Van den Hoonaard, Deborah, 131
veterans, 43–44, 46, 174, 253*n*19, 254*n*31. *See also* GI Bill
victimization, 8, 169–170. *See also* elder abuse and mistreatment
Villages programs, 156–158, 274*n*19
volunteering, 39, 156–158, 224, 228, 243–244

Wachterman, Melissa, 281*n*94
Warren, John Robert, 45
wealth (assets), 34, 163, 206
weathering hypothesis, 74, 75

welfare, 70, 72, 80, 172–175, 248*nn*17–18. *See also specific programs*
West Virginia, 286–287*n*75
widowhood: coping strategies for, 105; dangers of, 117; gender and, **22–23**, 23–24; intergenerational relationships and, 123; mortality rates and, 119; racial disparities in, 115; social networks and, 131, 133, 166; social roles and, 38–39; Social Security benefits and, 31–32, 221
Wilson, William Julius, 121
Winter, Laraine, 204
Wisconsin Longitudinal Study (WLS), 45, 145, 200, 253*n*14, 267*n*34
Wisconsin Study of Families and Loss (WISTFL), 201–203
Women's Health Initiative, 65
World Health Organization, 88
World War II, 43–44, 253*n*19